Gastroenterology
An Integrated Course

Gastroenterology
An Integrated Course

Editors

Iain E. Gillespie M.D., M.Sc., F.R.C.S. (Ed., Eng. and Glasg.)
Professor of Surgery, The University of Manchester; Honorary
Consultant Surgeon, Manchester Royal Infirmary

T. J. Thomson M.B., Ch.B., F.R.C.P. (Glasg. and Lond.)
Consultant Physician, Gastroenterology Unit, Stobhill Hospital,
Glasgow; Honorary Lecturer, Department of Materia Medica,
University of Glasgow

SECOND EDITION

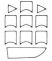

CHURCHILL LIVINGSTONE
Edinburgh London and New York 1977

CHURCHILL LIVINGSTONE
Medical Division of Longman Group Limited

Distributed in the United States of America by Longman Inc.,
19 West 44th Street, New York, N.Y. 10036 and by associated
companies, branches and representatives throughout the
world.

First Edition   1972
   Reprinted   1974
Second Edition   1977

ISBN 0 443 01457 4

Library of Congress Cataloging in Publication Data
Gillespie, Iain E.
    Gastroenterology.

    Includes index.
    1. Gastroenterology.   I. Thomson, Thomas James.
II. Title.   [DNLM: 1. Gastrointestinal diseases.
WI100 G257]
RC801.G54   1976   616.3   76–5864

Printed in Hong Kong

Preface to the Second Edition

In this second edition we have tried to take note of several criticisms raised by reviewers of the first edition. Many of the original authors have been able to contribute again, and each has been asked to look carefully through his text and, where necessary, update the material. In addition we are pleased to welcome two new contributors, Dr M. Ferguson and Professor J. H. Barber, the latter providing for us an interesting and important account of the special diagnostic and management problems encountered in general practice.

We also hope that the inclusion of a limited number of selected, mainly key review references, will be helpful to the reader, for guidance in obtaining further detailed information on specific topics.

It has been our aim to retain the original simple format of presentation and the objectives of the first edition of this book.

1977

I. E. G.
T. J. T.

Preface to the First Edition

Gastroenterology is one of the most appropriate subjects for an integrated approach. Many patients with gastrointestinal disorders require the help of general practitioners, physicians, radiologists, surgeons, pathologists, and, increasingly, experts from other medical disciplines. There is also a tendency for those with common and important diseases of the alimentary tract to be under the joint simultaneous supervision of physician and surgeon. Good examples are chronic peptic ulcer, haematemesis and melaena, and ulcerative colitis.

In Glasgow, as in many other Medical Schools, a considerable amount of integration has been introduced into the instruction on clinical subjects to medical students, and this volume is based on the main topics discussed during the gastroenterology section of the fourth year, main integrated clinical instruction course. All the authors have taken part regularly in these courses over the past six years, and have, therefore, experience of the topics which students find difficult to understand. Each has tried to give most emphasis in the text, to the disorders which occur most frequently in clinical practice, or which have a clearly defined aetiology and therapeutic approach. Where, in spite of much indirect evidence and speculation, we have an incomplete understanding of the cause or causes of a disease, the descriptive accounts are purposely brief.

It is hoped that the book will serve as a useful accompaniment to the instruction in an integrated gastroenterology course, to be supplemented by the student's personal additional notes. Blank pages have been inserted for this purpose at the end of the book.

The initiative for this volume came largely from Professor A. D. Roy, now of the University of East Africa at Nairobi, Kenya, and the Editors wish to acknowledge the considerable preliminary work which he did. We are also extremely grateful to our publishers, Churchill Livingstone, for impressive patience and excellent guidance on numerous occasions.

We are also greatly in the debt of Mr G. Donald and his staff of the Department of Medical Illustration at the Western Infirmary, Glasgow, particularly Mrs P. Miles, for the many line diagrams, and of Mrs E. Nimmo for typing the entire text.

1972   I. E. G.
                                                                 T. J. T.

Contributors

The Mouth, Tongue and Salivary Glands

Martin M. Ferguson, B.Sc., M.B., Ch.B., B.D.S.
Lecturer in Oral Medicine and Pathology, Glasgow Dental Hospital and School

T. Gibson, D.Sc., M.B., F.R.C.S.Ed., P.R.C.S.Glasg.
Director, Regional Centre for Plastic and Oral Surgery, Canniesburn Hospital, Bearsden, Glasgow

The Pharynx and the Oesophagus

John Hutchison, M.B., Ch.M., F.R.C.S.Glasg., F.A.C.S.
Consultant Surgeon, Royal Infirmary, Glasgow

The Stomach

Iain E. Gillespie, M.D., M.Sc., F.R.C.S.Ed., F.R.C.S.Eng., F.R.C.S.Glasg.
Professor of Surgery, the University of Manchester; Honorary Consultant Surgeon, Manchester Royal Infirmary

Sir Andrew Watt Kay, M.D., Ch.M., D.Sc., F.R.C.S.Ed., F.R.C.S.Eng., F.R.C.S. Glasg., F.R.S.E., F.R.A.C.S., F.C.S.(S.A.), F.A.C.S., F.R.C.S.(C.)
Regius Professor of Surgery, University Department of Surgery, Western Infirmary, Glasgow

T. J. Thomson, M.B., Ch.B., F.R.C.P.Glasg., F.R.C.P.Lond.
Consultant Physician, Gastroenterology Unit, Stobhill Hospital, Glasgow, and Honorary Lecturer, Department of Materia Medica, University of Glasgow.

G. P. Crean, Ph.D., F.R.C.P.Ed., M.R.C.P.Glasg.
Physician-in-Charge, the Gastrointestinal Centre, Southern General Hospital, Glasgow; Honorary Lecturer of Gastroenterology, University Department of Medicine, Western Infirmary, Glasgow

The Malabsorption Syndrome

W. C. Watson, M.D., Ph.D., F.R.C.P.Glasg., M.R.C.P.Lond.
Associate Professor of Medicine, University of Western Ontario, Canada

Henry I. Tankel, M.D., F.R.C.S.Ed., F.R.C.S.Glasg.
Consultant Surgeon, Southern General Hospital, Glasgow

The Biliary System and the Pancreas

Douglas H. Clark, M.D., Ch.M., F.R.C.S.Ed., F.R.C.S.Glasg.
Consultant Surgeon, Western Infirmary, and Gartnavel General Hospital, Glasgow

William Manderson, M.D., F.R.C.P.Glasg., F.R.C.P.Lond.
Consultant Physician, Royal Infirmary, Glasgow

Colin MacKay, M.B., Ch.B., F.R.C.S.Ed., F.R.C.S. Glasg.
Senior Lecturer in Surgery, University of Glasgow

The Liver
I. W. Dymock, M.B., Ch.B., F.R.C.P.Ed., F.R.C.P.Glasg.
Consultant Physician and Gastroenterologist, Stepping Hill Hospital, Poplar Grove,
Stockport, Cheshire

The Acute Abdomen (including Intestinal Obstruction)
David Miln, M.B., Ch.B., F.R.C.S.Glasg.
Consultant Surgeon, Stobhill Hospital, Glasgow
Ronald M. Ross, M.B., Ch.B., F.R.C.S.Ed.
Consultant Surgeon, Royal Alexandra Infirmary, Paisley

Intestinal Infections
K. A. Buchan, M.B., Ch.B.Ed.
Associate Professor (Pathology), University of Calgary, Canada
Peter McKenzie, M.B., F.R.C.P.Glasg., D.P.H.
Consultant Physician-in-charge, Department of Infectious Diseases, Belvidere Hospital,
Glasgow; Regional Adviser in Infectious Diseases

Crohn's Disease
T. J. Thomson
Stuart Young, M.A., M.B., Ch.B., F.R.C.S.Glasg., F.R.C.S.Ed.
Consultant Surgeon, Stobhill General Hospital, Glasgow.

Ulcerative Colitis
T. J. Thomson
Douglas Roy, M.B., F.R.C.S.Ed., F.R.C.S.Eng., F.R.C.S.Glasg.
Professor of Surgery, the Queen's University of Belfast, Institute of Clinical Science,
Grosvenor Road, Belfast

Tumours of the Intestine
Douglas Roy
F. D. Lee, M.D., M.R.C.Path.
Consultant Pathologist, Department of Pathology, Royal Infirmary, Glasgow

Diverticular Disease of the Colon
M. Kennedy Browne, B.Sc., M.D., F.R.C.S.Ed.
Consultant Surgeon, Royal Infirmary, Glasgow

The Anal Canal and Anus
Shedden Alexander, Ch.M., F.R.C.S.Ed., F.R.C.S.Glasg.
Consultant Surgeon, Ormskirk and District General Hospital, Ormskirk, Lancashire

Gastrointestinal Diseases in General Practice
J. H. Barber, M.D.Ed., M.R.C.G.P., D.Obst. R.C.O.G.
Norie-Miller Professor of General Practice, University of Glasgow

Contents

Chapter   *Page*

 1   The Mouth, Tongue and Salivary Glands   1

 2   The Pharynx and the Oesophagus   14

 3   The Stomach   37

 4   The Malabsorption Syndrome   76

 5   The Biliary System and the Pancreas   107

 6   The Liver   133

 7   The Acute Abdomen (including Intestinal Obstruction)   167

 8   Intestinal Infections   184

 9   Crohn's Disease   201

10   Ulcerative Colitis   208

11   Tumours of the Intestine   220

12   Diverticular Disease of the Colon   242

13   The Anal Canal and Anus   252

14   Gastrointestinal Diseases in General Practice   274

     Index   285

1. The Mouth, Tongue and Salivary Glands

Martin M. Ferguson and T. Gibson

INTRODUCTION

Embryologically, the oral mucosa, salivary glands and the enamel of the teeth are derived from an ingrowth of ectoderm, while the dentine, pulp and cement are mesenchymal in origin.

While some disorders are restricted to the mouth, certain systemic diseases have oral manifestations. The mouth constitutes the first part of the alimentary canal and as such may involved in diseases affecting other parts of the alimentary canal, e.g. Crohn's disease. However, when considering the embryological derivation of the oral mucosa, it is not surprising to find that numerous dermatological conditions extend into the mouth, e.g. pemphigus vulgaris, lichen planus and erythema multiforme.

Early clinical signs or symptoms may also occur in the oral cavity in association with immune disorders, nutritional deficiencies, endocrinopathies and diseases of the haemopoietic system.

DENTAL DISEASES

The structure of tooth and its supporting tissues is illustrated in Fig. 1.1. The external surface of the tooth is covered by enamel, which is non-vital and extremely hard. The underlying dentine is vital, and exposure of this tissue is painful.

Dental caries, periodontal disease and malocclusion are the three most common dental conditions encountered in practice. Although each is largely preventable, it is remarkable that all are increasing in prevalence in our community.

Dental caries

Dental caries, or decay, commences at localized areas on the outer surface of the enamel and progresses inwards to the dentine. The dentine is next destroyed and the carious process continues until it involves the neurovascular soft tissue within the tooth, i.e. the dental pulp. The richly innervated pulp tissue is enclosed in the rigid calcified

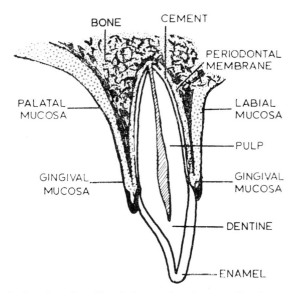

Fig. 1.1 Sagittal section of maxillary incisor tooth and surrounding tissues.

dentine; any increase in pressure due to inflammation produces pain.

The most widely accepted theory for the initiation of dental caries is that the oral bacteria, which are concentrated in deposits attached to the tooth surface, have the ability to convert carbohydrates into acid. This acid results in the demineralization of the tooth surface. Prevention of dental caries can be achieved by:

(a) reducing the intake of refined carbohydrates, particularly as snacks between meals,

(b) regular tooth brushing after meals along with the use of dental floss for cleaning the areas between teeth,

(c) increasing the resistance of the enamel to caries by the use of fluoride. Fluoride may be added to the drinking water to give a final concentration to 1 part per million in areas where the water supply does not contain an adequate amount. Such a concentration of fluoride does not cause any known diseases. Alternative measures are to take sodium fluoride tablets or have fluoride applied topically to the teeth.

(d) plastic sealants applied to the fissures of teeth to prevent any acid formed from coming in contact with the enamel.

SEQUELAE OF DENTAL CARIES

Once caries begins, cavity formation progresses to involve both the enamel and dentine. The decayed tissue is easily removed at this early stage and the tooth filled by the dental surgeon before the patient experiences pain. If the cavity remains untreated, sharp pain will be brought on by hot and cold substances as well as by exposure to sugar. It is usually still possible to fill the tooth at this stage.

Without treatment, the tooth may become painful for prolonged periods and be tender to touch or to percussion. A more radical treatment is now necessary in the form of removal of the affected pulp, i.e. root treatment, or extraction of the tooth. Still later, when the pulp infection has become established and spread of the infection has involved the adjacent periodontal membrane and alveolar bone, an acute dental abcess may develop at the apex of the root. This usually requires extraction of the tooth. Antibiotics alone are not sufficient for the treatment of a dental abscess.

Periodontal disease

Periodontal disease (gingivitis) is an inflammatory condition affecting the gingival mucosa initially, and subsequently involving the supporting tissues around the teeth, i.e. the alveolar bone and periodontal membrane (periodontitis).

As much as 99 per cent of the British population has varying degrees of periodontal disease, and at least as many teeth require to be extracted on account of periodontal disease as for dental caries. It is the commonest reason for tooth loss in those over the age of 35 years.

Chronic gingivitis is due to inadequate tooth cleaning, allowing the development of dental plaque; this consists of bacterial deposits which accumulate around the teeth and gums. Therefore, it is entirely a preventable condition. Later inflammatory changes are progressive damage to the supporting alveolar bone and periodontal membrane (chronic periodontitis) which lead ultimately to loosening and loss of the teeth.

The essential treatment of periodontal disease is to keep the gingival sulcus free from infection by removal of dental plaque and calculus (tartar). Minor surgery may also be required either to any pockets which have formed or to modify the bony socket margins.

The commonest form of acute gingivitis is acute ulcerative gingivitis (Vincent's infection), in which extensive ulceration of the gingivae, with bleeding, pain and halitosis, occurs. In addition there may be enlargement of the cervical lymph nodes, together with a mild or moderate constitutional disturbance. The aetiology of acute ulcerative gingivitis is still obscure: although smears taken from ulcers usually reveal increased numbers of *Borrelia vincenti* and *Bacillus fusiformis*, it has not been possible to transmit the disorder from one individual to another. Possibly a general or local lowering of resistance may be a predisposing factor.

Acute ulcerative gingivitis responds favourably to thorough mechanical cleansing of the teeth and gums, together with improved oral hygiene and removal of areas where food stagnation occurs. Only occasionally are these measures insufficient and systemic metronidazole or penicillin is necessary. Without long-term oral cleanliness, recurrence is almost certain.

Malocclusion

Between 40 and 50 per cent of British school children have some form of malposition or malocclusion of the teeth. Orthodontic correction is desirable not only from the aesthetic point of view, but also to prevent dental caries and periodontal disease occurring in areas of difficult access for cleaning. A further problem which tends to occur in association with certain types of malocclusion is temporomandibular joint pain and even arthritis.

Developmental disturbances affecting the teeth

Developmental anomalies affecting the teeth may occur during the phases of tooth initiation, morphodifferentiation, deposition of the hard calcified dental tissues or during eruption of the teeth themselves. Such disturbances in growth can affect the actual number of teeth as well as their form and structure.

Hypoplasia and hypocalcification of the teeth arise either from a genetic defect or from severe metabolic disturbances during childhood. This latter group includes viral infections and rickets. The usual defects are horizontally arranged hypoplastic pits or grooves across the crowns of the affected teeth. However, these teeth are not more prone to dental caries, and treatment, using plastic sealants, is carried out on aesthetic grounds.

Congenital syphilis produces a characteristic form of enamel hypoplasia with lateral tapering towards the incisal edge of anterior teeth, together with notching of the incisal edge (Hutchinson's teeth). The first molar teeth are also involved with globular masses of enamel replacing the normal cusps (mulberry molars). These appearances of the teeth are not absolutely pathognomonic of syphilis, as similar disturbances can also occur as a result of chronic mechanical pressure. Conversely, not all cases of congenital syphilis have these dental findings.

Tooth discolouration may arise from pigments circulating in the blood during tooth development, e.g. neonatal jaundice and congenital porphyria. Tetracyclines given either to the mother during pregnancy or to the child during the phase of dental development may cause permanent yellow to grey discolouration due to incorporation of the antibiotic into the teeth. Therefore, tetracyclines should be avoided both during pregnancy and up to the end of the sixth year, while the crowns of the permanent anterior dentition are calcifying.

ORAL MUCOSA AND TONGUE

The mouth is lined by stratified squamous epithelium which is keratinized in some areas (hard palate, dorsum of tongue and gingivae) and non-keratinized in others (buccal mucosa, soft palate, labial mucosa and floor of mouth).

Lesions affecting the oral mucosa can be localized or widespread throughout the mouth. If there is extensive mucosal involvement then the term 'stomatitis' is applied; disease of the tongue is 'glossitis', of the gums, 'gingivitis', and of the lips, 'cheilitis'.

Trauma

The oral mucosa is most commonly injured by the teeth: sharp edges of natural teeth or dentures may catch the mucosa and produce ulceration or a blow to the lips may cause the incisors to penetrate the labial mucosa and lips. In both circumstances the aetiology is fairly obvious and treatment is aimed at removal of a cause of repeated trauma. Should an ulcer persist in the absence of any apparent trauma or irritation, then it must be regarded as potentially neoplastic and a biopsy is desirable.

Recurrent aphthae

Recurrent oral ulcerations, or aphthae, usually occur on the non-keratinized oral mucosa and present as shallow, painful ulcers covered by white slough. The ulcers vary in size from 1 to 5 mm in diameter, and may appear either singly or in crops lasting five to fifteen days.

The aetiology of recurrent aphthae is unknown, although they are thought possibly to be more common in individuals with an atopic diathesis. Twenty per cent of patients presenting with what appears to be typical oral aphthae have an underlying systemic disorder, such as deficiency of iron, vitamin B_{12} or folic acid. A few women have aphthae which appear between ovulation and menstruation, and in these specific cases therapy with oral contraceptives or oestrogens is usually successful.

Treatment of the remaining cases of recurrent aphthae is empirical. Hydrocortisone pellets, triamcinolone in carboxy-methylcellulose paste, or a 0·2 per cent aqueous chlorhexidine mouthwash may be of benefit.

Glossitis and sore tongue

Many disorders may give rise to a painful or burning sensation in the tongue. Several nutritional deficiencies produce a red, tender tongue, which may in later stages become pale and atrophic. Dryness of the mouth, or xerostomia, can also cause discomfort of the tongue.

and not infrequently a superimposed candida infection aggravates the condition.

Geographic tongue, or benign migratory glossitis, is a benign condition which is characterized by the intermittent appearance of round erythematous atrophic areas surrounded by a white margin. The aetiology is unknown and there is no treatment other than to reassure the patient of the benign nature of the condition.

Non-infective granulomata

There are several benign, non-infective, inflammatory, hyperplastic lesions which develop in the tissues adjacent to the teeth. The name epulis was previously applied to all of these lesions, but this term should be discontinued.

A pyogenic granuloma represents an unusually intense hyperplastic inflammatory response in the gingivae. This is a swelling of up to 1 cm, with a deep red surface which tends to bleed easily, and which arises commonly during pregnancy. The treatment for pyogenic granuloma is local excision, together with improved oral hygiene. In the pyogenic granuloma associated with pregnancy, however, the lesion often subsides spontaneously following delivery.

A second type of granuloma occurs adjacent to the teeth, but this variety contains multinucleated giant cells and is termed 'peripheral giant cell granuloma'. Again the lesion is benign, and the treatment is local excision.

INFECTIVE GRANULOMATA

Syphilis

Oral syphilitic lesions can occur in all stages of the disease. A primary chancre is most commonly found on the lip or tongue, and presents as a firm nodule which ulcerates and becomes covered with a whitish slough. During the secondary stage 'mucous patches' may appear on the oral mucosa; these are multiple, superficial ulcers. Snail-track ulcers are another feature of secondary syphilis. The gummata of tertiary syphilis may develop intra-orally, being most common on the tongue and palate. Atrophic glossitis and white patches (leukoplakia) on the mucosa are further oral lesions of tertiary syphilis.

Tubercle

Tuberculous ulceration of the mouth is now a rare complication of pulmonary tuberculosis. The tongue is the commonest site, and the ulcer is irregular, indurated and painful.

ORAL INFECTIONS

Herpes simplex

Infection with this virus is the commonest cause of stomatitis in infants and young children, although it does occasionally occur in adults. In the primary infection, vesicular lesions develop on the palate, gingivae, dorsum of tongue and lips. The cervical lymph nodes become enlarged and tender. There is usually a mild constitutional upset, with the child becoming febrile and refusing food: this lasts for between a week and ten days. No specific treatment is normally required, but attention should be paid to an adequate fluid intake together with analgesics and sedatives where required, such as elixirs of paracetamol and promethazine.

Further episodes of secondary infections occur in a number of people, but these are nearly always confined to the lip and take the form of a 'cold sore'.

Herpes zoster

'Shingles' may occur in the regions supplied by the trigeminal nerve, giving rise to a rash and stomatitis. The earliest sign of the disease is pain in the area supplied by the affected branch of the nerve, followed soon by a vesicular eruption on mucosa and skin. The pain can be extremely severe and persist long after the skin and mucosal lesions have healed. In intractable cases, section of the nerve roots may be necessary.

Acute specific fevers

The vesicular eruption of the skin present in smallpox and chicken-pox may also occur on the oral mucosa. Koplik's spots, like white grains of salt on a bright red base, occur on the buccal mucosa in the prodromal phase of measles. In rubella, red macules may appear on the palate, but this is not common.

Candida infections (candidosis)

Oral infection with *Candida albicans*, a yeast-like fungus, is relatively common. This organism is a common inhabitant of the mouth, and becomes a problem only when there is a disturbance to the normal oral environment. Candida infection often occurs when there is suppression of the bacterial flora with antibiotic therapy. It is also a complication of corticosteroid treatment, particularly when antibiotics are used topically in the mouth. The appearance of an intra-oral candidal infection may herald the onset of diabetes mellitus, and this should be excluded in the absence of any other aetiology.

Candidosis may take several forms. The characteristic appearance is of a creamy, white patch with an erythematous base. The white patch is readily rubbed off, leaving a red, bleeding base, and the patch contains clumps of *C. albicans*, identifiable on microscopic examination. Chronic candidosis may be responsible for fiery red, sore gums beneath dentures, and white hyperplastic areas of the mucosa. In both of these conditions there is an infiltration of the candida into the tissues, where hyphal forms of the fungus are seen. Candida is also a common cause of angular cheilitis, with deep painful fissures developing at the angles of the mouth.

Treatment of candida is by nystatin or amphotericin B lozenges, together with local application of the antifungal cream to the fitting surface of the dentures or angles of the mouth where necessary. This should be continued for at least two weeks, and extended to two months in cases of chronic candidosis.

Drugs causing stomatitis

Agranulocytosis, due to bone marrow depression by chloramphenicol, phenothiazines and cytotoxic drugs can precipitate secondary infective oral ulceration and gingivitis. In erythema multiforme bullous reaction of the mucous membranes, with rapid ulceration, can be associated with ingestion of either barbiturates or sulphonamides.

Occasionally, patients with toothache illogically hold aspirin tablets against the gums in the region of a painful tooth; a chemical burn often results, with the appearance of a white area of necrotic tissue surrounded by an erythematous margin.

Leukoplakia

Leukoplakia is a clinical term for the appearance, on the oral mucosa, of a white patch which cannot be removed by scraping (cf. Candida) (Fig. 1.2). It most usually occurs in people over the age of 40 years, and is commonly of little consequence. However, a small but significant number do undergo malignant change and it is, therefore, best regarded as a premalignant condition. The leukoplakias which do develop most commonly into squamous carcinoma tend to be patchy with erythematous margins, and the descriptive term of 'speckled leukoplakia' is applied.

Although external stimuli, such as denture trauma, may be associated with the appearance of leukoplakia in some patients, the cause is not known. Careful investigation and follow up are essential: any obvious irritants should be removed, and a biopsy should be performed on any such white patch. The histology of most leukoplakias shows keratinization, hyperkeratosis, or changes in the stratified epithelial cell maturation pattern (dyskeratosis). When frankly malignant changes are revealed, the entire affected area must be completely excised.

Patients with leukoplakia should be kept under periodic review and repeat biopsy performed if any visible alteration occurs.

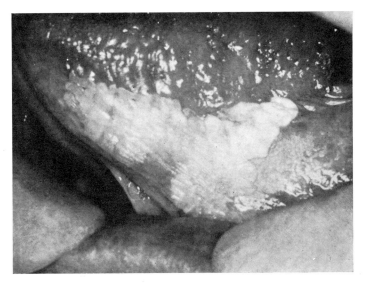

Fig. 1.2 Leukoplakia of tongue and floor of mouth.

Neoplasia

True benign tumours are rare in the oral cavity, although fibro-epithelial polyps or denture granulomata occur as a result of local trauma or irritation. The commonest benign neoplasm is the papilloma appearing as a warty swelling on the mucosa. It is treated by excision.

Squamous cell carcinoma is the commonest malignant tumour of the mouth (Fig. 1.3).

It occurs predominantly in men aged 50 or more, and the areas most commonly affected are the lateral borders of the tongue, the lower lip, the floor of the mouth and the lower alveolus. In some patients the tumour is related to chronic irritation from the sharp edge of a tooth, an ill-fitting denture or smoking, especially clay-pipe smoking; in some areas of India chewing the betel leaf is a predisposing factor. There appears to be an increased risk of this tumour in patients with tertiary syphilis. Oral cancer has become less common in Britain during the past 50 years and this has been related to such factors as changes in smoking habits from pipes to cigarettes, improved dental care and early diagnosis and treatment of syphilis. In many cases, however, there is no obvious predisposing factor.

Squamous cell carcinoma presents as an indurated swelling which may be ulcerated. Pain is not a feature in the early stages. Histological examination reveals a variety of appearances from invasive, well-differentiated, squamous epithelium with cell nest formation, to the more undifferentiated types. Treatment depends to some extent on the site. Carcinoma of the lip may be successfully treated by excision or by radiotherapy; it seldom metastasizes and has a good prognosis.

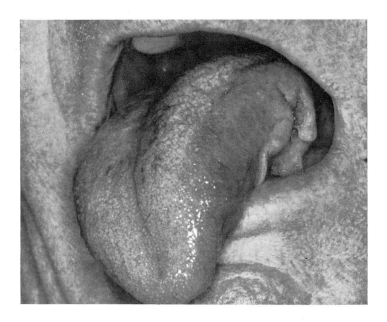

Fig. 1.3 Squamous carcinoma of tongue.

Carcinoma of the tongue may also be treated by radiotherapy or excision; metastases to the regional lymph nodes on either side of the neck are common, however, and block dissection of the nodes may be required. Carcinoma of the floor of the mouth metastasizes so frequently that it is best excised in continuity with the regional nodes on the same side. Wide excisions of mandible and maxilla may be required when the tumour is adherent to or involving bone. Techniques of reconstruction have improved to such an extent that it is possible to repair as primary procedures even quite major facial deformities. Patients need never be left drooling uncontrollably through defects after cancer ablation.

Tumours arising in the small salivary glands may appear on the palate, the tongue or the cheek mucosa. The histological pattern varies as described on page 13, but all have a marked tendency to recur unless excised very widely in the first instance. They are not radiosensitive.

DISEASES AFFECTING SALIVARY GLANDS

In humans, there are three pairs of major salivary glands (parotid, submandibular and sublingual), in addition to the many minor salivary glands situated in the oral mucosa. The volume of saliva secreted in 24 hours is in the region of 1·5 litres.

Saliva is a watery secretion containing mucoids, immunoglobulins, enzymes (especially amylase) and inorganic salts. It has several functions, including lubrication for mastication and speech and cleaning of the mucosa and teeth.

OBSTRUCTIVE CONDITIONS

Mucoceles

Mucoceles are mucus-containing cysts which occur superficially in the oral mucosa. They arise as a result of duct obstruction with retention of secretion. Treatment is by surgical excision or marsupialization. Although small mucous glands are present in all regions of the oral cavity except the anterior aspect of the hard palate, by far the most common site for these cystic lesions is the lower lip, and it is thought that they may be initiated by trauma. The term 'ranula' is used to describe the large mucous cyst which occurs in the floor of the mouth.

Calculi

Calculi occur most commonly in the submandibular gland or duct. Small stones cause occasional pain and transient swelling over the submandibular gland area during or just after eating. When they have been present for some time, infection supervenes, causing permanent enlargement of the gland. When the calculus is in the duct, simple surgical removal of the calculus is sufficient. When it is in the gland, excision of the gland plus the calculus is necessary. If acute sialoadenitis is present this should be controlled by antibiotic therapy before operation is performed.

INFECTION AND INFLAMMATION

Epidemic parotitis

Epidemic parotitis or mumps is the commonest inflammatory condition affecting the salivary glands. It is caused by a virus spread by droplet infection and affects mainly children and young adults. Glandular tissues are principally involved, the commonest being the parotid glands, but occasionally the submandibular salivary gland, the testicle, the pancreas or the ovary may be affected. The incubation period of mumps is about 18 days. Usually parotid swelling alone is the first feature, although the disease may begin with a constitutional disturbance for several days, followed by swelling of the parotid glands.

The diagnosis is made from the history and clinical presentation. A complement fixation test, which is usually positive one week after the onset of symptoms, may assist in making the diagnosis in atypical cases.

The treatment is symptomatic. Mouthwashes should be prescribed, as the mouth may be very dry on account of reduced salivary flow from the affected glands. Patients should be isolated until all glands are symptom-free and no enlargement is present.

Acute sialoadenitis

This condition most frequently involves the parotid glands. Acute parotitis tends to develop during severe febrile illnesses and after major surgical operations, especially if adequate attention is not given to the prevention of dehydration, elimination of infection and careful oral hygiene. Infection may reach the gland either ascending from the oral cavity or via the bloodstream during bacteraemia or septicaemia. This is a serious condition and requires prompt treatment with the appropriate antibiotics; surgical drainage is necessary when abscess formation has occurred within the gland capsule.

Chronic sialoadenitis

This may occur as a residual infection after acute parotitis but is often a complication of obstructive lesions of the submandibular gland or duct. Infection reaches the glands along the ducts, the commonest organisms being *Streptococcus viridans* and *Staphylococcus aureus*. Treatment is by appropriate antibiotic therapy after bacteriological examination of saliva from the duct orifice. Where calculi are present, surgical excision of the gland is indicated.

DEGENERATIVE CONDITIONS

Sjögren's syndrome

The features of this syndrome are dryness of the mouth, dryness of the eyes, combined with rheumatoid arthritis or other connective tissue disease. To substantiate the diagnosis of Sjögren's syndrome, two out of these three criteria must be present. The condition is most frequently found in female patients over 40 years of age. Characteristic histopathological changes occur in the salivary and lacrimal glands. Glandular tissue is replaced by massive infiltration of lymphocytes and plasma cells, with the resultant clinical signs of dryness of mouth and eyes. Diagnosis is made from the history and clinical examination, and there may be typical serological changes associated with connective tissue disorders. Treatment is symptomatic; glycerine mouthwashes help to relieve the dryness of the mouth.

Post-irradiation damage

Damage may follow irradiation of tumours in the upper alimentary or respiratory tracts. The salivary glands are particularly sensitive to radiation and the reduced salivary flow may be temporary or permanent. Glycerine mouthwashes or pastilles may give symptomatic relief.

TUMOURS

The neoplasm most commonly involving the salivary glands is the pleomorphic salivary adenoma. This tumour may occur in major or minor salivary glands, and common sites are the parotid and palatal glands. The pleomorphic adenoma has a characterisitic histological pattern with duct-like structures and a matrix which often consists of an amorphous mucoid substance, thought to arise from altered secretion of the glandular tissue.

As it grows, the surrounding tissue is compressed into a pseudo-capsule of the tumour, from which it can readily be enucleated. This should never be done since tumour cells are invariably present in the capsule and recurrence is inevitable. Although often regarded as benign since it does not metastasize, such a tumour is locally invasive and can cause great morbidity for many years unless radically excised in the first instance. In the parotid gland, excision is complicated by the presence of the facial nerve which requires careful dissection.

Every gradation in histological appearance can be found from the almost benign pleomorphic adenoma to the frankly malignant adeno-carcinoma, and such terms as cylindroma, adenocystic carcinoma and mucoepidermoid carcinoma are applied to specific types. All require radical excision to prevent recurrence. It is imperative to avoid cutting into the tumour at operation to prevent seeding in the wound.

It must be emphasized that any painless swelling developing slowly in the parotid gland or on the hard or soft palate is to be regarded as a salivary adenoma or one of its histological variants and widely resected. Tumours recurring after inadequate primary excision can rarely be totally eradicated without massive tissue ablation.

FURTHER READING

Cawson, R. A. (1968) *Essentials of Dental Surgery and Pathology*. London: J. & A. Churchill.
Dolby, A., ed. (in press) *Oral Mucosa in Health and Disease*. Oxford: Blackwell.
Shafer, W. G., Hine, M. K. & Levy, B. M. (1974) *Textbook of Oral Pathology*. London: W. B. Saunders.

2. The Pharynx and the Oesophagus

John Hutchison

DEVELOPMENT

There are three notable features of the embryological development of the upper alimentary tract (Fig. 2.1):

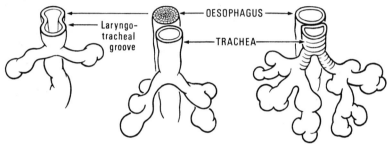

Fig. 2.1 Embryological development of oesophagus.

1. *Lengthening.* The oesophagus in particular elongates from a length of only 1 mm in the 35-day embryo, whilst the primitive solid rod of epithelial cells is vacuolated to become a tube lined by cuboido-columnar epithelium.

2. *Differentiation.* This occurs within the epithelial lining so that its cranial end, the primitive pharyngo-oesophageal region, comes to be lined by a stratified squamous epithelium, whereas a distal segment of variable length retains its columnar, gastric-like epithelium into late embryonic life and in some cases into adult life.

3. *Respiratory development.* The respiratory tract develops as a ventral bud from the primitive pharynx and branches out to form the trachea and bronchi, becoming lined by its own specialized epithelium.

An appreciation of these three important factors leads to an understanding of the congenital anomalies in this region. These include tracheo-oesophageal atresias and fistulae, mediastinal foregut cysts, hiatal hernia and anomaly of the lining of the lower oesophagus. This latter condition was erroneously referred to as congenital short oesophagus, and is now called Barrett's oesophagus.

PHYSIOLOGY OF SWALLOWING

Swallowing is a complex physiological act whereby food passes from

14

the mouth to the stomach. It is a highly co-ordinated muscular sequence which may be considered in separate stages: oral, pharyngeal
and oesophageal.

The oral stage is under voluntary control. A masticated bolus of food
is collected on the upper surface of the tongue, which rises at the tip
and a wave of contraction of the tongue passing backwards pushes the
bolus towards the pharynx. From this point the process becomes
involuntary; it is impossible to stop swallowing, and a series of reflexes
occur involving the cranial nerves V, IX and X, whereby the bolus is
propelled backwards and downwards. In the second phase, the pharyngeal constrictors squeeze the contents downwards into the gullet and
by simultaneous reflex actions the mouth, nasopharynx and respiratory
passages are occluded. The posterior part of the tongue is pressed upwards on the roof of the mouth, the soft palate elevated and the posterior wall of the nasopharynx bulges forward. Respiration is arrested
and the air passages are isolated by the elevation of the larynx. It is
almost impossible to swallow and inhale voluntarily at the same time.
During the third phase the bolus passes along the length of the oesophagus into the stomach. Three forms of oesophageal contraction are
described: primary, secondary and tertiary. With each conscious
swallowing effort, a primary peristaltic wave commencing at the upper
end of the oesophagus travels uninterruptedly to the cardia at a rate
of 5 cm per second, propelling food into the stomach. A secondary
peristaltic wave beginning at the level of the aortic arch occurs if the
primary wave fails to empty the oesophagus. Tertiary oesophageal
contractions are segmental and non-propulsive, playing little part in
the normal swallowing reflex. Oesophageal peristalsis is not necessary
for the swallowing of fluids in man, the initial phase of swallowing
together with the action of gravity being sufficient.

COMPETENCE OF THE CARDIA

A number of factors are believed to influence competence of the
cardia. These are the submucosal sphincter of the cardia, the angle
between the oesophagus and the stomach (the angle of His), the oblique
fibres of the oesophagogastric musculature, the crura of the diaphragm
and the positive intra-abdominal pressure on the abdominal segment
of the oesophagus. Probably the two most important factors are the
intrinsic submucosal sphincter, and the positive pressure exerted on
the abdominal part of the oesophagus.

VOMITING

Vomiting is a non-specific symptom which can be caused by a great
variety of stimuli. Irrespective of the cause, opening of the gastro-
oesophageal junction is an essential feature of the act of vomiting. The
pyloric sphincter contracts, the stomach and oesophagus, including the

gastro-oesophageal junction relax, and respiration is arrested with fixation of the diaphragm in the inspiratory position. The respiratory tract is isolated as in swallowing with closure of the glottis and elevation of the larynx. The contents of the stomach are then expelled by a violent contraction of the abdominal muscles. The stomach and oesophagus remain atonic throughout and in adults there is no reverse peristalsis.

It would seem that the essential feature during the act of vomiting is the elevation of the abdominal part of the oesophagus from the positive intra-abdominal pressure into the area of the negative intrathoracic pressure, the lower oesophagus and cardia being tented upwards. In this way closure of the cardia which prevents regurgitation under ordinary circumstances is prevented, and with the propulsive efforts of the abdominal musculature and the very marked increase of intra-abdominal pressure, the gastric contents are expelled upwards against gravity throughout the length of the oesophagus.

SYMPTOMS OF PHARYNGO-OESOPHAGEAL DISORDERS

1. *Dysphagia.* Difficulty in swallowing is the most important symptom, and usually indicates obstruction. Malignant tumours of the pharynx or oesophagus classically cause a progressive increase in dysphagia, difficulty being experienced first only with solid food, later with semisolids, and finally even with liquids. On the other hand, dysphagia can be intermittent in such conditions as achalasia, or the earlier stages of benign strictures of the oesophagus.

Difficulty with swallowing can be a symptom of various conditions such as bulbar paralysis, cerebro-vascular accident, muscular dystrophy or myasthenia gravis. It may also occur after oesophageal surgery or radiation. It is also a fairly common complaint in patients with hysteria.

Since the sensory innervation of the oesophagus is segmental, accurate localization of the level of hold-up is usual.

2. *Heartburn.* This symptom usually indicates regurgitation of irritant substances from the stomach into the oesophagus.

3. *Waterbrash.* This term describes the release of an excessive volume of salivary secretion into the mouth. It is commonly associated with heartburn.

4. *Regurgitation.* When a considerable amount of fluid escapes proximally from the stomach, or collects above an obstructive lesion in the gullet, the liquid wells up into the pharynx and, especially during the night, may be inhaled, leading to respiratory symptoms.

INVESTIGATIONS OF PHARYNX AND OESOPHAGUS

Clinical examination includes routine physical examination, abdominal examination for hepatic enlargement and palpation of cervical nodes, since the lymphatics of the pharynx and the upper oesophagus drain to cervical lymph glands. Special investigations are chest X-ray, barium swallow and endoscopy with biopsy and possible cytology. The principal aids to diagnosis are:

1. *X-ray.* X-ray of thorax and barium swallow examination provide useful information. The radiological examination of the lower oesophagus, cardia and fundus of the stomach may require careful positioning of the patient to produce reflux from the stomach to the oesophagus and to demonstrate hiatal herniation, or lesions of the cardia and fundus.

2. *Endoscopy.* The nasal, oral and hypopharyngeal regions can be examined by direct endoscopy under local anaesthesia and biopsies taken.

The inspection of the interior of the oesophagus, oesophagoscopy, is now performed using fibrescopes. These instruments are easy and safe to pass, have excellent illumination and a clear magnified image.

The fibre-oesophagoscope is graduated to 60 cm so that it can be can be passed through the cardia. On withdrawal, it gives a clear view of the proximal stomach and cardia. Small biopsies and brush biopsies are easily obtained, and attachments for automatic photography are available.

The Negus metal oesophagoscope (Fig. 2.2) was the choice in this country for many years but its use is potentially dangerous. Its main use nowadays is for the removal of foreign bodies and the dilatation of strictures. This latter procedure is, however, now easily and safely carried out by the use of the Eder-Puestow dilators. A guide wire is first passed along a channel in the fibrescope and through the stricture. After withdrawal of the fibrescope, hollow bougies are then safely passed over the guide wire.

Fibrescopes may be passed under general or local anaesthesia.

3. *Pressure recording.* Studies of oesophageal pressures and motility waves have been shown to produce recognizable wave patterns in several conditions, including achalasia, and oesophagitis, and further application of wavometric techniques may help our understanding of the sphincters and muscle walls of the oesophagus and cardia.

DISEASES OF THE PHARYNX

PHARYNGITIS

Inflammation of the pharynx may be acute or chronic.

Acute pharyngitis

Acute pharyngitis is most commonly due to an infecting agent, e.g. haemolytic Streptococcus, which also involves the tonsils. Trauma such as occurs on swallowing a foreign body or irritating substances may also cause acute pharyngitis.

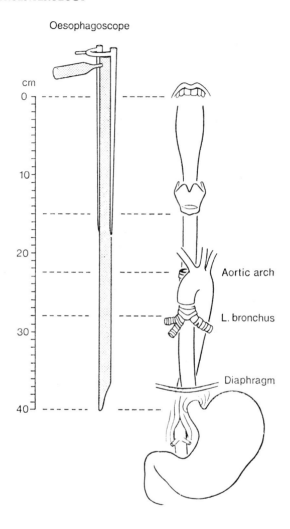

Fig. 2.2 Diagram of levels in the oesophagus when tip of the rigid oesophagoscope is introduced to different lengths measured from the incisor teeth.

The main symptom is pain on swallowing and, in the presence of infection, there may be constitutional disturbance, fever and tender enlargement of the anterior cervical lymph nodes.

Treatment

In the presence of infection the appropriate antibiotic, e.g. penicillin in the case of streptococcal infection, should be given. Simple analgesics such as aspirin may be required for the relief of pain.

Chronic pharyngitis

This is most commonly caused by irritant substances passing repeatedly over the pharyngeal mucosa. Tobacco smoke, dust in the inspired air, hot or spicy food or drink and especially alcohol are all culprits in this respect. There is often an associated laryngitis.

The patient complains of painful dysphagia, the diagnosis is made from the history and the granular erythematous appearance of the pharyngeal mucosa.

Treatment

This consists of avoidance of both the irritant substance and hot food or liquid.

FUNCTIONAL DISORDERS OF SWALLOWING

The term 'globus hystericus' is used to describe the sensation of having a lump in the throat but without true dysphagia. The patient swallows frequently because this relieves the globus symptom, although the compulsive desire to swallow may cause some discomfort. The condition is often relieved by swallowing food, in contrast to pharyngitis and other organic lesions in which swallowing is painful and may result in spasm.

Functional dysphagia is a purely psychiatric disorder in which there is no organic lesion but there is a very real difficulty in swallowing and severe malnutrition may result.

The important issue in all of these cases is to carry out a full investigation to exclude organic lesions such as sideropaenic dysphagia, pulsion diverticulum or achalasia.

Treatment includes the reassurance of a full investigation, antispasmodics and the use of a mercury bougie.

PHARYNGEAL TUMOURS

Benign tumours

Simple tumours of the pharynx are relatively uncommon. They give rise to pressure effects or haemorrhage. Treatment is by excision.

Malignant tumours

Malignant tumours of the pharynx are of greater clinical importance. There are two main groups, those arising from above the larynx, and the postcricoid group.

Histologically epilaryngeal tumours are more often squamous carcinomata but transitional-cell types may occur. They usually occur in men of older age-groups and upper cervical lymph node involvement is common. The treatment of choice is radiotherapy.

By contrast, postcricoid tumours occur in middle-aged women usually as a complication of sideropaenic dysphagia. They are of transitional-cell type, invasive in character and lymphatic spread occurs early.

The symptoms are dysphagia, which may be associated with pain in the neck, jaw and ear, and not uncommonly the tumour directly involves the cranial nerves. The patient may give a history of ill-health associated with chronic anaemia. It is therefore very important when investigating such patients to consider the possibility of the Brown-Kelly-Patterson syndrome and to inspect the pharyngo-oesophageal region.

Treatment

Treatment may be by radical resection which involves a prolonged and multistage operation associated with high morbidity and mortality. It is seldom justified. X-ray therapy gives better overall results with much less disturbance to the patient.

RETROPHARYNGEAL ABSCESS

Retropharyngeal abscess in either acute or chronic form is now a rare occurrence. The acute abscess is readily recognized by inspection of the posterior pharyngeal wall. Treatment is by per-oral incision. The chronic abscess is almost invariably tuberculous and points in the side of the neck. Evacuation of this is effected through an incision behind the sternomastoid muscle.

DIVERTICULA

These are considered along with oesophageal diverticula on page 28.

DISORDERS OF THE OESOPHAGUS

Reflux oesophagitis

Reflux oesophagitis may be defined as an inflammatory reaction resulting from the irritation of the squamous epithelium of the gullet by regurgitated juices. It is important to note that only squamous epithelium is affected in this way. In the earlier stages the epithelial lining is congested, but later the surface becomes ulcerated. If this condition is untreated, progressive intramural inflammation may lead to fibrosis and perioesophagitis with stricture formation.

Many factors are responsible, including incompetence of the cardia, increased intra-abdominal pressure and possibly excess gastric acid secretion.

Incompetence of the cardia is most commonly associated with sliding hiatal hernia (p. 21). Occasionally there is incompetence without herniation, possibly due to developmental abnormality. Resection of the cardia or plastic procedures at this site disturb the closing mechanism. Intubation either for gastric aspiration or for feeding also prevents closure of the cardia so that a recumbent patient may develop ulceration during the postoperative period. Increased intra-abdominal pressure develops during pregnancy and in association with adiposity, constipation, stooping and coughing.

Acute oesophagitis occurring in the neonate due to the existence of a congenital sliding hiatal hernia with gross incompetence may result in severe haemorrhage.

Symptoms

The chief complaint is heartburn, which may amount to severe pain both in the retrosternal and interscapular regions. It is due to irritation of the mucosal lining, and also to abnormal spastic contractions of the gullet. With ulceration, bleeding may occur and it may be severe, while in other cases chronic haemorrhage may result in anaemia. Intermittent dysphagia may occur due to spasm without organic stenosis, but persistent increasing dysphagia indicates organic stricture formation.

Diagnosis

Diagnosis is established by barium swallow, oesophagoscopy and biopsy. Chronic stricture more often occurs in older patients in whom differentiation from malignant disease becomes difficult.

Treatment

The treatment of oesophagitis in the majority of cases consists of conservative measures. These include weight reduction and antacids and the avoidance of large meals. The patient is advised to avoid stooping and also to raise the head of the bed on 20 cm blocks. If these measures fail and a sliding hiatal hernia is present, surgical repair should be advised.

Sliding hiatal hernia

In this condition the cardia with a pouch of stomach is elevated through the hiatus (Figs. 2.3 and 2.4). The oesophagus is of normal length, evidenced by the ease with which the herniation can be reduced at operation.

Sliding hiatal hernia may be congenital. Some neonates present with gross herniation, but the majority of these will recover by the simple method of being nursed in the sitting position, indicating that there is no congenital shortening of the gullet.

On the other hand, the major incidence of hiatal hernia as a clinical problem is in the fifth to the seventh decades, suggesting that whatever developmental fault may exist, the major aetiological factors are acquired. It is accepted that gastro-oesophageal competence depends on a number of factors, e.g. a physiological sphincter mechanism at the cardia, the oblique entrance of the oesophagus into the stomach, the positive intra-abdominal pressure exerted on the abdominal part of the oesophagus.

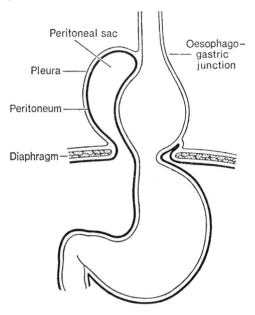

Fig. 2.3 Diagrammatic representation of the basic anatomical defects in sliding hiatal hernia.

Symptoms

Sliding hiatal hernia is of little clinical importance unless it is associated with gastro-oesophageal incompetence, and reflux. The symptoms are those of reflux oesophagitis described on page 20. A large thoracic pouch may cause pain due to loculation and obstruction. It may lead to some degree of respiratory embarrassment due to its size and to associated pulmonary collapse, or it may be the seat of gastric ulceration with severe bleeding, but these are uncommon complications.

Treatment

Twenty per cent of patients with hiatal hernia have associated conditions such as duodenal ulcer, gallstones, gastric ulcer or myocardial disease. It is therefore important that full investigation be carried out before it is assumed that the symptoms are entirely due to the reflux. Hiatal hernia and reflux oesophagitis should be treated conservatively as described for oesophagitis (p. 20). The majority of patients will respond to such measures. Indications for surgical treatment are clear:

1. Failure to relieve symptoms of oesophagitis by medical treatment
2. Persistent or severe bleeding
3. Stricture formation.

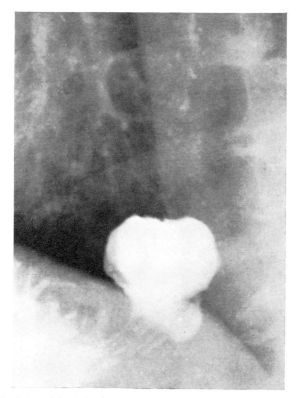

Fig. 2.4 Typical radiological appearances of sliding hiatal hernia on barium meal examination. Demonstration of the hernia usually requires some procedure to increase temporarily intra-abdominal pressure, and thereby fill the herniated portion of stomach with barium. (See also Fig. 2.3.)

It is wrong to adopt an over-conservative approach to this problem. The final stage of reflux associated with hiatal hernia in which a fixed oesophageal stricture develops is a condition more often encountered in older people and operative treatment is difficult and carries considerable risk. It is therefore proper to take the view that a hiatal hernia which is causing symptoms not relieved by medical treatment, should be considered for surgical reduction.

Surgical treatment. The surgical treatment aims at reduction of the hernia and restoration of gastro-oesophageal competence.

Satisfactory repair of the hiatus can be achieved by an abdominal, a thoracic, or a combined abdomino-thoracic approach. The main advantage of the abdominal approach is that other intra-abdominal disorders may be more easily corrected if necessary. The thoracic approach is more satisfactory for mobilization of the chronically inflamed retracted oesophagus. In the majority of cases the hernia is easily reduced into the abdomen with an adequate length of oesophagus, and the hiatus closed by sutures placed usually behind the oesophagus. There is no direct surgical means of creating a competent sphincter, but when the cardia is reduced into the abdomen, and the lower oesophagus comes under the influence of the positive intra-abdominal pressure, competence is restored. The wide hiatus can be reduced to a normal size and the oesophago-gastric angle restored. A variety of technical procedures has been described to prevent recurrence, and each has its advocates.

Para-oesophageal hiatal hernia

This is an uncommon condition accounting for about 5 per cent of all hiatal hernias. The fundus of the stomach herniates upwards alongside the oesophagus, laterally and anteriorly (Fig. 2.5). The cardia remains in its normal position and is usually competent so that the symptoms associated with gastro-oesophageal reflux are absent.

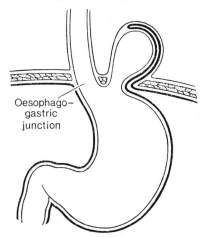

Oesophago–
gastric
junction

Fig. 2.5 Diagrammatic representation of the basic anatomical defects in para-oesophageal hernia.

When the gap in the diaphragm is extensive, a large part of the stomach may roll up into the thorax so that the greater curvature and even the greater omentum and colon are contained in the sac. It is sometimes difficult to distinguish this condition radiologically from that of eventration of the diaphragm.

Severe pain may develop because of distension within the thoracic pouch which has become loculated and obstructed. The pain is relieved by belching or vomiting. Pain and bleeding may occur due to ulceration usually situated at the constriction where the hernia passes through the diaphragm; if the hernia is large, there may be pain in the back and dyspnoea associated with cardiorespiratory embarrassment. Surgical reduction and repair give good results and should be performed whenever the diagnosis is made, thus avoiding the more serious complications.

Lower segment of oesophagus lined with columnar epithelium (Barrett's oesophagus)

In this condition, a variable length of the lower oesophagus retains a colummar-cell lining. The mode of development of the oesophageal mucous membrane already described (p. 14) readily explains how this anomaly occurs. It is a reasonably common condition, but may produce no symptoms. If, however, it is associated with incompetence and sliding hiatus hernia the resulting reflux will lead to peptic oesophagitis above the junction of the squamous and columnar epithelium, producing all the sequelae described on page 34, but at a higher level. Many of these cases will respond to conservative measures as described under reflux oesophagitis, but if medical treatment fails it will be necessary to restore competence at the cardia and to repair the hiatal hernia if present.

The term 'congenital short oesophagus' was used for many years to describe this condition, because it was recognised in children, leading to high stricture. However, it is now accepted that it may present for the first time at any age.

Functional disorders of the oesophagus

These include three conditions of uncertain aetiology: achalasia of the cardia, diffuse spasm, and tertiary contractions.

ACHALASIA OF THE CARDIA

This condition, formerly named cardiospasm, is believed to result from failure of a segment of lower oesophagus to relax in response to recurring peristaltic waves. The relationship between achalasia and diffuse spasm (p. 26) is uncertain.

Achalasia may occur at any age. The presenting symptom is dysphagia which gradually increases in severity. Although there is no satisfactory explanation, the patient may state that it is easier to swallow solids than fluids. As the condition progresses, the dysphagia becomes persistent and severe. When symptoms have continued, retention and stagnation of food within this large gullet may lead to ulceration and infection. Regurgitation, especially in the recumbent position, can cause inhalation into the respiratory tract; in such circumstances the main complaint may be of recurring chest infection.

The diagnosis is usually established by the history and barium swallow (Figs. 2.6 and 2.7). Endoscopy should be performed to exclude tumour, or simple stricture.

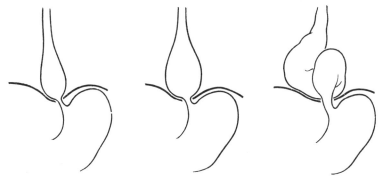

| Moderate Dilatation | Marked Dilatation | Elongation & Tortuosity |

Fig. 2.6 Diagram of three different grades of severity of achalasia of the cardia.

In early cases relief may be obtained by dilating the narrow segment, either by simple bouginage or by a hydrostatic dilator. The majority, however, require operation and the most popular procedure is anterior cardiomyotomy (the modified Heller operation), in which the longitudinal and circular muscle fibres are divided over a length of 5 cm extending over the lower oesophagus, cardia and proximal part of the stomach. This operation is performed either through an upper abdominal or thoracic incision, and is followed by rapid relief of symptoms. After this procedure oesophageal reflux occasionally occurs, and this may result from disturbance of the hiatus caused at operation.

DIFFUSE SPASM

This is a rare condition in which well-defined areas of spasm occur throughout the length of the oesophagus. There may be associated pain which can simulate that of cardiac origin.

Diffuse spasm may be difficult to treat. Relief can usually be obtained by intermittent bouginage, but it may be necessary on occasions to perform an extended myotomy throughout the length of the gullet.

TERTIARY CONTRACTIONS

They appear as a series of irregular incoordinated contractions of the oesophagus which do not aid the normal process of swallowing. They are seen in some patients with reflux oesophagitis, and may be found in elderly people with no apparent oesophageal disease. The term 'corkscrew oesophagus' is descriptive of an extreme degree of this condition. The diagnosis is essentially a radiological one. No treatment is required.

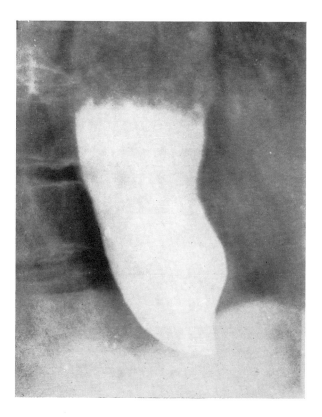

Fig. 2.7 Typical X-ray appearances of achalasia of the cardia on barium swallow examination. (See also Fig. 2.6)

Sideropaenic dysphagia (Brown-Kelly-Patterson syndrome or Plummer-Vinson syndrome)

Chronic iron-deficiency anaemia is commonly associated with degeneration of epithelial structures leading to koilonychia, atrophic glossitis and superficial gastritis. Similar changes may occur in the mucosa of the pharynx and upper oesophagus giving rise later to stenosis and dysphagia. The combination of iron-deficiency anaemia, superficial glossitis and dysphagia is known as the Brown-Kelly-Patterson or Plummer-Vinson syndrome. The condition may occur prior to the development of overt anaemia, in association with a low serum iron, and is therefore described as sideropaenic dysphagia.

Changes in the mucous membrane of the upper oesophagus and pharynx may proceed to ulceration and fibrosis resulting in scarring and deformity. This in turn leads to stenosis and sometimes to web or diaphragm formation. These changes may be seen on barium swallow and endoscopy (Fig. 2.8). Mucosal biopsy reveals atrophy with deficiency of the iron-containing enzyme, cytochrome oxidase. The aetiological importance of the enzyme deficiency is not established. Dysphagia in this condition is due to spasm in the earlier stages and later to the effects of organic stricture. The syndrome, which is almost always found in females in the fourth, fifth and sixth decades, is a precancerous condition; about 15 per cent of such patients will develop postcricoid carcinoma.

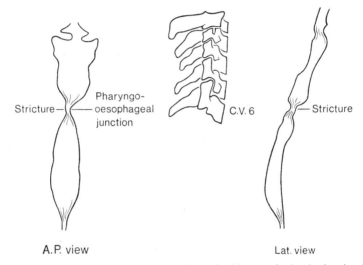

A.P. view   Lat. view

Fig. 2.8 Diagram of usual outlines of stricture in sideropaenic dysphagia, showing characteristic level in relation to cervical vertebrae.

The treatment is by adequate iron replacement; dysphagia is relieved by dilatation of the stricture during endoscopy. A careful follow-up is necessary to maintain a normal level of serum iron, to relieve dysphagia and to recognize the early appearances of malignant change.

Pharyngo-oesophageal diverticula

There are three types (Fig. 2.9):
 1. Pharyngo-oesophageal (pharyngeal diverticulum)
 2. Thoracic (midoesophageal diverticulum)
 3. Epiphrenic (supradiaphragmatic diverticulum).

Pharyngo-oesophageal. A pharyngeal diverticulum arises in the midline posteriorly, between the oblique and transverse fibres of the

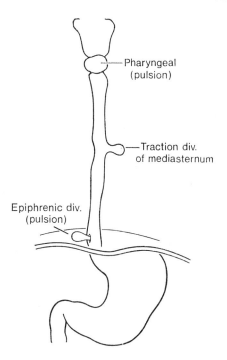

Fig. 2.9 Three commonest sites at which pharyngo-oesophageal diverticula develop.

inferior constrictor muscle of the pharynx. It is of pulsion type and occurs through a weak part of the pharyngeal wall just above the transverse fibres of the cricopharyngeus muscle which form the pharyngo-oesophageal sphincter (Fig. 2.10). Depending on its size, the pouch may cause dysphagia, effortless regurgitation of food, or fullness on one side of the neck, usually the left. The initial presentation may be one of the complications, which include ulceration, perforation, fistula formation or aspiration pneumonitis. The condition is best treated by a one-stage surgical resection of the pouch through an incision in front of the sternomastoid muscle.

Thoracic. Diverticula at the midoesophageal level may develop either spontaneously, or as a result of traction associated with chronic inflammatory disease, particularly tuberculosis of the tracheal and tracheobronchial lymph glands. Symptoms seldom arise from the primary condition, but oesophagobronchial or oesophagomediastinal fistula, or haemorrhage may occur.

Epiphrenic. The epiphrenic diverticulum occurs at the lower end of the oesophagus and usually bulges to one side of the gullet. It seldom gives rise to troublesome symptoms, but may on occasion reach a considerable size, and cause dysphagia with retention and bleeding.

Treatment is by one-stage resection usually through a right-sided lower thoracotomy.

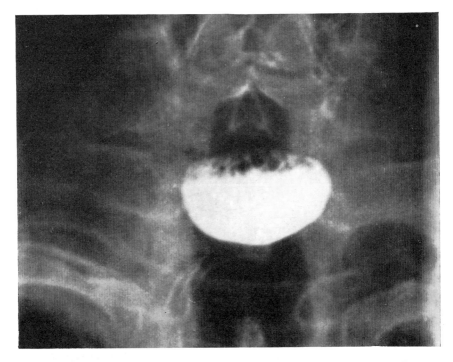

Fig. 2.10 Typical X-ray appearances of pharyngeal diverticulum on barium swallow examination: antero-posterior view.

Tumours of the oesophagus

BENIGN TUMOURS

Simple epithelial tumours such as papilloma or adenoma are extremely rare. The commonest benign tumour is the leiomyoma, which occurs usually in the lower oesophagus as a submucosal intramural swelling. It may protrude into the lumen and become pedunculated, causing obstruction. The only symptom is dysphagia and diagnosis is established by barium swallow and endoscopy. Treatment is surgical removal, either by enucleation of the tumour or by resection of a segment of the oesophagus and end-to-end anastomosis.

MALIGNANT TUMOURS

Carcinoma of the oesophagus is a disease of the later decades of life, 75 per cent of sufferers being over 60 years of age. The incidence in males is three times that in females. It is much less common than gastric carcinoma. In the western region of Scotland, with a population of three and a half millions, an average of 150 new cases of carcinoma of the oesophagus present annually.

As the tumour may extend over several centimetres of the oesophagus it is difficult to state precisely the incidence at different levels, but approximately 25 per cent are in the upper third, 45 to 50 per cent in the middle, and 25 to 30 per cent in the lower third. Eighty-nine per cent of all cancers of the oesophagus are of the squamous-cell type. The remainder, which are adenocarcinomata, arise either from the mucus-secreting glands of the gullet or from columnar-cell epithelium at the lower end.

Carcinoma of the oesophagus extends both longitudinally and circumferentially, producing either a bulky polypoidal growth blocking the lumen, or a stricture. Tumour growth may also penetrate the wall to involve the trachea, bronchi, aorta or mediastinum.

Initially lymphatic spread of carcinoma of the oesophagus is to the adjacent glands draining the appropriate segment, but when the disease is more advanced, glands at a more distant site may also become involved. The principal drainage of the pharynx and upper oesophagus is to the cervical glands. The middle portion drains directly to the para-aortic glands, and the lower third to the glands around the cardia, the lesser curve of the stomach, and coeliac axis.

Clinical diagnosis

The important symptom of this disease is dysphagia, which sometimes occurs as an acute incident associated with an attempt to swallow a large or solid bolus, but more commonly is of gradual onset. Not only is the patient unable to have the pleasure of taking fluid and food, but because of the associated starvation the general health deteriorates. When, however, the obstruction becomes complete and the patient is not even able to swallow his own saliva, there is the added distress of continual regurgitation and, in the recumbent position during the night, the danger of inhalation into the respiratory tract. A patient who complains of dysphagia, even as an isolated incident, should be fully investigated by X-rays and endoscopy; otherwise he may continue for several months accommodating to the increasing difficulty and eventually present with an inoperable tumour. The diagnosis of carcinoma of the oesophagus may be more difficult when the presenting symptoms are primarily those of anaemia due to blood loss from the tumour. The patient may not volunteer the symptoms of dysphagia.

The differential diagnosis lies between carcinoma and other causes of oesophageal obstruction. Chronic stricture secondary to reflux oesophagitis usually follows a history of heartburn. Achalasia usually occurs at an earlier age than carcinoma, and X-ray findings are quite different (Fig. 2.11; cf. 2.7). However, one must keep in mind the possibility of the coincidence of carcinoma with either simple stricture or achalasia. Dysphagia due to extrinsic pressure is uncommon, but it may result from mediastinal involvement in advanced bronchial carcinoma, or from enlarged mediastinal lymph nodes.

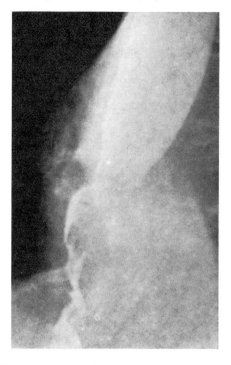

Fig. 2.11 Typical X-ray appearances of carcinoma of lower end of oesophagus.

Investigations and assessment for treatment

It is essential to examine the neck for enlarged lymph nodes. Further important investigations are X-ray screening with barium swallow, chest X-ray and oesophagoscopy. A definitive diagnosis cannot be made on X-ray examination alone. The possibility of malignancy should never be excluded without endoscopy and biopsy.

Oesophagoscopy (p. 17). At this examination the level of the upper end of the lesion is determined in centimetres from the incisor teeth, and the diagnosis established by the histological examination of specimens removed from the lesion.

Assessment for surgery. Certain factors preclude radical surgery in this disease. These include involvement of lymph nodes or the liver, or advanced cardiorespiratory insufficiency. Candidates for surgery should have careful assessment of their nutritional state, and any anaemia, protein deficiency or electrolyte abnormality corrected.

Treatment

The possible forms of treatment are:
1. Radical resection
2. Radical X-ray therapy
3. Palliative measures including: (*a*) short-circuit operations, (*b*) intubation of the tumour, and (*c*) palliative X-ray therapy.

Pharyngo-oesophageal lesions and those of the upper third of the oesophagus are best treated by irradiation. The prolonged and complicated measures necessary to remove such tumours surgically yield disappointing results and are seldom justifiable.

Lesions of the middle third may be treated by any of the methods listed, although, where technically feasible, we prefer surgical resection. Lesions of the lower third of the oesophagus and of the cardia, whether squamous or adenocarcinoma, are probably best treated by resection, whether this is a radical or a palliative procedure.

Radical resection. For both middle and lower third tumours the aims are to divide the oesophagus, ideally 5 cm above the upper limit of obvious tumour, and transect the stomach well below the lower limit. The remaining oesophagus and stomach are then anastomosed, usually end-to-end.

The actual operative approaches differ depending on the site of the tumour. For middle third lesions the abdomen is first explored to determine whether metastases are present or absent. If absent, the oesophageal mobilization is performed through a separate high right-sided thoracic incision. For lower third tumours, if the abdominal exploration shows that resection is technically possible, the further oesophageal mobilization is approached by extending the abdominal incision into the lower left pleural cavity.

Radical X-ray therapy. Tumours of the upper and middle regions may also be treated by irradiation from an external high-energy source such as radioactive cobalt. The irradiation can be focused on the oesophageal region from various angles, thus minimizing damage to more superficial tissues.

Palliative treatment. The object of palliative treatment is to relieve dysphagia. If surgical removal, either radical or palliative, is not possible there are two alternatives: X-ray therapy or intubation.

Squamous and undifferentiated tumours respond to X-ray therapy, and this is a valuable method of palliation in the upper and middle third lesions. A recognized and serious complication of this treatment, however, is development of a fistula between the oesophagus and the trachea or bronchus.

The insertion of an indwelling tube through the malignant stricture is a satisfactory method of relief in advanced cases although this is only of short-term benefit. Plastic tubes, such as Celestin or Mousseau-Barbin patterns are usually employed nowadays. Insertion involves laparotomy and gastrotomy with the attendant risks in a patient in poor physical condition. Nevertheless, relief of dysphagia may extend over several months. There is no longer any place for the operation of gastrostomy in the treatment of carcinoma of the oesophagus.

Prognosis and results

Operative mortality for tumours of the middle third is around 25 per cent and for the lower third and cardia about 10 per cent. About one-third of patients who survive operation will live for two years and 5 to 10 per cent will live for five years, the survival figures for patients with lesions of the lower third being better than those for the middle third.

Simple strictures of the oesophagus

Simple strictures of the oesophagus occur as a late result of physical or chemical trauma, but the commonest cause is ulceration caused by continued gastro-oesophageal reflux. Chemical agents such as corrosive fluids, and physical trauma resulting from impacted foreign bodies or from instrumentation may lead to ulceration with subsequent stricture formation. Many cases are adequately treated by bouginage, which, if necessary, can be repeated at intervals over a long period of time (Fig. 2.12). In these circumstances the patient himself may be taught to pass bougies.

Treatment of stricture following oesophageal reflux

Prevention of stricture formation by the treatment of reflux oeso-

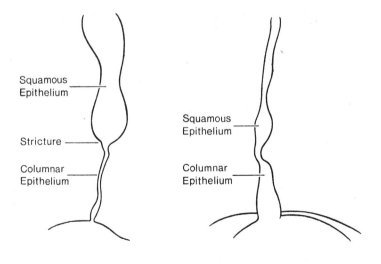

BEFORE Dilatation   AFTER Dilatation

Fig. 2.12 Benign stricture of oesophagus: diagrammatic explanation of X-ray appearances in Figure 2.13.

phagitis (p. 20) is of prime importance. Should the patient present with a stricture he requires full investigation by X-ray (Fig. 2.13), endoscopy and biopsy to determine the nature of the lesion. When the diagnosis of simple stricture has been established it may be effectively treated by bouginage. The patient should also be advised on the medical treatment of reflux oesophagitis. In those who also have a hiatal hernia, surgical repair of the hernia is indicated.

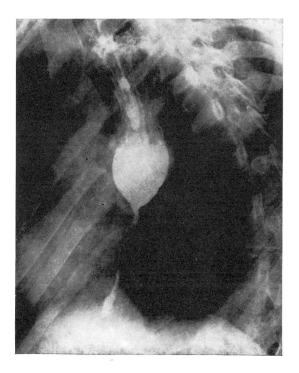

Fig. 2.13 Benign stricture in Barrett's oesophagus: X-ray appearances on barium swallow before and after dilatation by bougies. (See also Fig. 2.12)

Rarely all other methods of treatment fail and resection of the stricture is required. Continuity may be re-established by bringing up a jejunal loop, the upper end of which is anastomosed to the oesophagus above, and the stomach below, the diaphragm.

Foreign bodies impacted in the oesophagus

These occur most commonly in children under three years of age, the site of hold-up being most frequently at the cricopharyngeal sphincter. Other sites are at the level of the aortic arch and at the gastro-oesophageal junction. Diagnosis is based on the history, X-ray examination and endoscopy. Not all foreign bodies are radio-opaque and the use of gastrografin may be helpful in identifying the object. Endoscopy will locate the foreign body and may permit its removal.

Perforation of the oesophagus

Perforation usually results from injury, either at endoscopy or bouginage, or from swallowing a foreign body. Injury during oesophagoscopy occurs usually either at the pharyngo-oesophageal junction or at the lower end of the oesophagus.

Spontaneous perforation of the apparently normal oesophagus may rarely occur.

If perforation is suspected, X-rays of neck and chest should be taken, and a careful watch kept for the development of surgical emphysema in the neck. Fortunately many patients with minimal tears will settle without operative interference. Oral intake is forbidden and the patient is treated by intravenous fluids and parenteral antibiotics. Larger perforations should be repaired.

'SPONTANEOUS' RUPTURE OF THE OESOPHAGUS

Rarely, rupture can occur in an apparently normal oesophagus. This is nearly always associated with retching, vomiting or coughing after the ingestion of large quantities of food and/or alcohol. As a result there is a rapid rise in the intraluminal pressure which causes a tear. Mediastinitis, pneumothorax and pleural effusion may occur, usually on the left side. In some cases the pleural involvement may be delayed and a developing empyema leads to the retrospective diagnosis of spontaneous rupture.

The classical picture is that of sudden and dramatic collapse with pain coming on after a bout of vomiting and coughing. The differential diagnosis includes many abdominal and thoracic emergencies, such as perforated peptic ulcer and coronary artery thrombosis.

Early thoracotomy with closure of the perforation is indicated. If operative treatment is delayed beyond 12 hours and primary closure becomes impossible, a water-seal drainage of the pleural cavity and mediastinum is required.

FURTHER READING

Cohen, S. (1974) Diseases of the esophagus. In *Gastrointestinal Pathophysiology*, ed. Brooks, F.P. New York, London, Toronto: Oxford University Press.
Payne, W. S. & Olsen, A. M. (Eds.) (1974) *The Esophagus*. Philadelphia, Lea & Febiger.
Wells, C., Kyle, J. & Dunphy, J. E. (Eds.) (1974) The pharynx and oesophagus. In *Scientific Foundations of Surgery*. London: Heinemann.
Wells, C., Kyle, J. & Dunphy, J. E. (Eds.) (1974) The effects of surgery of the oesophagus. In *Scientific Foundations of Surgery*. London: Heinemann.

3. The Stomach

Iain E. Gillespie, Sir Andrew Watt Kay, T. J. Thomson and G. P. Crean

PEPTIC ULCER

This subject includes the common duodenal ulcer, the rather less common gastric ulcer, the still less frequent recurrent ulcer after a gastric operation and, rarest of all, the ulcer occurring in the Zollinger-Ellison syndrome caused by a gastrin-secreting tumour in the pancreas.

Although the pattern of peptic ulcer, the sex incidence, the ratio of duodenal to gastric lesions, and the frequency and severity of complications have apparently undergone changes over the past few decades and are probably still changing at the present time, peptic ulcer in general is still a large health problem in this country; various estimates, which admittedly are approximations, have suggested that as many as one in ten of our population suffers at some time or other during his or her lifetime from ulcer-type dyspepsia. It has been suggested that various social factors may influence the incidence of peptic ulcer, but we believe that the continual and often profound changes in social structure of our population make comments based on arbitrary social gradings of little value. Epidemiological studies of large groups of patients with peptic ulcer have shown a slight relative preponderance of blood group O in those with duodenal ulcer, but knowledge of a particular patient's blood group does not assist in either diagnosis or management of an individual patient. While we still do not know the precise cause or causes of peptic ulcer, much is known about the natural history of the disease, and the basic principles of both medical and surgical treatment are fairly generally agreed.

It is probable, but not conclusively proven, that all ulcers begin as breaks in the lining mucosa of the affected part of the upper gastro-intestinal tract, and that proteolytic digestion by gastric juice containing acid and pepsin is essential for the continuance of the lesion. It seems likely that the initial damage to the mucosa can result from various harmful influences and that the relative contribution of each may vary from one individual ulcer patient to another. Thus there is some indirect evidence which suggests that there is relative vagal over-activity in duodenal ulceration and disordered function of the pyloric antrum in gastric ulcer. Recurrent ulcers after gastric operations might then also be explained by a failure to control adequately the primary defect. Ulcers in the Zollinger-Ellison syndrome are attributed to the excessive output from the pancreas of the hormone gastrin which in turn stimulates the acid-secreting cells of the stomach; this is one of the strongest pieces of evidence in favour of a disorder of acid secretion being directly responsible for ulceration.

The pathology of ulcers is so well known that it is not necessary here to do more than summarize the appearances.

Acute ulcers. These rarely come under clinical scrutiny unless they bleed or perforate. They tend to be shallow and rarely penetrate deeper than the muscularis mucosae.

Chronic ulcers. Chronic ulcers, in an active phase, penetrate the muscle coat, and the fibrous tissue-lined crater may contain a slough. A peptic ulcer is rarely static, and in the healing phase the crater is reduced in size by contraction of its fibrous tissue base and by the growth of granulation tissue which may become covered by a thin layer of epithelium growing in from the margins. Repeated episodes of scarring may lead to much deformity and, in the case of pyloric or duodenal ulcer, to organic stenosis and impaired gastric emptying.

Clinical presentation

Although duodenal and gastric ulcers possibly arise from different pathological processes, the symptoms and signs with which they commonly present are almost indistinguishable. It was formerly taught that there were certain distinguishing diagnostic features, but most clinicians find that although it is usually easy to make the diagnosis of peptic ulcer, it is often difficult to decide whether the ulcer is in the duodenum or in the stomach. In this country duodenal ulcer is 10 to 15 times commoner than gastric ulcer and this difference is more marked in males. On chance alone therefore, it is much more likely that a patient presenting with typical symptoms will prove to have a duodenal ulcer.

The principal and almost invariable symptom of a peptic ulcer is upper abdominal pain. This is usually located in the epigastrium and described as a boring, gnawing, or nagging sensation. Indeed, many patients do not use the term 'pain', with its implication of severity, to describe the symptom and prefer the term 'discomfort'. The severity varies from patient to patient and, in each individual, may vary considerably from time to time. It is characteristic of the pain that it tends to occur when the stomach is empty, and is therefore more noticeable an hour or two after the previous meal, or just preceding the following meal which commonly provides prompt, if temporary, relief. The explanation for this relationship with eating food, and drinking milk, is that at least one of the factors causing the pain is exposure of nerve endings in the ulcerated stomach or duodenal wall to acid gastric juice; food or milk absorbs this acid and so relieves pain. It might be expected that a gastric ulcer would be exposed to acid gastric juice at an earlier stage after a meal than the more distally located duodenal ulcer, and indeed it was formerly taught that the pain of gastric ulcer was experienced on average between half and one hour after a meal, whereas that of duodenal ulcer did not occur until approximately two hours after eating. There is, however, such a wide variation in the interval between a meal and the onset of ulcer pain that it is not usually possible to distinguish the two types of ulcer on this basis. Furthermore, some peptic ulcer patients are not aware of a constant relationship between the eating of meals and the onset of pain or discomfort.

Irritation of the ulcer by acid gastric juice may also be the explanation for many peptic ulcer patients being wakened by pain in the early hours of the morning; it is thought that acid gastric secretion may continue after the stomach has emptied following the last meal of the day. When the pain is sufficiently severe to interfere with sleep, the patient often discovers for himself that eating a small snack or even drinking a glass of milk will be sufficient to give enough relief to enable him to return to sleep.

Radiation of the pain from the epigastrium through to the back may in some instances indicate that the ulcer has penetrated beyond the confines of the gastric or duodenal wall to involve structures in the retroperitoneal tissues. A gastric ulcer may erode gradually into the body of the pancreas and a posterior duodenal ulcer may penetrate into the tissues above the head of the pancreas in the region of the common bile duct and perirenal tissues.

Typically, the ulcer patient suffers daily recurring pain for one or more weeks and then the symptoms gradually subside, leaving him completely symptom-free for several weeks, months or (rarely) years. Physical or psychological stresses sometimes appear to have initiated recurrences of symptoms, but there is usually no acceptable explanation for them. The periodic nature of symptoms is so characteristic of the disease that relentless upper abdominal pain which occurs daily and persists for months is almost certainly not due to peptic ulcer.

Rest in bed can almost invariably be expected to relieve the pain of peptic ulcer within a few days and, as well as being a useful therapeutic manoeuvre, it is sometimes used as a diagnostic test.

Heartburn, flatulence, and vague 'indigestion' are among other symptoms complained of by peptic ulcer patients, many attributing these to the ingestion of fatty foods. Fat intolerance, traditionally associated with gallbladder disease, is often complained of in peptic ulcer disease. There is no ready explanation for this finding, apart from the long-established belief that fatty foods are in some way less easy to digest than other foods.

Vomiting is not a common complaint in peptic ulcer patients. Formerly, the occurrence of vomiting was said to be commoner in those with gastric ulcer than with duodenal ulcer, but this statement does not bear careful scrutiny. When vomiting does occur it is usually of recently ingested, partly digested food and, since it usually relieves ulcer pain, some patients may deliberately induce vomiting to obtain relief. The occurrence of copious, persistent vomiting in patients with long-standing duodenal ulcer suggests the onset of some degree of obstruction to gastric emptying from scarring in the region of the duodenal ulcer. This condition has been for many years called pyloric stenosis, but it is not strictly narrowing of the pylorus itself and it would be more accurate to use the term duodenal stenosis. The vomiting in this condition is remarkable not only for its large volume, but also for the tendency of the vomitus to contain food which has been swallowed many hours or even days previously.

Although a patient's weight may vary from time to time throughout the course of his illness, marked weight loss in duodenal ulcer is usually found only with the development of stenosis. It results from the reduction in the amount of food reaching the absorptive areas of the small intestine and from the copious loss of fluid consequent on repeated vomiting. Patients with gastric ulcer may lose weight due to diminution in appetite during relapse. In these circumstances full investigations are required to exclude gastric carcinoma (page 69).

Clinical examination

The likely existence of peptic ulcer is usually suspected on the history alone. In most patients the only abnormal physical signs are tenderness and muscle 'guarding' on moderate pressure on the upper abdomen. With duodenal ulcer the tenderness, which may be slight even in relapse, is commonly sited slightly above and to the right of the umbilicus; in gastric ulcer it varies with the site of the ulcer. A succussion splash may be elicited on gently rocking the trunk from side to side on the examination couch. This sign can be elicited in normal individuals after a particularly heavy meal, and so it is not of pathological significance unless it is present three to four hours after a meal, when it provides evidence of delayed gastric emptying. This delay is usually the result of duodenal stenosis, but it occurs occasionally in peptic ulcer patients even in the absence of organic narrowing when there is oedema and spasm related to an ulcer situated near the gastric outlet.

The diagnosis of a peptic ulcer is usually confirmed by a barium meal examination. Some ulcers will be more readily seen on screening during the examination. Others are only detected on inspection of the X-ray films. Ulcers vary in size from time to time, and at the time of an initial barium meal it may have been too small to be clearly demonstrated. When typical ulcer symptoms persist, a second barium meal may reveal a proportion of these ulcers which were previously undetected. The typical X-ray appearances of a gastric ulcer are shown in Fig 3.1 and of a duodenal ulcer in Fig. 3.2.

When barium meal examination fails to reveal an ulcer in the stomach or duodenum, but characteristic symptoms of peptic ulcer continue, endoscopic examination with a flexible fibre-optic gastroduodenoscope is indicated. An ulcer in the stomach or duodenum which has remained undetected on radiological examination may be identified by this method.

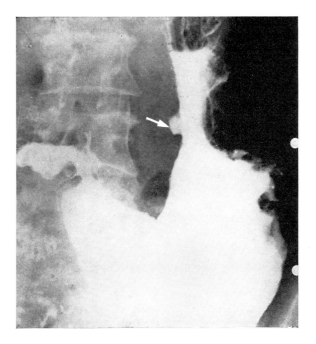

Fig. 3.1 Typical X-ray appearance of benign gastric peptic ulcer.

A considerable amount of attention has been given to the measurement of gastric acid secretion both under basal conditions and after maximal stimulation with histamine or the synthetic gastrin-like pentapeptide, pentagastrin. To what extent do these measurements further the diagnosis of peptic ulcer? In the present state of our knowledge they are of limited value in routine clinical practice. It is true that the total absence of any acid response following maximal stimulation precludes the presence of peptic ulcer. It is also true that, on average, duodenal ulcer patients have double the maximal gastric acid response of normal subjects whereas gastric ulcer patients have normal or slightly lower than normal maximal acid responses. There is, however, a large overlap in the range of values in both groups of patients and in normal subjects so that such measurements of acid response are unlikely to further the diagnosis in the majority of cases (Fig. 3.3). The single, rare disorder in which the measurements of basal and maximally stimulated acid secretory responses are of prime importance is the Zollinger-Ellison syndrome; the finding of unusually high 'basal' levels, with a relatively small further increment in acid response following maximal stimulation, is characteristic in this condition (p. 65).

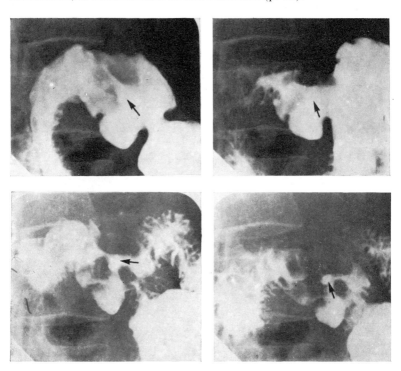

Fig. 3.2 Typical X-ray appearance of chronic duodenal ulcer.

With good radiology and endoscopy, if necessary repeated, most ulcers should be confidently identified, and it is now very rare for diagnosis to be made only at laparotomy. There is often, however, a surprising lack of correlation between the size of an ulcer and the symptoms which it can cause, and at operation it may be necessary to open the pyloro-duodenal junction to identify a small ulcer.

Medical treatment

The ready availability of numerous antacids or other gastric preparations and the publicity given to them in the press, television, and other advertising media make it easy for patients to embark on an initial self-prescribed therapeutic trial. It is impossible to know how many of these are completely effective, but it seems likely that some patients who develop peptic ulcers manage to control the symptoms satisfactorily until spontaneous healing takes place. Of those who consult family doctors, many will again obtain adequate relief from following a simple conservative regime. A minority of patients, who fail to respond to various measures to be outlined, eventually require operation.

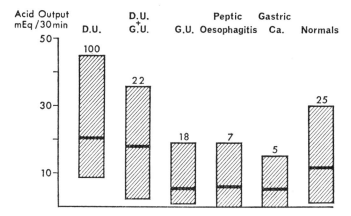

Fig. 3.3 Augmented histamine response in different disease groups (means and ranges). The solid horizontal lines represent the means and the shaded areas the ranges for all responses in each group (D.U. = duodenal ulcer; G.U. = gastric ulcer; Ca. = carcinoma). Although the responses of the duodenal ulcer patients on average are greater than those of the other groups, there is too much overlap between one group and another for the maximal acid response to be of reliable diagnostic assistance in the majority of instances.

We believe that the dietary and other measures prescribed should be basically simple to follow, and should not involve a major upheaval of the patient's daily routine. Complicated instructions are not likely to be followed satisfactorily, and indeed there is a lack of evidence that any elaborate advice is of proven therapeutic value. The main principles of conservative management are now discussed.

Diet

A great variety of dietary regimes have been prescribed in the past on the most slender evidence, and there is little reason to believe that the quality of the foods selected is of great importance. In contrast, the regular timing of meals is important in controlling symptoms. The patient should be advised to have something to eat approximately every two hours during the day; this minimizes fluctuation of the intragastric acidity. It is of course not necessary for the patient to eat a large meal at each two-hour interval, and small snacks consisting of biscuits and a milk-containing drink will usually be sufficient. In addition, a snack is also advised immediately before going to sleep at night. Patients will often say that a particular item of diet seems to induce pain and, if so, it seems only reasonable to advise the avoidance of this particular foodstuff. On the other hand, there seems no good reason to restrict the choice of foods in any other way and a varied diet will ensure an adequate intake of minerals, protein, vitamins and other essential substances.

What advice should be given about smoking and alcohol? There are several good reasons for advising any patient to give up cigarette smoking, and peptic ulcer patients are no exception. There is evidence that the cessation of cigarette smoking will accelerate the rate of healing of gastric ulcers, but there is no factual evidence with regard to duodenal ulcer. Alcohol is known to stimulate gastric acid secretion and, when taken in excess, may cause a diffuse inflammation of the gastric mucosa. It is doubtful whether it is necessary to forbid the taking of alcohol, but patients should avoid spirits, particularly when fasting.

Drugs

Antacids. Most patients find that one or other of the numerous antacid preparations will give effective symptomatic relief. The most popular remedies contain various combinations of aluminium hydroxide, phosphate, silicate or glyconate; magnesium trisilicate, hydroxide, or carbonate; calcium carbonate. There is considerable variation in the apparent effectiveness of single drugs and mixtures from one individual to another. Again, a patient may switch with benefit from one preparation to another, because the one which he was originally taking seemed to lose its effectiveness. For this reason it seems unreasonable for the medical adviser to hold strong preferences for particular antacid preparations, and if a patient is not experiencing satisfactory relief from the first choice, a trial with another agent may well be more successful.

Symptomatic relief cannot always be explained by a neutralizing effect on the gastric acid, for it is often surprising how rapid and prolonged is the relief obtained from a dose of an antacid preparation which is chemically unable to neutralize more than a small amount of the acid secreted. Consequently, it is our usual practice to advise a patient to take his antacid preparation only when required for symptomatic relief rather than to try, valiantly but without hope of success, to achieve permanent neutralization of the gastric contents by taking frequent large doses. There is no reason to prescribe antacids before or after meals, or at fixed times throughout the day.

Antacid preparations containing magnesium have a mild laxative action, whereas aluminium hydroxide may have the opposite effect on the bowel, and these mild side-effects may dictate the choice of preparation in a particular patient. The possible occurrence of systemic alkalosis, when very large doses of sodium bicarbonate have been ingested over a short period of time, should be borne in mind.

Anticholinergic drugs. These also enjoy considerable popularity, although they are not usually so immediately effective in relieving pain as are the antacid medicines. If given in adequate dosage, sufficient to cause slight side-effects such as dryness of the mouth, it can be shown that these drugs will reduce gastric acid and pepsin secretion, and also diminish gastric motility. For this latter reason the anticholinergic drugs have often been referred to as 'antispasmodics', and there is some evidence that muscular spasm may contribute to peptic ulcer pain in some subjects. There are available many anticholinergic agents whose actions are basically those of the belladonna alkaloids, atropine and hyoscine. One side-effect of these drugs, dryness of the mouth due to diminution in salivary flow, has already been mentioned but other anticholinergic effects may also be apparent, such as slight blurring of vision, and difficulty in emptying both the bladder and the bowel. In some patients these side-effects may prove unacceptable, and any interference with visual acuity might pose a real hazard in certain occupations. Glaucoma, prostatism and duodenal stenosis constitute definite contraindications to the use of anticholingergic agents.

Sedatives. Knowledge that rest in bed will regularly result in a remission from peptic ulcer symptoms has been extended to the belief that sedation might also have a beneficial effect. There has also been a widely held view that many patients with peptic ulcer are of an unduly worrying, anxious and agitated personality. However, there is no good evidence that the regular use of sedatives will achieve more satisfactory remission or protect patients against further relapses, and the tendency to add small doses of sedatives or tranquillizers to other gastric pharmaceutical preparations is to be deplored. However, such drugs may well be beneficial in a selected minority of peptic ulcer patients who display signs of hyperexcitability, anxiety or introspection and for whom there would be every reason to prescribe such medication even in the absence of the ulcer; when indicated these drugs should be prescribed separately and in a dose suitable for the particular patient.

Various inhibitors of gastric secretion. In recent years there have become available for experimental evaluation a number of potent inhibitors of gastric secretion, and there is understandable interest in their possible role in the treatment of peptic ulcer, especially duodenal ulcer. These include the hormones secretin and cholecystokinin, the peptides of less certain status, e.g. gastric inhibitor peptide, vasoactive intestinal peptide, urogastrone, and various 'enterogastrones'. All of these must be given parenterally, and perhaps of even greater interest are two groups of substances which exert their powerful suppressant effect on gastric secretion after oral administration—a) certain prostaglandins, and b) histamine H_2-receptor antagonists, e.g. metiamide and cimetidine. The possibility of effective pharmacological control of gastric hypersecretion seems nearer, and it remains to be seen whether this will satisfactorily relieve ulcer symptoms.

Specific agents. From time to time the claims of a new 'ulcer cure' are extolled. In view of the natural tendency of peptic ulcers to remit and relapse at unpredictable intervals, there are enormous difficulties in the evaluation of such agents. Nonetheless, a responsibility rests on those undertaking the management of large numbers of patients with peptic ulcer to submit new and potentially useful drugs to critical controlled trial. Two substances which have recently shown considerable promise in such trials are extracts of liquorice. It is interesting that simple liquorice preparations have been used in folklore medicine for many years for their alleged healing properties. The two pharmacological preparations in which interest has been most recently focused are carbenoxolone sodium and deglycyrrhizinated liquorice. Both have been shown to accelerate the healing of gastric ulcers as measured by precise, standardized barium-meal techniques, and both are currently undergoing more extensive evaluation. The former compound exhibits fluid-retaining properties in therapeutic dosage, but when these are prevented by thiazide diuretics, the therapeutic value of the drug with regard to peptic ulcer appears to be unimpaired. The possible development of hypokalaemia must be borne in mind. The deglycyrrhizinated liquorice preparation has no such fluid-retaining properties. These drugs are known to prolong the life of gastric mucosal cells, to increase local mucus production and reduce the back-diffusion of hydrogen ions across the gastric mucosa, but how these, or other actions, relate to ulcer healing is uncertain.

PSYCHOLOGICAL ASPECTS OF PEPTIC ULCER

Opinions vary from, on the one hand, the belief that virtually all peptic ulcers are caused by psychological disturbances, to the view that any mental disturbance is a consequence of the ulcer rather than the cause. There is no doubt that psychological factors may from time to time aggravate the symptoms and precipitate relapses. Psychological factors are, however, difficult to measure with any precision, and until real advances are made in quantitative measurement it seems impossible to evaluate the role of psychological factors in the aetiology, and the role of psychotherapy in the treatment of peptic ulcer.

Surgical treatment

INDICATIONS FOR ELECTIVE OPERATION

The commonest reason for advising operation in patients with peptic ulcer is the failure of the simple conservative measures outlined to control the symptoms adequately. It is difficult to lay down a hard-and-fast rule on the duration of history beyond which operation should be advised automatically, since patients vary considerably in the periodicity of their ulcer dyspepsia. The majority of duodenal ulcer patients coming to operation have had symptoms for more than five years, and many give a history going back more than 20 years. Factors other than simply the length of time over which symptoms have persisted are generally taken into consideration in reaching a decision for operation in a particular patient.

When a patient complains that antacids and other medical measures are no longer effective, it seems unreasonable to delay operative treatment even if the history is relatively short. On the other hand, the patient who enjoys long remissions of up to a year at a time, and can fairly readily control his relapses by a simple antacid preparation, may never be advised to have surgical treatment unless he develops some complication.

Loss of time from work because of ulcer symptoms is another important indication for operative treatment; this applies mainly to young and middle-aged men with families dependent on their continuing in regular employment.

Repeated interruption of sleep by typical ulcer pain, increasing evidence of radiation of the pain through to the back, and a strong family history of peptic ulcer all raise the likelihood that operation will be required sooner or later. The previous occurrence of a complication such as perforation (p. 53) or haemorrhage (p. 54) increases the likelihood of the recurrence of either complication, a consideration which favours a decision to advise surgical treatment.

The possible development of malignant change is a matter for concern in only the gastric ulcer patient; a duodenal ulcer does not undergo malignant change, but it should be emphasized that the duodenal ulcer patient is not immune to gastric cancer.

Finally, when the occupation of the patient may take him for prolonged periods of time away from accessible medical care, e.g. in the case of deep-sea merchant seamen, it may be advisable to relax the criteria for elective operation.

TYPES OF OPERATION

Since the approach to the surgical treatment of duodenal ulcer differs from that to gastric ulcer, each will be considered separately.

Duodenal ulcer

It has already been mentioned that duodenal ulcer patients will be found to secrete, on average, twice as much gastric acid as a group of normal subjects, and there is therefore a belief that this hypersecretion of acid is causally related to the ulcer. Even in those duodenal ulcer patients whose secretory responses fall within the normal range, it is postulated that they still have a 'relative' hypersecretion with regard to the resistance of the duodenal mucosa. The common aim of most elective operations for duodenal ulcer is therefore to reduce permanently the capacity of the stomach to secrete acid, and also pepsin. The objective can be achieved in at least four ways.

1. The vagus nerves can be severed as the main trunks pass the lower end of the oesophagus, thereby abolishing the stimulating impulses which are brought to the stomach by way of these nerves. This procedure, truncal vagotomy, not only diminishes gastric secretion, but also alters gastric motility and causes delay in gastric emptying, and therefore a 'drainage' procedure—either gastrojejunostomy or pyloroplasty (Fig. 3.4)—is required at the time of vagotomy.

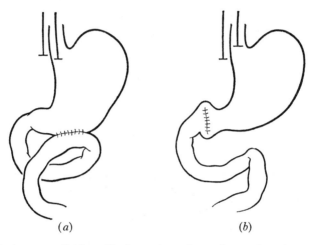

(a)   (b)

Fig. 3.4 Vagotomy, division of both anterior and posterior vagal trunks at the lower end of the oesophagus, requires the addition of a 'drainage' procedure to allow satisfactory emptying of the stomach. The two commonest 'drainage' procedures are (*a*) gastrojejunostomy and (*b*) pyloroplasty.

A more limited vagal denervation (selective vagotomy) can be achieved by selectively dividing the main nerves below the origins of the coeliac branch of the posterior trunk, and the hepatic branch of the anterior trunk, these two preserved branches going to supply non-gastric areas of the upper gastrointestinal tract, e.g. gallbladder, small intestine and pancreas...

Still further restriction of the denervation to solely the acid/pepsin secreting proximal portion of the stomach is the aim of highly selective vagotomy—or proximal gastric vagotomy (Fig. 3.5)—in which the individual terminal branches going to the proximal stomach are divided, preserving the main trunks (of Latarjet), travelling along the lesser curvature to supply the antrum and pyloric region. Since motility and gastric emptying are less disturbed there should be no need for a 'drainage' procedure to accompany this operation. Further time is needed to evaluate the relative merits of these different patterns of vagotomy.

2. Excision of the antrum (antrectomy) may be performed, thus

removing the source of the hormone gastrin which is normally released by food in the stomach.

3. A combined vagotomy and antrectomy will abolish both the nervous and hormonal modes of stimulation to the gastric acid cells.

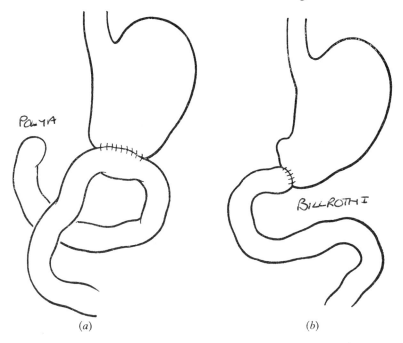

(a) (b)

Fig. 3.5 Partial gastrectomy, in addition to removal of the antrum, involves excision of a substantial portion of the mucosa which secretes acid and pepsin. (a) For duodenal ulcer the Polya (gastrojeunal) anastomosis is required to give adequate protection against recurrent ulcer. (b) The Billroth I (gastroduodenal) anastomosis is preferred for benign gastric ulcer.

4. Removal of a substantial portion of the acid- and pepsin-secreting mucosa (partial gastrectomy) diminishes gastric secretion by removing the 'target glands' and the pyloric antrum. Following gastric resection, gastrointestinal continuity may be restored by anastomosing the gastric remnant to the duodenum or to the first loop of jejunum (Fig. 3.5). For some unexplained reason the recurrent ulcer rate after a partial gastrectomy for duodenal ulcer with gastroduodenal (Billroth I) anastomosis is much higher than with gastrojejunal (Polya) anastomosis.

Antrectomy alone, which has generally been found insufficient to protect duodenal ulcer patients against recurrence of further ulceration, is no longer practised. This would suggest that disorders of antral gastrin production are not a common cause of duodenal ulcer. Each of the other three procedures achieves substantial reduction in the secretion of acid and pepsin and ensures cure of duodenal ulcer in the majority of patients. In reaching a decision about which procedure to prefer, at least three factors other than the theoretical ones should be taken into consideration, namely the immediate mortality risk, the possibility of recurrent ulcer, and morbidity from postoperative sequelae.   P S 9

First, with regard to mortality, current evidence suggests that vagotomy operations are less hazardous than the other procedures, and it is likely that the introduction of any form of gastric resection is the factor which increases the risk, albeit slightly.

Secondly, the lowest recurrent ulcer rates would appear to result from the combined operation of vagotomy with antrectomy, and only slightly higher rates occur after partial gastrectomy. From the current published literature, vagotomy with a simple drainage procedure would appear to carry the highest recurrent ulcer risk, probably in the region of 5 per cent.

Thirdly, partial gastrectomy has a higher incidence of such postoperative sequelae as loss of weight, anaemia, malabsorption, and 'the dumping syndrome' (p. 59) than the other procedures. Vagotomy with a simple drainage procedure would appear to be more acceptable in this respect at present, but it should be noted that this operation has not been evaluated over as lengthy a period of years as has gastrectomy and the results of long-term studies will be of the greatest interest.

In summary, vagotomy with a simple drainage procedure, or one of the more selective patterns of vagotomy, would appear to be the safest procedure, and many surgeons feel it is justified to accept a higher risk of recurrent ulcer as the price for a lower mortality. Combined vagotomy with antrectomy has not yet become generally popular, in spite of the encouraging low incidence of recurrent ulcer. This is probably because of some anxiety that patients may be liable to the sequelae both of gastric resection, and of vagal denervation.

Of the various complications which may follow these gastric operations (p. 59), one of the most controversial is diarrhoea following vagotomy. A reduction in the incidence of this problem was one of the main hopes of the more selective types of vagotomy (Fig. 3.6). Although initial reports suggest that this may have been achieved it remains to be seen whether they control gastric secretion as adequately as truncal vagotomy plus a 'drainage' procedure, with an equivalent or better overall incidence of post-operative sequelae.

Recurrent ulcer following vagotomy is usually the result of incomplete nerve section. Indeed, the surgeon's inability to guarantee complete nerve section may prove an obstacle to the general acceptance of vagotomy. A number of methods of testing for intact nerve fibres have been developed and should continue to be explored. The test in most general use for assessing completeness of vagotomy after the operation is the determination of the gastric acid response to the intravenous injection of 0·2 units per kg of soluble insulin which induces hypoglycaemia and thereby stimulates the vagal nuclei. A positive response, indicating the persistence of some intact fibres, is denoted by an increase in acid concentration at any time within two hours of the insulin injection of 20mEq/litre or more over the basal levels. Should the basal secretion be totally anacid, an increase in acid concentration of 10 mEq/litre or more at any time within the two hours after insulin is sufficient to indicate a positive response. It is desirable that surgeons should check the completeness of their vagotomies by using such a test.

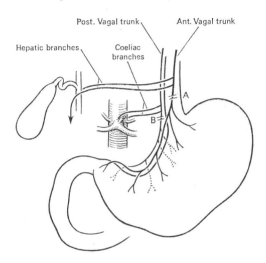

Fig. 3.6 Distribution of vagal nerves. The vagus nerves have many branches. It is possible to divide only those branches going finally to the stomach, leaving intact those travelling to other intra-abdominal organs. This is the basis of 'selective vagotomy' procedures. In the diagram, A and B are points of section in selective vagotomy.

Gastric ulcer

Most surgeons treat gastric ulcer by partial gastrectomy, with a gastroduodenal anastomosis (Fig. 3.5b). The line of gastric transection usually passes just proximal to the gastric ulcer itself, and as much stomach as possible is conserved. The presence of a normal or slightly subnormal acid production in gastric ulcer precludes the need to reduce gastric secretion by an extensive resection. The results of gastrectomy are good, and recurrence of ulceration is extremely rare. Postgastrectomy sequelae, as will be discussed, do occur, but they are generally less frequent than following gastrectomy for duodenal ulcer. Although there has been no strong dissatisfaction with this surgical approach, there have been recent trials of vagotomy with a drainage procedure, and even of a drainage procedure alone, and some early encouraging results are claimed. One of the main objections to this new approach is the failure to remove a malignant ulcer. Even when a biopsy of such an ulcer is taken at operation, doubt may persist regarding the nature of the lesion. For this reason the widespread use of procedures which do not involve excision of the ulcer cannot yet be advocated.

Recurrent ulcer

The diagnosis of recurrent ulcer is often difficult. The patient may present with periodic symptoms, in many ways similar to his original ulcer dyspepsia. Often, however, the site of the pain differs, being located at a lower level, and perhaps to one or other side, rather than epigastric. Again, there may not be a clear relationship between pain and the taking of meals, and the relief from milk or an antacid may not be obvious. The history may be predominantly one of vomiting, or of recurrent blood loss into the alimentary tract. Symptoms may arise within a few months of the original operation or, occasionally, after many years. Because of structural alterations in the upper gastro-intestinal tract following operation, radiological signs are often difficult to interpret, and it may not be possible to clearly identify the ulcer crater. However, most recurrent ulcers can now be visualised by a skilled endoscopist using one of the highly manoeuvrable fibre-optic gastro-duodenoscopes now available. The ulcer is usually on the distal side of the stoma or pyloroplasty.

The great majority of recurrent ulcers follow operations done for chronic duodenal ulcer. A short course of medical treatment, along the lines outlined for primary duodenal or gastric ulcer, should be tried in the first instance. If satisfactory control of symptoms is achieved the question of further surgical treatment can be deferred. Experience has shown, however, that most patients will request, and merit, further operation. The following policy, aimed at further reduction of gastric acid output, is suggested. If the first operation has been a partial gastrectomy, the addition of truncal vagotomy is recommended. If the original operation included vagotomy, the possibility of this having been incomplete should be entertained. Pre-exploration insulin tests, repeated if necessary, should be performed. If a positive response is obtained, indicating the persistence of some intact vagal fibres, re-exploration of the lower end of the oesophagus should be made, either by an abdominal approach or by left thoracotomy. The former approach, which we prefer, permits identification of the recurrent ulcer, assessment of the stoma and full abdominal exploration. It is usually discovered that the missed vagus fibres at the original operation have lain in the tissues behind the oesophagus, and it is rare that an anterior fibre has escaped division. If an obvious nerve trunk is found at the re-exploration, the division of this should theoretically be sufficient to cure the recurrent ulcer. On the other hand, should the re-exploration reveal no further nerve fibres, or the insulin test confidently indicates that the first vagotomy has been complete, it would seem reasonable to add a limited gastric resection, thus ensuring complete removal of the gastrin-producing pyloric antrum.

Finally, the possibility of the Zollinger-Ellison syndrome (p. 65) should be borne in mind at exploration for recurrent ulcer, and extensive exploration of the pancreas for a possible tumour should be made.

COMPLICATIONS OF PEPTIC ULCER

Perforation

The majority of perforations of either duodenal or gastric ulcers present in characteristically dramatic fashion. There is sudden onset of generalized severe abdominal pain. Respiratory movements are severely limited; the abdomen is characteristically rigid, and silent to auscultation. Most perforations can be diagnosed confidently without any auxiliary aids; where there is genuine reservation, a straight X-ray film taken with the patient erect may reveal the presence of free gas within the peritoneal cavity showing as a traslucent crescent between the liver and diaphragm shadows. Simple suture of the perforation at the earliest opportunity continues to be the most widely used surgical treatment and there is every reason to believe that this is the safest and wisest course in routine surgical practice. More than half of the patients who have a simple suture of perforation will eventually require a further elective operation for recurrence of chronic ulcer symptoms, and for this reason, some surgeons recommend an immediate definitive operation for the ulcer at the time of perforation. A few small series of patients treated by immediate vagotomy and drainage, or by immediate partial gastrectomy have been reported with apparently encouraging results. This approach should be restricted to patients in whom there is a long history of increasing dyspepsia before the perforation, who have been otherwise fit and are preferably under the age of 55, and in whom the operation can be done within eight hours of perforation. A further requirement is that there has been minimal peritioneal contamination. Until further evaluation of this treatment has been made, it would seem wise to restrict it to this highly selected group of patients. Meantime, we advocate the practice of simple closure of the perforation as the primary procedure, since it is a quick, safe, and effective way of dealing with the acute emergency.

Duodenal stenosis

The occurrence of organic stenosis with obvious dilatation of the stomach, retention vomiting, and marked succussion splash is an indication for surgical treatment. If the patient is in severe fluid and electrolyte depletion, and in particular if there is marked hypokalaemic alkalosis, pre-operative correction is required. In keeping with current views on the aetiology of duodenal ulcer, the operation of choice is a vagotomy with a simple drainage procedure. The provision of adequate gastric drainage is mandatory and gastrojejunostomy is generally preferred to pyloroplasty, particularly when the greater curvature of the dilated stomach is located in the pelvis.

HAEMATEMESIS AND MELAENA

The commonest cause of acute gastrointestinal bleeding in Great Britain is peptic ulceration, which may be oesophageal, gastric, duodenal, stomal or rarely, related to ectopic gastric mucosa. Chronic duodenal ulceration accounts for more than one-third of cases, while about one-quarter are due to bleeding from acute ulcers or erosions of the stomach or duodenum. Such superficial mucosal lesions appear to be increasing in incidence, many being associated with drugs known to increase the risk of bleeding. Other sources of bleeding from the gastrointestinal tract include hiatal hernia, carcinoma of the stomach, gastro-oesophageal varices in portal hypertension, and less common conditions such as hereditary vascular disorders, trauma and haemorrhagic diseases. All of these must be kept in mind when dealing with haematemesis and/or melaena.

Clinical management
When a patient presents with acute gastrointestinal haemorrhage, three questions arise:
1. Where is the source of haemorrhage?
2. Is blood transfusion indicated?
3. Is surgical treatment required?

Source of haemorrhage

A full history should be taken from the patient and a relative, with special enquiry regarding previous history of dyspepsia and the results of barium meal examination which may have been done. It must be remembered that a chronic peptic ulcer may be present in the complete absence of symptoms of dyspepsia. Furthermore, although a patient may be known to have a chronic peptic ulcer the site of haemorrhage may be an acute erosive gastritis. Detailed enquiry should be made about the recent ingestion of drugs, especially salicylates. Many patients do not appreciate that some proprietary compounds contain acetylsalicylic acid, which is known to cause gastric haemorrhage. The doctor will find it useful to have available a list of the commonly used preparations which contain aspirin, and to ask the patient or a close relative about each of these. Alcohol and phenylbutazone are also worthy of special mention in this respect. A history of vomiting and retching preceding the haematemesis or melaena will raise the possibility of tearing of the mucosa at the oesophagogastric junction, caused by the strain of vomiting.

Loss of appetite, easy satiety and epigastric distension after meals, in association with loss of weight, should raise the possibility of gastric carcinoma. That the source may be from gastro-oesophageal varices is suggested by a profuse flow of blood welling into the mouth without active retching or vomiting. Even in the absence of this lead a history of chronic ingestion of alcohol or of previous attacks of jaundice, should be sought. Any haemorrhagic diathesis should be asked about and, in the rare case of hereditary haemorrhagic telangiectasia, the source of haemorrhage can be strongly suggested by obtaining a family history of bleeding from mucous membranes, for example, epistaxis.

PHYSICAL EXAMINATION

A specific search should be made for icterus, cervical lymphadenopathy and evidence of hepatic parenchymal insufficiency, such as liver palms, spider naevi, flapping tremor and, in males, gynaecomastia and testicular atrophy. Telangiectasis may be seen on the buccal mucosa or on the nasal vestibule. The abdomen should be examined for an intragastric mass, hepatomegaly and/or splenomegaly.

A suggested practical course of management with indications of the priorities for the various diagnostic and treatment procedures is outlined on page 58. The following remarks merely describe the different diagnostic measures which may be used, not necessarily in sequence. The insertion of a nasogastric tube not only allows detection of continued or recurrent bleeding, but may assist in identification of the source of haemorrhage.

At this stage, there may be strong presumptive evidence of the source of haemorrhage, but it should be noted that the presence of a known lesion such as duodenal ulcer does not mean that this is necessarily the source of bleeding. Endoscopic examination may identify the presence of fresh blood or clot adherent to an ulcer or erosion in the upper alimentary canal. X-ray after the ingestion of a small quantity of barium or gastrografin can be done within 24 hours of the haemorrhage, provided shock is absent. Special techniques have been developed for doing this while the patient remains in bed and, in many cases of chronic gastric or duodenal ulcer, the lesion can be identified. In spite of carrying out all of these investigations, circumstances may arise when the source of haemorrhage can only be identified on exploratory surgical laparotomy.

Is blood transfusion indicated?

There are some well-defined circumstances when blood transfusion should be given. One is following on massive haemorrhage where the clinical signs of pallor, perspiration, tachycardia, hypotension and possibly gasping respiration give a clear indication that replacement of circulating blood volume is mandatory. Rapid infusion of at least 2 litres of blood is required. A useful guide to the volume of blood required can be obtained by monitoring the central venous pressure through an intravenous catheter. Recurrent or continuing bleeding constitutes a second indication for blood transfusion. Confirmation of the occurrence of such haemorrhage may present a problem. Inspection for fresh blood of samples of gastric contents aspirated via an indwelling nasogastric tube; a rise in pulse rate and fall in arterial blood pressure suggest further bleeding. Recording of central venous pressure is also of value in these circumstances.

During the first 24 hours following a haematemesis or melaena, a simple measurement of the haemoglobin level or the packed cell volume may be misleading as a guide to the volume of blood lost. Serial readings are required, as two to three pints of blood may escape from the intravascular compartment without significant immediate changes in these measurements.

There is no evidence to support the view that blood transfusion aggravates the tendency to recurrent bleeding from peptic ulceration by raising the blood pressure at the site of haemorrhage. On the contrary, there are dangers associated with prolonged anoxaemia and hypotension, which can be prevented by the appropriate transfusion. Following bleeding, the patient can be restless or even delirious due to cerebral ischaemia, and it is known that cerebral thrombosis may develop in such circumstances. Similarly, angina pectoris or myocardial infarction may develop. These complications are more common in elderly patients whose cerebral and coronary circulations are already compromised before the onset of haemorrhage. The function of the kidneys is also at risk during the phase of anoxaemia and hypotension. There is a fall in the glomerular filtration rate, which causes a rise in the level of the serum urea which may be further aggravated by dehydration and the absorption of blood products from the lumen of the small intestine. Severe hypotension, if uncorrected, may result in permanent renal damage and acute uraemia. Yet another strong indication for blood tranfusion is in the patient who is likely to require surgical treatment to arrest the haemorrhage. Particularly when this is the case, every attempt should be made by judicious transfusion to maintain normal levels of haemoglobin, blood volume and blood pressure.

When the decision has been taken to transfuse the patient several rules must be carefully observed. Blood for infusion must be accurately cross-matched, and in the case of an acute massive haemorrhage time may be bought by infusing up to 1 litre of 5 per cent dextrose in water or by using plasma while the cross-matching is being carried out. In the average case, the first litre of blood can be infused over a period of about four hours and thereafter the rate of transfusion should be governed by the changes in arterial blood pressure and pulse rate. It is essential, especially in elderly patients, to avoid overloading the circulation, as evidenced by a rise in central venous pressure and the development of fine crepitations at the pulmonary bases. Monitoring of the central venous pressure during transfusion provides the most precise method of preventing this complication.

In some centres increasing success in controlling bleeding from the upper gastro-intestinal tract is claimed to follow vigorous oral antacid therapy, aimed at achieving virtually complete neutralization of the gastric contents.

Is surgical treatment required?

There is no unequivocal answer to this question except in the rare situation when acute, massive, continuing haemorrhage is endangering life and the immediate necessity is to stop the bleeding. In the much more common situation several factors are taken into account when a decision regarding surgical operation is being made. Continuing haemorrhage or recurrence of bleeding while under observation is a strong indication for surgical treatment. It has been shown that the mortality, which is about 2 per cent in relation to the first bleeding, rises to about 20 per cent in patients who have had subsequent haemorrhage during the same attack. The age of the patient is also important in the assessment of need for operation. The mortality from haematemesis or melaena increases with age, and rises substantially in patients over 60 years of age, and therefore operation is more often required in this older age group. Although profuse haemorrhage may arise from an acute gastric erosion, the indications for surgical treatment are usually less when this is the diagnosis than when the source of bleeding is a chronic gastric or duodenal ulcer. Surprisingly, the length of history of chronic peptic ulceration does not correlate with the severity of the haemorrhage and the subsequent course. The presence of coincident disease, for example, myocardial ischaemia, bronchitis and emphysema, or chronic renal disease, especially in the middle-aged and elderly patient, may so increase the risks from surgery that there is extreme reluctance to undertake operation unless there is a direct threat to life from continued severe blood loss.

It is only after taking a complete history and making serial observations on clinical examination and special investigations that a final decision can be made in the individual case regarding the need for surgical operation.

The form of surgical operation may be decided only at laparotomy, being determined by the nature and site of the lesion which is found. There are, however, certain general principles which are applied. In the case of chronic gastric ulceration, partial gastrectomy is the operation of choice. When the ulcer is situated in the body of the stomach, should the conditions be favourable, the surgeon may perform a wedge re-section thus avoiding possible sequelae of a subtotal gastrectomy. In the case of duodenal ulceration, undersuture of the ulcer may be performed, followed by pyloroplasty and vagotomy, or alternatively a partial gastrectomy of the Polya (gastrojejunal anastomosis) pattern may be used. A greater problem arises when the site of ulceration has not been identified even after full investigation including exploratory laparotomy. In this event, a wide gastrotomy, and if necessary duo-denotomy, is performed to allow examination of the gastroduodenal mucosa. If bleeding is from one or two isolated erosions it may be arrested by direct suture, but if the erosions are numerous excision of the involved area may be required.

Treatment of haematemesis/melaena

The treatment can be summarized as follows. The patient should be reassured. Only if required in the individual should sedation be given, in the form of diazepam by intramuscular injection. His position in bed should be governed by his clinical state. If there is no shock he can be comfortably supported by pillows, but in the presence of hypoten-sion the pillows are removed and the foot of the bed should be raised. Venous blood is cross-matched with stored blood, and initial measure-ments of haemoglobin and packed cell volume are made. The blood pressure and pulse rate are recorded at half-hourly intervals. Thirst can be relieved by giving sips of water, or ice to suck. Intravenous infusion of plasma or 5 per cent dextrose in water may be required in an emergency for the treatment of shock while blood is being cross-matched. Blood transfusion is given if indicated. A nasogastric tube is passed to allow sampling of the gastric contents. Endoscopy and X-ray examination should be used in appropriate circumstances. The patient should be given a bland, semisolid diet as soon as he will take it. The total intake of fluids should be such as to provide a urinary output of at least 1500 ml per day; this will commonly mean an intake of about 3 litres in 24 hours. When there is any suspicion of continuing or recurrent bleeding the need for surgical operation must be kept under constant review.

Drug therapy is not invariably required, but an antacid such as magnesium hydroxide can be offered should dyspeptic symptoms arise. The patient may be allowed up when the bleeding is known to have ceased for a few days, provided the level of haemoglobin is at least 10 g per 100 ml. Ferrous sulphate in a dose of 200 mg three times a day by mouth should be given during the convalescent phase in order to replenish any deficiency in the iron stores of the body.

A patient who has suffered from haematemesis or melaena is especi-ally at risk from drugs which contain aspirin and he should be specifi-cally warned to avoid the use of these in the future.

As has already been stated on page 57, an episode of bleeding increases the chance of recurrence at a later date and also the likelihood of the patient requiring elective surgical treatment.

POSTGASTRECTOMY SYNDROMES

Within the last few years, the surgical treatment of peptic ulceration has changed. There have been increasing attempts to preserve as far as possible normal gastrointestinal continuity and to minimize resection of stomach. One aim of this change in policy has been to reduce the incidence of undesirable sequelae which have occurred following on the operation of partial gastrectomy. The name 'postgastrectomy syndromes' has been classically given to these upsets, but all forms of gastric surgery may give rise to some of these disorders. They could be more correctly named the 'postgastric-operation syndromes', but the simple term 'postgastrectomy' has established itself in the medical literature and is likely to remain.

Part of the difficulty presented by this group of disorders is the great range and variability of symptoms, and the complex interrelationships between them. It is rare to encounter a patient complaining only of a single symptom, and the relative contributions of one disability or another to the total clinical picture may be very difficult to unravel.

For discussion purposes the different features of postgastrectomy disorders may be classified as follows:
1. Mortality
2. The early postprandial syndrome—the dumping syndrome
3. The late postprandial syndrome—hypoglycaemic attacks
4. Bilious vomiting
5. Stomal ulceration
6. Biliary stasis
7. Nutritional sequelae
8. Postoperative bowel disturbance.

1. Mortality

This varies to some extent with the experience and the ability of the surgeon. Analysis of reports of large series of cases reveals a mortality of above 5 per cent following the operation of partial gastrectomy and of 0·1 to 0·5 per cent when the operation has been that of vagotomy and a drainage procedure.

On the other hand no difference in immediate risk to life has been reported from controlled trials of these different procedures by experts in gastric surgery.

2. The early postprandial syndrome

The term 'dumping' is, by common usage, restricted to this group.

The basic disorder is the precipitate unloading of 'unprepared' food into the jejunum. There are two elements to this symptom complex, an intestinal one and a vasomotor one. The intestinal element gives rise to exaggerated peristalsis, epigastric discomfort, abdominal fullness and nausea, vomiting and diarrhoea. The vasomotor element comprises general weakness, light-headedness, palpitation, pallor and perspiration. These vasomotor symptoms have been attributed to a fall in circulatory plasma volume secondary to sudden movement of fluid from the blood under the osmotic attraction of the hypertonic contents of the bowel. Autonomic imbalance and disturbance of serum electrolytes may play a part as may also serotonin release. The attack typically occurs five to thirty minutes after eating, particularly a carbohydrate meal, and may last as long as an hour. The symptoms may subside if the patient lies down. They may be precipitated by instilling hypertonic fluids into the jejunum. When one remembers the importance of the stomach as a reservoir and as a physiological mechanism for passing on metered amounts of material into the small intestine, it is tempting to ascribe the symptoms of dumping to the reduction in size of the stomach resulting from partial gastrectomy. It is evident, however, that this cannot be the explanation in all cases, as the syndrome can be found in patients after non-ablative gastric procedures, such as gastrojejunostomy.

Treatment

The treatment of the dumping syndrome may be considered under three headings:

Diet. The patient is advised to take frequent small meals, the diet containing protein and fat, but less carbohydrate than previously.

Drugs. These have not been shown to be of proved therapeutic value, although some have advocated the use of serotonin antagonists.

Surgical treatment. In patients with disabling symptoms further surgical operation may be necessary. The purpose is to delay the passage of food into the jejunum. There is a variety of possible procedures, including (*a*) conversion from gastrojejunal to gastroduodenal anastomosis, (*b*) narrowing of the anastomotic junction, (*c*) increasing the gastric reservoir capacity by plastic procedures involving the use of jejunum, and (*d*) interposing a jejunal loop (antiperistaltic) between the stomach and the jejunum.

3. Late postprandial syndrome—hypoglycaemic attacks

These occur as a result of rapid gastric emptying and subsequent rapid absorption of monosaccharides from the jejunum, giving rise to hyperglycaemia, exaggerated insulin release and consequent hypoglycaemia. The symptoms develop two and a half to three hours after eating and can be minimized or avoided by eating every two hours or taking glucose on appearance of symptoms.

4. Bilious vomiting

This disorder occurs almost exclusively after operations which involve the creation of a gastrojejunal anastomosis, with therefore an afferent segment of upper small intestine conducting the bile and pancreatic secretion towards the stoma. The characteristic symptoms are epigastric discomfort after meals and relief from vomiting of bile. It has also been called the afferent loop syndrome because it is believed to be associated with distension of the afferent loop particularly when this is long. The character of the vomitus is important in establishing the diagnosis. It is dark green or greenish-brown in colour and does not contain food. Such patients quickly learn that the only method of preventing the symptoms is to stop eating and therefore weight loss is common.

The treatment is reconstructive surgery designed to shorten or remove the afferent loop. The various techniques include conversion to a gastroduodenal type of anastomosis, internal decompression by an enteroenterostomy, or a Roux-en-Y procedure (an end-to-end anastomosis between gastric remnant and jejunal segment similar to the oesophagojejunal anastomosis in Fig. 3.8)—see page 73.

5. Recurrent ulceration—see page 52.

6. Biliary stasis

It has been suggested that after partial gastrectomy or vagotomy with drainage there may be an increased incidence of biliary disease, and this may be due to stasis of bile.

7. Nutritional sequelae

Of all the operations designed to prevent recurrent duodenal ulceration, pyloroplasty and vagotomy might be expected to cause the least anatomical and physiological disturbance. The incidence of syndromes such as dumping, bilious vomiting, heartburn and flatulence is probably less after this operation than after gastrectomy. One might expect relatively little change in the digestion and absorption of food after this operation, but prolonged carefully controlled follow-up of patients after all the various gastric operations will be necessary before the full consequences of nutritional deficiencies can be assessed in relation to the particular type of procedure.

The nutritional sequelae which require to be considered are as follows.

LOSS OF WEIGHT

The most important single cause of weight loss after partial gastrectomy is diminished caloric intake. Some patients find that they are unable to eat large meals and they may adopt unusual dietary habits following operation. Steatorrhoea has been described in 30 to 40 per cent of patients with a Polya type of anastomosis or with a vagotomy and drainage procedure, but malabsorption of fat is uncommon after a Billroth I resection or simple gastrojejunostomy. Hypoproteinaemia is not usual unless there is associated disease, such as a stagnant loop of bowel, jejunal diverticulosis or chronic pancreatic insufficiency.

ANAEMIA

For many years anaemia has been known to follow partial gastrectomy and in large series of cases the incidence has been reported as between 40 and 50 per cent. The blood status of a large group of patients followed for many years after vagotomy and drainage procedure still awaits definition. The major cause of anaemia is iron deficiency. This results from one or more of the three factors, malabsorption of iron, inadequate intake and excessive loss of iron from the alimentary tract. Although the absorption of inorganic iron in liquid form in fasting postgastrectomy patients is usually normal, malabsorption of iron in the food may result from the reduced secretion of acid in such patients. As the duodenum is known to be an important site for absorption of iron, the loss of duodenal absorptive surface after those operations which bypass the duodenum may be relevant. Rapid gastric emptying and intestinal hurry could also interfere with normal absorption of iron. Poor dietary intake of iron will obviously aggravate any deficiency and there have been reports of such patients in whom the iron content of the diet has been less than 10 mg per day. Loss of blood from the alimentary tract must be considered if there is erosive gastritis, particularly in patients taking salicylates orally, stomal ulceration, hiatus hernia, oesophagitis, or other factors such as haemorrhoids.

Iron deficiency can be treated by inorganic iron salts, such as ferrous sulphate 200 mg three times a day. It is important to continue with therapy for several months in order to replenish the iron stores in the body. The question of prophylaxis is discussed on page 64.

Following partial gastrectomy, subnormal levels of vitamin B_{12} have been found in 20 per cent of patients. At least 5 per cent will show clinical evidence of such a deficiency in the form of megaloblastic anaemia or a neuropathy. The major cause of deficiency of vitamin B_{12} is malabsorption due to failure of secretion of intrinsic factor which results from atrophy of the gastric remnant. Such malabsorption can be corrected by giving intrinsic factor. In a small proportion of postgastrectomy patients the deficiency is due to the blind loop syndrome, the stagnation of intestinal contents in a diverticulum or bypassed segment, where bacteria prevent the absorption of vitamin B_{12} by competing for the vitamin-intrinsic-factor complex. In such patients malabsorption of vitamin B_{12} is not corrected by intrinsic factor, but improves after treatment with the appropriate antibiotic or surgical removal of the 'blind loop'.

As many as 45 per cent of patients after partial gastrectomy have been shown to have subnormal levels of serum folate, but the deficiency is usually mild and it is not associated with haematological abnormality. The incidence does not increase with time following the operation and the main cause is probably inadequate dietary intake. It must always be remembered that any associated disease, such as idiopathic steatorrhoea, chronic infection or malignancy might aggravate the deficiency of folate and, in severe cases, such diagnoses should be excluded. Treatment of the dietary deficiency can be readily accomplished by giving folic acid orally in tablet form in a dose of 5 to 10 mg per day.

BONE DISEASE

Osteomalacia. Symptomatic osteomalacia occurs in between 1 and 3 per cent of patients following partial gastrectomy; it rarely appears until more than five years after the operation. It is commoner after a Polya gastrectomy than after a Billroth I type, and the patients usually complain of skeletal pain and weakness of the muscles. Pseudofractures may be seen in the pelvis and along the edges of the scapulae. There is no single diagnostic biochemical test, but if the product of the fasting levels of serum calcium and serum phosphate in mg per cent is less than 30 and if there is also a raised level of the serum alkaline phosphatase this is very suggestive of osteomalacia. The diagnosis can be confirmed by biopsy of bone, which will show osteoid seams broader than 12 μm in an undecalcified section. The treatment of established osteomalacia consists in giving vitamin D 50,000 units daily and calcium supplements up to 8 g per day, under strict biochemical control to avoid overdosage.

Osteoporosis. The diagnosis of osteoporosis depends on X-ray appearances, and assessment of patients seven years after operation has shown an incidence more than twice that expected in a control population. The cause of osteoporosis is uncertain, but histological examination shows the bony trabeculae to be thin and the osteoid seams narrow or absent. Oral calcium and anabolic steroids have been recommended but they are of uncertain benefit.

Prophylaxis

It is clearly desirable to minimize the chances of postoperative symptoms wherever possible. There are several factors which should demand attention before operation. Anaemia should be corrected if present. A history of looseness of bowel motions would be a strong influence against the choice of an operation involving vagotomy, as this may be followed by distressing diarrhoea. Should malabsorption be suspected, appropriate screening tests (p. 83) should be carried out before operation. After gastrectomy a case can be made for routinely prescribing supplements of iron, vitamin D and calcium, in view of the known high incidence of deficiency of these substances, which increases with the passage of time. Whether or not supplemental therapy is given, it is essential that all patients after gastric surgery for peptic ulceration should be reviewed at regular intervals, e.g. annually, so that the insidious onset of the deficiency syndromes can be detected and treated at the earliest possible moment.

8. Postoperative bowel disturbance

Transient upset of bowel function is common after most gastric operations, and usually the tendency is towards greater frequency and increased fluidity of the motions. In most patients regularity is restored in a few weeks, and although the bowels may move on average a little more often than before the operation this is generally regarded as an acceptable bonus of the operation rather than a disability. In a minority diarrhoea, usually of an intermittent pattern, persists as a troublesome symptom.

Several factors might contribute to the cause of the diarrhoea. The reduction in gastric acid secretion after vagotomy or gastrectomy may alter the bacterial content of the upper small bowel, or interfere with production, metabolism or absorption of bile or pancreatic juice constituents. Vagal denervation may impair small bowel absorption. Gastrojejunostomy or gastrectomy may result in bypass of the physiologically important source of pancreatic-stimulating hormones in the duodenum, and therefore impaired enzymatic digestion of a meal. The various anatomical rearrangements may alter gastrointestinal motility.

As commented on page 50, most stress has been laid on the possibility that vagal denervation is an important underlying cause of the diarrhoea, and both selective and highly selective vagotomy, which although denervating the stomach spare the branches going to the rest of upper gastrointestinal tract apart from the stomach, have been advocated to prevent the diarrhoea. Adequately controlled trials of the various procedures are, however, required to ascertain whether these modifications do achieve a significant reduction in the disorder. Diarrhoea is a surprisingly difficult symptom to define and to measure with any precision, and this is probably the main reason for the controversy regarding incidence after different operations.

Symptomatic measures such as the oral administration of codeine phosphate or diphenoxylate hydrochloride may diminish the number of loose motions, but often these are not effective. It is particularly difficult to arrange a medication schedule when the symptom is unpredictably intermittent. Alterations in diet are usually also unsuccessful, although if the ingestion of a certain food substance seems to precipitate attacks it would, of course, be wise for the patient to try the effect of exclusion of this item from the diet. Rarely one of the causes of malabsorption described in Chapter 4 will present in someone who has had an ulcer operation, and such a possibility should be kept in mind.

When diarrhoea is severe and fails to respond to simple measures the possibility of further operation may be considered. Sometimes dramatic relief can be obtained by the substitution of a gastroduodenal anastomosis or pyloroplasty for a gastrojejunal anastomosis. The interposition of a segment of jejunum between gastric remnant and duodenum is a further possibility, as is also the reversal of a short segment of ileum. Unfortunately these revisional procedures are not always successful, and they require further careful assessment.

ULCEROGENIC TUMOUR OF THE PANCREAS

(NON-β-CELL TUMOUR OF THE PANCREAS)

The Zollinger-Ellison syndrome

This rare disorder is named after the two surgeons who first described it in 1955. A tumour of the pancreatic islet tissue produces large quantities of gastrin, which in turn causes marked gastric hypersecretion, leading to severe peptic ulcer disease and diarrhoea. Peptic ulceration, besides being severe, often occurs in unusual sites such as the jejunum or oesophagus. It occurs most commonly between the ages of 30 and 60, but no age is immune; men are affected slightly more often than women, but the difference is slight compared to the striking sex difference in the incidence of the usual type of peptic ulcer. The history is usually short and the ulcers may be surprisingly large or multiple. The ulcer symptoms themselves are indistinguishable from those due to ordinary peptic ulcer, but they are unusually severe and persistent, there is little or no periodicity and conventional treatment does little to alleviate them. Bleeding and perforation are common, and either may be the presenting symptom. Perhaps the commonest presentation is that of severe recurrent ulceration following a standard operation for peptic ulcer, the syndrome not having been recognized at the time of the original operation. Excess production of gastric secretion is almost invariable, and volumes in excess of 1000 ml may be recovered during continuous aspirations for 12-hour periods. A characteristic feature is that the administration of an exogenous stimulus, such as histamine or pentagastrin, does not increase the secretory rate much above 'resting' or 'basal' values, since the stomach is already continuously secreting at or near maximal rates because of the high levels of endogenous gastrin in the circulation.

A curious feature of the syndrome is that 25 per cent of patients with ulcerogenic tumour of the pancreas also develop functioning adenomas

of one or more of the other endocrine organs, the glands most commonly affected being the parathyroids, the pituitary and the adrenals. This
syndrome of multiple endocrine adenomas, or the polyglandular
syndrome, is familial and individual members of an affected family may
present with different combinations of endocrine disorders such as
acromegaly and hyperparathyroidism or hyperparathyroidism and the
Zollinger-Ellison syndrome.

Pathology

Although the majority (60 per cent) of ulcerogenic tumours are
malignant, both the tumour and its metastases are slow growing;
although many large metastases may be present the primary tumour
itself is often surprisingly small. In about 10 per cent of cases the
tumour is ectopically located in the mucosa of the duodenal loop;
rarely there is diffuse adenomatosis of the islet tissue throughout the
pancreas. Gastrin-producing cells (G-cells) similar to those normally
in the pyloric antrum, have been identified by immunofluorescence
in the pancreatic tumours. There may, in fact, be a second type of the
syndrome arising from hyperplasia of the antral G-cells. There is
gross hypertrophy of the gastric mucosa, and cell-counting techniques
have shown that the parietal and peptic cell populations of the stomach
are enormously increased.

Diagnosis

The following features should raise the suspicion of the syndrome:
(1) patients presenting with ulcers in an unusual site (e.g. in the duodenum distal to the cap, in the jejunum or in the oesophagus); (2)
those presenting with the combination of ulcer symptoms and diarrhoea; (3) the rapid recurrence of ulcer symptoms after operation; (4)
unusually coarse gastric mucosal folds on barium examination; (5) an
unusually large basal acid secretion. Since the tumour secretes large
amounts of gastrin into the circulation the diagnosis may be established
by assay of the patient's blood for gastrin-like activity. The principle
of such an assay is to compare the effect of the patient's serum against
that of known amounts of gastrin in stimulating gastric acid secretion
in an experimental preparation such as the anaesthetized cat or rat.
Bioassays for the detection of gastrin are tedious to perform and do not
give fully quantitative results, and greater sensitivity, reproducibility
and accuracy are obtained in radioimmunoassay, which is now available in several centres.

Treatment

Medical treatment is ineffective. Ideally the condition should be
cured by removing the pancreatic tumour, but unfortunately this may
not be successful for the following reasons. The tumour is often malignant and metastases are already present in half the patients coming to
operation; there may be several small primary tumours in the pancreas;

or there may be diffuse hyperplasia of the islet tissue throughout the gland. So long as functioning tumour remains, any residual acid-secreting mucosa is dangerous since further ulceration is almost bound to follow, and the patient is exposed to life-threatening risks from perforation or haemorrhage. In addition to resection of as much of the pancreatic tumour as possible, therefore, total gastrectomy is strongly advised to remove all traces of gastric mucosa.

GASTRITIS

There is confusion in the use of the term 'gastritis'. Differences in interpretation exist between clinician and pathologist. Strictly speaking, the term implies histological inflammatory changes in the gastric mucosa, but such appearances are not uncommon in individuals who are completely free of all symptoms.

On histological grounds gastritis may be regarded as **acute** or **chronic** and for practical purposes it can be accepted that symptoms are caused only by the acute form.

Acute gastritis

The commonest form of acute inflammation of the gastric mucosa is that caused by the ingestion of irritant materials—*exogenous gastritis.* Perhaps the most frequent irritant is alcohol; others include drugs such as aspirin and phenylbutazone, and strong corrosives. Acute gastritis may also occur during the course of specific infection such as diphtheria or influenza—*haematogenous gastritis*; a particularly severe variety of this form of gastritis may occur during the course of septicaemia.

The symptoms of acute gastritis, whatever the cause, include anorexia, nausea and retching and a dull epigastric ache. The pathological changes consist of congestion of the mucosa, and desquamation of the uppermost cell layers; shallow ulceration may occur. As the superficial layers of the gastric mucosa can regenerate within 48 to 72 hours, it seems unlikely that a single attack or even several attacks of acute gastritis can lead to permanent histological changes in the stomach.

Chronic gastritis

In chronic gastritis the histological changes include infiltration of the gastric mucosa with inflammatory cells such as plasma cells and neutrophils and eosinophil polymorphs; these changes are accompanied by some degree of glandular atrophy, and there may be also patchy intestinal metaplasia. Chronic gastritis may be classified according to the extent of these histological changes into three grades of severity:

1. Chronic superficial gastritis
2. Chronic atrophic gastritis
3. Gastric atrophy.

Diagnosis

It is extremely doubtful whether chronic gastritis gives rise to clinical symptoms and therefore the diagnosis can only be established by finding typical changes on biopsy; even these may be of patchy distribution, so that blind biopsy may be misleading. Gastric atrophy may be suspected on barium meal examination because of diminished size of the gastric rugae. Acute or chronic gastritis may be recognized at gastroscopy although the gastroscopic findings do not always correlate with the histological appearances; a low output of gastric acid in response to maximal stimulation with histamine or pentagastrin also suggests the diagnosis of gastritis.

The cause and significance of chronic gastritis

The incidence of chronic gastritis increases with age. It is commoner in women than in men and there is a high incidence in patients with long-standing iron-deficiency anaemia; it is also commoner in those who drink or smoke heavily. The possible causes include recurrent exposure of the gastric mucosa to mechanical or chemical trauma. It has also been suggested that recurrent regurgitation of bile into the stomach may lead to gastritis. Circulating antibodies active against parietal cells are found in the serum of a proportion of patients with chronic atrophic gastritis, suggesting that this condition may be due to a disturbance of immunological mechanisms. Such antibodies are found in the majority of patients with pernicious anaemia and in many of their relatives. Parietal cell antibodies occur also in patients who develop chronic gastritis in association with other autoimmune diseases such as thyroiditis and idiopathic adrenal insufficiency, but it is not known whether the antibodies are the cause or an effect of the gastritis, and many patients with severe chronic gastritis do not have parietal cell antibodies.

The clinical significance of chronic gastritis is uncertain. There appears to be a definite association between gastritis and iron-deficiency anaemia, and it is generally accepted that the gastritis is a cause of iron deficiency, either because of decreased absorption or because of bleed-. ing from the atrophic mucosa. Severe atrophic gastritis may lead to pernicious anaemia, due to failure of secretion of intrinsic factor. It is not known, however, whether the gastric atrophy of classical pernicious anaemia is merely an advanced stage of a slowly evolving chronic gastritis or whether it is different in kind to other types of chronic gastritis. There is an undoubted relationship between chronic gastritis on the one hand, and gastric ulcer, gastric carcinoma and gastric polyposis on the other; some degree of gastritis is almost always present in these conditions. In the case of gastric ulcer the gastritis may be localized to the ulcer-bearing area of mucosa. The question whether chronic gastritis precedes the development of gastric carcinoma or gastric polyposis, or whether the gastritis is the result of these conditions cannot be answered with certainty; there is a body of opinion supporting the view that gastritis precedes carcinoma and may even predispose to it.

Treatment

The treatment of acute gastritis is symptomatic. Gastric irritants are withheld, any underlying systemic illness is treated and bland diet and possibly antacids are prescribed.

The treatment of chronic gastritis varies depending on the suspected cause of the disorder. Iron-deficiency anaemia, if present, should be completely corrected. Chemicals such as alcohol and drugs which are known to irritate the gastric mucosa should be avoided. In the presence of chronic atrophic gastritis, a test of absorption of vitamin B_{12} should be performed and, where necessary, appropriate therapy instituted.

CANCER OF THE STOMACH

There is a marked variation in the incidence of stomach cancer throughout the world. At present, Japan would seem to have the highest rate, Great Britain occupies an intermediate position, and it is less common in North America. A dramatic decrease in the incidence of the disease in the United States of America over the past 30 years seems to be continuing, and this is almost certainly due to some environmental changes rather than to genetic factors. Although many hypotheses have been proposed to explain the various geographical differences and the changing patterns in individual countries, we still have no definite knowledge of a specific cause of the disease. In Scotland, gastric cancer is almost twice as common in men as in women: in men its incidence is exceeded only by that of carcinoma of the bronchus; in women gastric cancer is the fifth most common malignant tumour.

More than 95 per cent of the cancers which develop primarily in the stomach arise from the glandular mucosa and are adenocarcinomas. Very occasionally rare types of sarcoma develop in the stomach, such as lymphosarcoma and, more rarely still, leiomyosarcoma, but it is most unlikely that the diagnosis of these unusual tumours will be made before exploratory operation. Although, theoretically, adenocarcinoma could arise from any part of the gastric mucosa, it is much commoner to find it in certain parts of the stomach than in others. The commonest site is in the pyloric antrum, the next the middle of the stomach, and least frequent the cardia. By the time patients seek medical advice a high proportion of them have the tumour occupying a large part of the stomach, and at that stage it may not be possible to determine from which part of the stomach the tumour originated.

The vast majority of cancers arise without any previous gastric disorder being diagnosed, or even suspected. In a small proportion of patients, however, there may have been a previously existing benign gastric peptic ulcer. For a long time the relationship between benign gastric ulcer and the development of gastric carcinoma has been a controversial matter, and argument on the frequency of the association continues. A fair summary of the present position is that both the proportion of benign gastric ulcers which eventually become malignant, and the proportion of gastric cancers which have arisen from benign gastric ulcers, are small, probably less than 2 per cent in both cases. The co-existence of a chronic duodenal ulcer and a gastric cancer is extremely rare. Less rare, however, is the development of a gastric cancer some years after the successful surgical treatment of a duodenal ulcer.

The majority of patients with gastric cancer will succumb to the disease. The principal reason for this bad prognosis is delay in diagnosis due to the insidious onset, and the mildness and vagueness of the presenting symptoms. Often, patients have no symptoms until the disease is beyond the limits of cure. A sizeable portion of the stomach wall can be replaced by tumour before the patient feels anything amiss with his health. When he does present to his doctor, the complaint may be of some slight diminution in the appetite, epigastric fullness after a small meal, or some ill-defined sensation in the upper abdomen, a bad taste in the mouth, unpleasant eructations, or perhaps some slight and unaccountable loss of weight. Ulceration of the gastric mucosa by tumour often causes recurrent minor bleeding from the stomach, and this may result in anaemia with consequent pallor, tiredness, breathlessness on exertion, light-headedness, or even signs of early congestive cardiac failure such as ankle swelling towards the end of the day. When presented with a middle-aged person, particularly a male, with unexplained anaemia, the likelihood of carcinoma of the stomach should certainly be kept in mind. Abdominal pain is not a usual symptom of carcinoma of the stomach.

It is unusual for a patient to present to his doctor because of an obvious change in the contour or consistency of his abdomen, but occasionally when the disease has reached an advanced stage before causing symptoms, the presenting complaint may be of a hard lump in the upper abdomen or a generalized increase in abdominal girth due to the development of ascites.

Vomiting may occur, but is usually late unless the tumour happens to arise near the pyloric end of the stomach, thereby causing some degree of obstruction to gastric emptying. It is sometimes to the patient's advantage if this occurs, because the symptom enforces urgent investigation and treatment at a time when the tumour may be at a relatively early stage and so may have a higher chance of cure. The vomitus usually contains retained food, and may be brownish in colour due to small quantities of altered blood.

When there is any suspicion of gastric cancer a full clinical examination should include detailed palpation of the relaxed abdomen and a rectal examination, and a sample of blood should be taken to determine whether there is any sign of anaemia, or elevation of the E.S.R. Examination of the abdomen may well reveal no abnormality, and indeed the detection of a palpable tumour is often an indication that the disease is beyond the stage of cure. In a thin patient a small, bobbin-like tumour at the pyloric end of the stomach may be quite readily palpable and yet still be sufficiently localized for adequate removal by operation. The right hypochondrial region should also be examined to determine whether there is any obvious enlargement of the liver, such as might result from the presence of metastases. If there is a malignant effusion in the peritoneal cavity this may be detected by the usual signs of shifting dullness to percussion, or a transmitted thrill across the abdomen. Information sought on rectal examination includes both the possible presence of palpable deposits of malignant tissue in the pouch of Douglas, which would render the tumour incurable by operation, and the presence of altered blood in the rectal contents. Rarely, palpation of the left supraclavicular fossa may reveal metastatic lymph node enlargement.

Whether clinical signs are present or absent, once the suspicion of gastric carcinoma is raised a barium meal examination should be performed. The majority of gastric carcinomas will cause an irregular filling defect at the corresponding part of the gastric outline and thus give confirmation of the diagnosis (Fig. 3.7). Occasionally, when the lesion is small and especially if the outline is similar to that produced by a simple peptic ulcer, the radiologist may not be certain of the diagnosis. Under these circumstances, endoscopy with one of the currently available flexible direct-viewing gastroscopes is desirable. Usually the combination of radiological and endoscopic findings will establish the diagnosis; on those rare occasions in which there is still uncertainty after both procedures, and if strong clinical suspicion continues, exploratory operation should be advised.

Two further diagnostic techniques which have been advocated are measurement of gastric acid secretion and exfoliative gastric cytology. It was formerly thought that the majority of patients with gastric cancer had achlorhydria. This is now known not to be true, and indeed it is quite possible to obtain normal gastric acid secretory responses, both under basal and maximally stimulated conditions, in the presence of a gastric tumour. Certainly the more advanced the gastric carcinoma the less will be the acid secretion, as might be expected from the destruction of normal glandular mucosa. Since the presence of acid in the gastric secretion, however, does not exclude the possibility of gastric cancer, there seems no real diagnostic value to be obtained by such tests. With regard to the examination of sediment from gastric washings for possible clumps of malignant cells, this has not generally been found to be a useful procedure. Several centres in different countries throughout the world continue to make a special study of this technique, and various modifications in the obtaining of samples and in their interpretation continue to appear. Considerable training and experience are, however, required of the histopathologist who becomes a cytopathologist, and this factor alone has militated against the general adoption of the procedure.

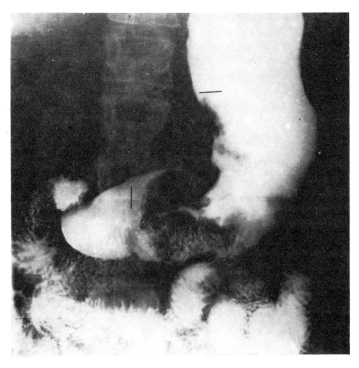

Fig. 3.7 Carcinoma of stomach shown as large filling defect (between two line marks) on barium meal examination.

In the treatment of gastric cancer the main hope of cure or useful palliation continues to rest with surgery. There is no indication that chemotherapy or radiotherapy has any real contribution to make in this particular field. The surgical objective is to remove all obvious malignant tissue and restore gastrointestinal continuity. Unfortunately, only about one-third of patients coming to operation are found to have tumours which appear to be capable of being removed completely; in the remainder it is possible to perform palliative procedures at most.

When it is hoped that the operation may be curative, the aim is to remove the tumour with a wide margin of apparently uninvolved gastric tissue proximal and distal to the tumour mass, and to include in continuity with the piece of stomach being resected the segments of mesentery containing any involved lymph nodes. For tumours in the distal stomach this usually comprises a radical but subtotal partial gastrectomy with the greater part of the greater and lesser omenta; gastrointestinal continuity is restored by a gastrojejunal anastomosis. For resectable tumours arising in the proximal segments of the stomach either a subtotal proximal resection may be performed, continuity being restored by anastomosing the oesophagus to the antrum directly; an alternative procedure is to perform total gastrectomy closing the duodenal stump, and bringing up a loop of jejunum to unite with the oesophagus, either as a loop or as a Roux-en-Y type anastomosis (Fig. 3.8). There was formerly a vogue for performing total gastrectomy in virtually all patients with carcinoma of the stomach in the hope of improving the rate of cure, but the mortality and morbidity rates for total gastrectomy were so forbidding that most surgeons in this country have returned to the preference for a subtotal resection wherever possible. It seems that this return to the less radical procedure has not been accompanied by a noticeable deterioration in the overall results of surgical treatment.

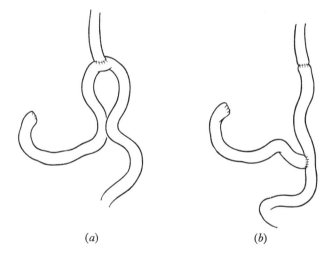

(a)   (b)

Fig. 3.8 Total gastrectomy. After total removal of the stomach the lower end of the oesophagus can be anastomosed either (a) to the antimesenteric side of a loop of jejunum or (b) end-to-end to a divided portion of jejunum, and further anastomosis of proximal divided intestine at a lower level.

The factors which render a carcinoma of the stomach inoperable are the presence of distant metastases in the liver or elsewhere within the peritoneal cavity, and the penetration of tumours from the stomach into other organs, such as the pancreas, the undersurface of the liver or the retroperitoneal tissues around the aorta. Even when the tumour has spread outside the confines of the stomach, however, it is still worth while removing the primary tumour from the stomach if this is technically feasible, as this will often provide useful palliation, with improvement in such symptoms as nausea, vomiting, foul eructations, unpleasant taste in the mouth, and loss of appetite. When the tumour causes obstruction in the pyloric region and yet is inoperable, it is often possible to bypass the tumour by a gastrojejunostomy, making the gastric opening several centimetres proximal to the uppermost border of obvious tumour. The temporary palliation achieved is often not impressive and some surgeons feel that this is not worth while. On the other hand, there is an understandable reluctance to do nothing at all at laparotomy, and the decision rests with the individual surgeon.

What is the outlook after operation? We can define immediate mortality as deaths occurring for any reason within 30 days of the operation. Even in those in whom the operation is hoped to have been curative there is an immediate mortality risk of approximately 20 per cent. This is much higher than the mortality risk of a partial gastrectomy for benign peptic ulcer, and is a reflection both of the more radical nature of the procedure and of the poorer state of health of the cancer patient. Secondly, what is the survival of these patients? A commonly used statistic in malignant disease is the five-year survival rate. This is an arbitrary measurement and whereas it may be meaningful for a particular group of malignant disease it is less so for others. There is virtually no five-year survival following palliative procedures or simple laparotomy, although rarely one hears of a patient who does have prolonged survival in spite of bad prognostic signs. Even after the most favourable gastric resection the five-year survival is probably less than 10 per cent. This means that in nine out of each ten patients in whom the surgeon thinks he may have a chance of having removed all the tumour he has in fact failed to do so. Further follow-up of the few survivors after five years from the date of operation continues to show evidence of late recurrence even beyond this time.

It can be concluded that treatment of gastric carcinoma is unsatisfactory and most of the effort expended in diagnosis and treatment, and the discomfort tolerated by the patient, is in the long run of little avail. There are, however, one or two encouraging indications that the results from operation would be likely to show a real improvement if the disease could be detected at a much earlier stage than is customary, but the insidious nature of the onset of symptoms makes it very difficult to see how much earlier diagnosis could be achieved in the majority of patients. The early detection of a significant number of gastric tumours would require large-scale screening of the entire asymptomatic middle-aged population and, even if a suitably simple and accurate screening technique was available, the administrative difficulties inherent in such a scheme are obvious.

FURTHER READING

Cox, A.G. & Alexander-Williams, J. (Eds.) (1973) *Vagotomy on Trial.* London: Heinemann.

Gregor, O. (1972) Epidemiology of gastric cancer. In *Recent Advances in Gastroenterology,* ed. Badenoch, J. & Brooke, B.N. Edinburgh: Churchill Livingstone.

Smith, R. (Ed.) (1975) *Surgical Forum—Gastric Surgery.* London, Boston: Butterworths.

Wastell, C. (Ed.) (1974) *Chronic Duodenal Ulcer.* London: Butterworths.

4. The Malabsorption Syndrome

W. C. Watson and Henry I. Tankel

The malabsorption syndrome includes a large number of conditions in which ingested food is incompletely absorbed. The primary fault may be impairment of either digestion or absorption. The digestive end-products of the main foodstuffs are:

Fats   —fatty acids, monoglyceride and glycerol
Proteins   —amino acids
Carbohydrates—monosaccharides (glucose, fructose or galactose).

Water, minerals and vitamins are not digested before absorption, but may need to be liberated from a bound state in the carrier food or conjugated with another substance (e.g. vitamin B_{12}).

DIGESTION

Cooking is an essential first step in the digestion of many foods since it initiates the depolymerization of celluloses and proteins.

Mastication grinds and lubricates food prior to swallowing, while salivary amylase causes some starch digestion.

GASTRIC DIGESTION

The stomach is a food reservoir with a variable rate of emptying: slow after a fatty meal, faster after carbohydrate. Its churning activity ensures adequate mixing of dietary liquids, solids and gastric juice. It secretes acid, pepsins, mucus and intrinsic factor. It absorbs water and alcohol and has a role in acid-base balance. It reduces dietary iron to the ferrous form. The most important digestive function of the stomach is the acid-pepsin digestion of protein to long- and short-chain peptides.

DUODENAL DIGESTION

Gastric chyme enters the duodenum in regulated amounts at a bolus rate of 3 per minute. Contact with the duodenal mucosa leads to the secretion of: cholecystokinin, which causes the gallbladder to contract; secretin and pancreozymin, which stimulate the exocrine secretion of the pancreas. Chyme now mixes with a number of substances all of which promote digestion.

Pancreatic bicarbonate neutralizes the acid and facilitates the action of the bile salts and specific enzymes. The optimum pH for enzyme activity in the small bowel is between 6·0 and 7·6.

Bile salts are detergents and have both an emulsifying and solvent effect on dietary fats. In dilute solutions they exist as unassociated molecules, or monomers. At higher concentrations they form poly-molecular aggregates (micelles) and the concentration at which this occurs is called the 'critical micellar concentration'. It is about 2 to 4 mmol.

Lipase digests triglycerides to diglycerides, monoglycerides, fatty acids and glycerol. Tri- and diglycerides remain in the oil phase while the monoglycerides and fatty acids enter the interior aliphatic region of the micelle. The micelle breaks down at the epithelial cell membrane, releasing the fatty acids and monoglycerides for absorption.

Amylase digests starch to maltose, a disaccharide.

Trypsin digests peptides to amino acids.

Meanwhile adjustments in osmolarity are taking place to make the intestinal chyme isotonic.

An additional source of digestive enzyme is the succus entericus, the juice secreted by the cells of the intestinal epithelium.

Digestive enzymes. These substances promote chemical hydrolysis, that is they split composite substances into basic units by the insertion of a water molecule at the bond. The reverse of the process is esterification.

ABSORPTION

The substances presented to the intestinal epithelium for absorption are:

Water
Vitamins
Minerals
Electrolytes
Glycerol
Monosaccharides
Disaccharides
Amino acids
Probably some small-chain peptides in adults and intact colostrum protein in infants
Fatty acids
Monoglycerides
Cholesterol
Bile salts
Miscellaneous substances such as food pigments, artificial colouring agents, drugs and alcohol.

FUNCTIONAL ANATOMY OF THE INTESTINAL MUCOSA

The functional unit of the intestinal mucosa is the villus (Fig. 4.1). The columnar epithelium renews itself every one or two days, new cells moving up from the base of the villus to be shed at the tip and digested. Microvilli line the villus surface and form the 'brush border', which can be seen by high power of ordinary light microscopy. There are about 1000 microvilli per square millimetre of surface area. The central core of the villus consists mainly of the lymphatic and vascular network which nourishes the villus and removes absorbed substances, and mononuclear cells which play an important role in direct and immunological defence mechanisms.

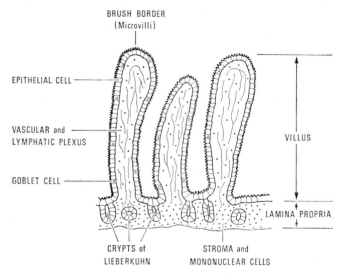

Fig. 4.1 Diagrammatic representation of the villus. The epithelial cells develop from the crypt cells. The Paneth cell is found among the crypt cells.

The substances which are to be absorbed must somehow pass across the surface membrane of the epithelial cells and microvilli. Whether the mechanism involved is one of active transport or passive diffusion, individual molecules must be moved across a membrane barrier. The forces responsible for this movement are either osmotic or electrical.

The epithelial cell contains many enzymes and some co-enzymes. It secretes peptidases into the succus entericus. These contribute to peptide digestion. Two important groups of enzymes act at, or very close to, the brush border. These are the disaccharidases (maltase, sucrase and lactase) which split the appropriate disaccharides into their constituent monosaccharides, and alkaline phosphatase which, as well as participating in phosphorylation, may also have some part to play in the electrophysical transfer of molecules across the membrane. Neither of these two groups of enzymes is secreted into the lumen. They act at their location in the cell.

Within the cell there are enzymes responsible for the resynthesis of triglycerides. These come into the general category of esterifying enzymes.

A special mechanism, pinocytosis, has been suggested for the absorption of particulate fat. It implies that the fat particles are engulfed by amoeba-like extrusions of the cell membrane and carried into the cell. There is as yet no absolute proof of this mechanism.

After absorption water-soluble substances such as carbohydrates, amino acids, water-soluble vitamins, short- and medium-chain fatty acids and even medium-chain triglycerides pass via the portal venous system to the liver. Fat-soluble substances, and in particular the chylomicrons which are formed in the epithelial cell, pass via the mesenteric lymphatics through the thoracic duct to enter the systemic circulation at the internal jugular vein.

SPECIAL ABSORPTION MECHANISMS

Most nutritional substances, ingested in reasonable amounts, are almost completely absorbed, irrespective of need. The main exception is iron, whose absorption is carefully regulated and restricted to about 10 to 20 per cent of the amount ingested. Iron requires a special transport substance called apoferritin, and for a long time it has been supposed that the amount of this substance available in the duodenum for iron transport was roughly proportional to the body's requirement. Recently this concept has been challenged and it has been suggested that the amount of apoferritin is determined in some way by the amount of iron available for absorption.

Vitamin B_{12} is dependent for its absorption on the presence of intrinsic factor in the gastric mucosa. It is not certain whether intrinsic factor acts by releasing the vitamin from its carrier foodstuff, or whether it acts as a co-factor facilitating absorption. There is considerable interest in the possibility that there may also be a gastric mucosal 'intrinsic factor' assisting iron absorption.

SITES OF ABSORPTION

Apart from the exceptions to be mentioned below, most substances are absorbed from the duodenum and proximal jejunum. There is a large absorption reserve. People are surviving in good health after resection of the entire small bowel distal to the first few inches of jejunum. Vitamin B_{12} and bile salts are absorbed from the terminal ileum. Water and electrolytes are absorbed throughout the small and large bowel. Calcium absorption occurs throughout the small bowel and this requires the presence of vitamin D.

Malabsorption may occur because of abnormality in any of the structures or functions described above.

Impairment of digestion occurs when there is deficiency of the gastric–pancreatic–gallbladder function. Inadequacy of the acid–pepsin mechanism is surprisingly unimportant, but surgical procedures which impair the reservoir and churning capacity of the stomach (such as subtotal or partial gastrectomy) or which bypass the duodenum (such as gastrojejunostomy or Polya gastrectomy) lead to faulty mixing of foods with bile, bicarbonate and pancreatic enzymes.

Malabsorption may occur with the Zollinger-Ellison syndrome. There are at least three possible reasons for this. The excessive acid secretion may produce an unphysiologically low duodenal pH with inactivation of enzymes, or it may exhaust the duodenal secretin/cholecystokinin mechanism. Hypergastrinaemia of itself may promote excessive intestinal water and electrolyte loss. The abnormal secretion of other gastro-intestinal hormones, especially the vasoactive intestinal peptides, is an occasional cause of this kind of diarrhoea-malabsorption.

Complete absence of intrinsic factor, as in pernicious anaemia, leads to malabsorption of vitamin B_{12}.

Pancreatic failure is a further cause of malabsorption (p. 125).

Bile-salt deficiency may be due to failure of bile salts to reach the duodenum, as in diseases causing obstructive jaundice, or diminished reabsorption of bile salts because of disease or resection of the distal ileum.

Malabsorption arising from disease of the small intestine itself may be due to one or more of the following types of disorder.

Sequestration of substances in the lumen

Vitamin B_{12} may be sequestered and utilized by bacteria or helminths. Pathological concentrations of bacteria occur in conjunction with blind loops or multiple diverticula. The helminth best known to utilize the vitamin is the fish tapeworm *Diphyllobothrium latum*.

Dietary calcium may be lost because it forms insoluble soaps with unabsorbed fats, and some of the fat-soluble vitamins, such as carotene and vitamin K, may also be lost with excreted fat.

Reduction in absorbing surface

Diminution in the length of the bowel occurs for the following reasons:
1. Resection after volvulus, intussusception, injury, superior mesenteric artery occlusion, or for the treatment of pathological conditions of the bowel, such as Crohn's disease.
2. Enteroenteric or enterocolic fistula secondary to granulomatous or

neoplastic disease of the small or large bowel (rarely gastrocolos-tomies have been performed in error for gastroenterostomies).

Even when the bowel is of normal length the effective absorbing area may be grossly reduced by diseases which diminish the number, size and functional capacity of the villi and microvilli. Important examples of such conditions are coeliac disease, sprue, secondary amy-loidosis, Crohn's disease, ulcerative colitis and neoplasm. Transient villus damage can be caused by intestinal infections, drugs such as nitrogen mustard, and radiotherapy for pelvic disorders.

Reduction in epithelial enzyme activity

This may be congenital or acquired. Alactasia with lactose into-lerance is an example of the former. Because the disaccharidase enzyme lactase is absent from the epithelial cell the hydrolysis of lactose to glucose and galactose fails to occur. The unabsorbed lactose causes osmotic diarrhoea and is split by bacterial fermentation into lactic acid and carbon dioxide.

The enzymes are also affected in a non-specific way by diseases which damage or reduce the number of epithelial cells. Severe protein or iron deficiency may affect enzyme function, and it is possible that the malabsorption which is sometimes seen following the administration of neomycin is due to enzyme inhibition. Intestinal ischaemia secondary to mesenteric vascular disease may cause malabsorption through enzyme effects.

Intestinal alkaline phosphatase deficiency occurs under experimental conditions in the hypoadrenal rat, but it is not yet established that this is the cause of the malabsorption which sometimes occurs in Addison's disease.

Mesenteric lymphatic obstruction

The most important condition causing this is reticulosis, especially lymphosarcoma. The absorption mechanism is not primarily involved in these patients, but because fat cannot leave the cell the absorption mechanism becomes 'saturated' in some way and fat transfer across the membrane is reduced. Depending on the principal site of obstruction to the lymphatic system fat may leak out into the chest or abdomen producing a chylous pleural or peritoneal effusion.

CLINICAL PRESENTATION

Patients who have malabsorption may present with three kinds of symptoms.

Symptoms due to malabsorption

These include diarrhoea, abdominal distension, flatulence and discomfort due to increased bulk of intestinal contents and gas production.

Diarrhoea is by no means the commonest presentation in such patients. Even so, a history of pale, frequent, loose, bulky, offensive, porridgy stools which stick to the side of the lavatory pan or float on the water and flush away with difficulty, invariably indicates steatorrhoea. The pallor of the stools is due to the reducing action of unabsorbed glucose which discharges the colour of the bile pigments. Steatorrhoea can be present without such florid abnormalities of the stool.

Explosive diarrhoea with abdominal distension following the ingestion of certain foodstuffs, especially milk, points to malabsorption due to impaired digestion of lactose, or to intestinal hypermotility stimulated in some way by food allergy.

Symptoms due to secondary deficiencies

Specific symptoms which may point to vitamin, electrolyte or mineral malabsorption are shown in the following table.

Symptom	Deficiency
Anaemia	Iron, folic acid, vitamin B_{12}
Tetany, bone pain	Calcium
Glossitis, dermatitis	Nicotinic acid
Paraesthesia	Thiamine
Bruising, bleeding tendency	Vitamin K
Weakness	Potassium, sodium

Anaemia is usually of iron-deficiency type in children and macrocytic in adults. Mixed or dimorphic anaemias are more common in young adults. The macrocytic anaemia of malabsorption is usually due to folic acid deficiency, and provided the patients are eating a good diet and not in the third trimester of pregnancy, impaired folic acid absorption can be inferred. Unlike vitamin B_{12}, folic acid deficiency does not arise from increased bacterial utilization within the bowel.

Weight loss is a non-specific symptom which only suggests malabsorption if associated with more specific symptoms.

Symptoms due to the primary disease

Presentations which may suggest the pathology responsible for malabsorption are:

Presentation	Disease
Lymphadenophy	Reticulosis, especially lymphosarcoma
Polyarthritis	Rheumatoid arthritis with amyloidosis
Polyarthritis with pigmentation	Whipple's disease
Subacute intestinal obstruction	Crohn's disease
Boring central abdominal pain	Pancreatitis
Severe, persistent dyspepsia	Zollinger-Ellison syndrome
Abdominal angina	Mesenteric ischaemia
Obstructive jaundice	Biliary cirrhosis, pancreatic neoplasm

EXAMINATION OF THE PATIENT

Signs which may be directly attributable to malabsorption are weight loss, anaemia, abdominal distension with tinkling bowel sounds, hypoproteinaemic oedema, glossitis, stomatitis, carpopedal spasms, absent tendon reflexes and cutaneous bruising.

Adult patients of small stature with established rickets should be suspected of having malabsorption, especially if they are significantly smaller than their siblings, since this suggests that the reasons for their poorer skeletal development are intrinsic and not environmental.

The presence of eczema, dermatitis herpetiformis, and sometimes rosacea should raise suspicions of malabsorption.

CONFIRMATION OF MALABSORPTION

Faecal fat excretion

Steatorrhoea, or excessive fat in the stools, is accepted as absolute evidence of malabsorption, and estimation of the faecal fat is the most important single test in establishing malabsorption. Everyone is agreed that for an adult eating a normal diet with a daily fat intake of 50 to 150 g, a faecal fat loss of more than 7 g per day is abnormal. Some consider that more than 5 g per day is excessive. This means that a daily faecal fat loss of 5 to 7 g has to be interpreted along with other data.

Accuracy of collections is more important than strict balance studies. Stools should be collected over two consecutive periods of 3 days or continuously for 4 to 6 days. It is possible to perform faecal fat studies on ambulant out-patients. On admission to hospital, even patients with steatorrhoea sometimes become temporarily constipated.

There is no satisfactory substitute for the estimation of daily faecal fat loss for proof of steatorrhoea. The estimation of total fat as a percentage of dry faeces is unpleasant and sometimes misleading. The estimation of split and unsplit fat in faeces is largely irrelevant. The use of isotopically-labelled fats has not become established and levels of plasma lipid after a fat load are dependent on too many variables for accurate interpretation. The best technique for faecal fat estimation requires hydrolytic conversion to free fatty acids and subsequent chemical titration. By this method the upper limit of normal in our laboratory is 15 mEq per day.

Other forms of faecal examination

Inspection and microscopic examination of the stools are both valuable. The typical stool appearance described earlier is unmistakable. When fragments of undigested food are visible this suggests either extreme hypermotility or fistulous short circuits. If a patient is jaundiced the stools may be pale and greasy due to the inadequate digestion of fat, secondary to deficiency of bile salts or pancreatic lipase. Diagnoses suggested by this presentation include cancer of the head of the pancreas, impacted gallstones and primary biliary cirrhosis.

Microscopic examination of the faeces may reveal fat globules and undigested meat fibres. This points to maldigestion arising from pancreatic or biliary disease. Incidentally, and particularly in a tropical environment, stool examination may give the specific diagnosis by identification of parasites.

Tests of carbohydrate absorption

Tests of hexose (glucose, fructose or galactose) or disaccharide (lactose or sucrose) absorption require the administration of a test dose of the substance to the fasting patients and the estimation of blood levels at standard intervals. Except where specifically indicated, it is usual to measure the total reducing substances, expressing the results as blood or urine sugar.

Xylose absorption test

D-xylose is a relatively inert pentose which is absorbed by the small intestine without digestion, passes through the liver, and is totally excreted by the kidneys. Measurement of the amount of D-xylose excreted in the urine after an oral test dose therefore gives an indication of the absorptive capacity, mainly of the upper small bowel. In the standard test 5 g are given orally and the urine collected for 5 hours thereafter. This dose does not cause nausea or diarrhoea. Provided there is adequate renal function the test is abnormal if less than 1·2 g of xylose is present in the 5-hour collection.

Glucose absorption test

A flat blood sugar curve after an oral dose of glucose usually points to malabsorption, but in some normal individuals glucose metabolism may be so rapid that this pattern of blood sugar curve may be present without there being malabsorption.

In the rare conditions of hereditary glucose and galactose malabsorption the oral administration of glucose or galactose causes diarrhoea with a flat blood sugar curve, whereas fructose is well tolerated and gives a normal rise. Today the main use of the glucose tolerance test is in the interpretation of tests of disaccharide absorption.

Disaccharide absorption test

When the enzyme lactase is deficient, lactose cannot be split to its constituent monosaccharides so that an oral dose of lactose causes diarrhoea with abdominal distension and discomfort, associated with a low or flat blood sugar curve. The administration of the equivalent amounts of glucose and galactose produces a normal rise in blood sugar, and there is no diarrhoea.

Lactase deficiency is the commonest of these disorders, but sucrase/isomaltase deficiency also occurs and then the relevant test substance is sucrose.

Special absorption tests of limited usefulness

ABSORPTION OF VITAMIN B_{12}

The Schilling test can be used, not only to demonstrate malabsorption of the vitamin, but also to indicate the cause. Urinary excretion of more than 12 per cent of an oral dose of vitamin B_{12} labelled with isotopic cobalt (^{58}Co) denotes normal absorption. Excretion of less than 5 per cent usually indicates pernicious anaemia, and results between 5 and 12 per cent suggest malabsorption due to other causes. If the test is repeated giving hog intrinsic factor with the oral dose of labelled vitamin B_{12}, absorption will improve in patients who have pernicious anaemia or total gastrectomy, and be unaffected in the others.

Since therapeutic doses of the vitamin are used in the test it should only be done after such essential preliminary investigations as bone marrow aspiration and measurement of serum level of the vitamin.

IRON ABSORPTION

Malabsorption of dietary iron can be inferred if a patient taking an adequate diet has an iron-deficiency anaemia with low serum iron levels or depleted body stores provided that chronic or recurrent haemorrhage has been excluded. Conversely, iron absorption can be assumed if in association with increased oral intake of iron there is a reticulocytosis with rising haemoglobin and serum iron levels. Quantitative studies of iron absorption require the use of ^{59}Fe. The radioisotope is used mainly to investigate factors affecting iron absorption and seldom simply to demonstrate malabsorption.

There is a useful distinction between the effects of coeliac disease and pancreatic insufficiency on iron absorption. Iron is poorly absorbed in the former, but normally or even excessively absorbed in the latter.

CALCIUM ABSORPTION

Provided a patient is on a known dietary intake of calcium, malabsorption can be demonstrated by estimation of the faecal calcium. A normal adult ingesting about 1 g of calcium per day absorbs about one-third. In practice, hypocalcaemia (less than 9 mg/dl) in a patient with steatorrhoea is assumed to denote malabsorption of calcium.

A useful radioisotope test of calcium absorption is one in which plasma radioactivity is measured after an oral dose of $^{47}CaCl_2$. Peak plasma activity, expressed as a percentage of dose per litre of plasma, occurs 1 hour after administration and separates three clinical groups: normal (1·69 ± 0·5), calcium malabsorption (0·80 ± 0·07) and increased absorption (2·85 ± 0·11).

14C-GLYCOCHOLIC ACID BREATH TEST

Bile salts are deconjugated in the gut by bacteria. The amount of deconjugation can be sufficient to interfere with fat digestion. This occurs in small bowel disorders which cause stasis and subsequent bacterial overgrowth. Examples are jejunal diverticula, blind loops and scleroderma.

Excessive bile salt deconjugation can be demonstrated by the oral administration of 14C-glycocholic acid. If bacteria are present in excess, 14C-glycine is split off, absorbed, metabolized and the labelled carbon is excreted in the breath as $14CO_2$. Aliquots of the expired gas are collected in vials and measured for radioactivity.

The final diagnosis is made by considering clinical features together with the results of special investigations. Sometimes the response to therapy has diagnostic significance.

Clinical features of diagnostic importance

Some of these are indicated in the section on symptoms due to the primary disease. By themselves they are seldom sufficient to establish the diagnosis and need to be supported by special tests. For example, while intermittent, colicky, lower or central abdominal pain with perhaps mucus or blood in the stools, and with a mass in the right iliac fossa may strongly suggest Crohn's disease, the clinician will wish to see the characteristic radiological appearances of the follow-through barium examination before committing himself to the diagnosis.

Abdominal angina is another 'typical' symptom which requires amplification by lateral aortography before the diagnosis of mesenteric ischaemia can be accepted. Some of these clinical syndromes will be described later.

When malabsorption follows surgical procedures for the treatment of peptic ulcer, or bowel resections for one of the many reasons given later, this information usually contains the diagnosis.

Enlarged lymph glands, skin lesions, polyarthritis, pigmentation and jaundice are clues to the primary pathology. A history of residence in a tropical country may suggest sprue or infestation, but malabsorption in association with infection by *Giardia lamblia* has been encountered in patients who have never been abroad.

Thyrotoxicosis, diabetes mellitus and Addison's disease are endocrine conditions which are occasionally the apparent cause of malabsorption, and clinical features suggesting these conditions should be noted.

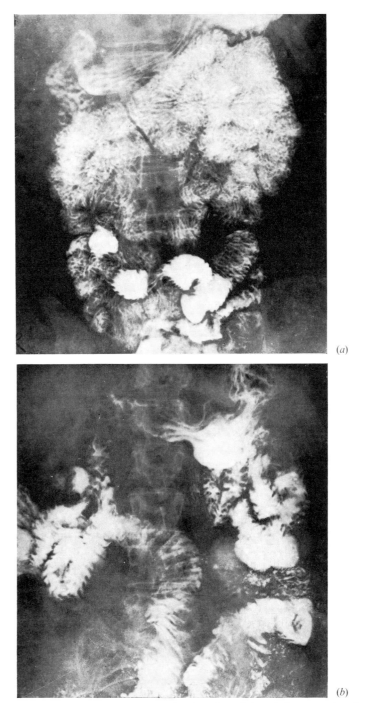

(a)

(b)

Fig. 4.2 (a) Normal follow-through examination of small bowel demonstrating the regular, 'feathery' pattern of the barium column. Compare this with (b) the pattern in malabsorption, in which the barium column is broken up in solid segments. There is also dilatation of the bowel lumen.

Special investigations

RADIOLOGY

X-ray appearances may be non-specific or diagnostic. Figure 4.2 shows a normal barium follow-through examination of the small bowel alongside a film of a patient with severe malabsorption. The characteristic abnormal features are the loss of the feathery pattern of the barium, distension of the bowel lumen with an increase in fluid content, and increased flocculation of the barium with segmentation and clumping of the barium column. The clumping of the barium into solid looking blocks is sometimes called 'moulage', a term which refers to the appearance of wax moulds. These X-ray appearances are evidence for malabsorption and are sometimes used by paediatricians as a screening test in suspected cases.

Occasionally the incidental finding of osteomalacia may direct attention to possible malabsorption.

Specific diagnoses revealed by radiology include:

1. *Calcific pancreatitis.* Pancreatic calcification is seen on straight views of the abdomen. This condition is rare in the United Kingdom, but not uncommon in Central and South Africa.

2. *Fistulae or blind loops which may be surgical or pathological.* Examples are gastroenterostomy, duodenocaecal fistula due to cancer of the caecum, gastrocolonic fistula due to gastric cancer or erroneous surgical anastomosis.

3. *Bowel resection*—for a variety of reasons.

4. *Intestinal ischaemia*—suggested either by a lateral abdominal film showing aortic calcification or proved by a lateral aortogram showing occlusion of the superior mesenteric artery.

5. *The 'string sign' of Crohn's disease of the terminal ileum.*

6. *Jejunal diverticulosis.*

BIOPSY

The introduction in 1956 by Crosby and Kugler of a biopsy capsule which could be swallowed by the patient, fired at any point in the stomach or small bowel, and immediately retrieved with the piece of tissue, was a major advance in the investigation of small bowel disease. While it is possible to obtain tissue from any part of the small bowel, for reasons of comparability and reproducibility it is usual to standardize the biopsy technique so that tissue is obtained from the first 30 cm or so of the jejunum. This means that it is essential to locate the biopsy capsule by radiology before firing it.

The piece of tissue may be examined in three ways: (1) by hand lens or dissecting microscope, to obtain information about 'surface anatomy' of the intestinal mucosa; (2) by routine light microscopy, using various specific tissue and histochemical staining techniques as well as the standard haemotoxylin and eosin; (3) by enzyme analysis of tissue homogenates, particularly for disaccharidase activity.

Abnormalities demonstrated by these methods may be specific or non-specific.

Specific abnormalities

Diagnoses which may be made on the basis of histological abnormality include:

Whipple's disease. Villi of relatively normal height contain masses of macrophages filled with a glycoprotein which stains with the periodic-Schiff reagent. The columnar cells of the epithelium are normal. Dilated lacteals may be present.

Amyloid disease. This is usually secondary to some chronic disorder such as rheumatoid arthritis. As well as the non-specific appearances of villus atrophy, staining by Congo red will show typical amyloid material in the walls of small blood vessels.

Intestinal lymphosarcoma. The villi appear normal but there is dilatation of the lacteals sometimes with microcyst formation. Intestinal reticulosis is occasionally found in association with the coeliac syndrome. In this case the mucosal appearances will be those of partial villus atrophy.

Giardiasis. Heavy infections with the protozoa, *Giardia lamblia* may be detected either by examination of stool samples, by microscopic examination of duodenal aspirate or of smears made from small bowel mucosa obtained by biopsy.

Diagnoses which may be made on the basis of enzyme deficiency include:

Alactasia. This is the commonest of the disaccharidase deficiencies. The histology is normal.

Sucrase-isomaltase deficiency. This is a very rare deficiency.

As the range of enzyme assays is extended it is possible that more clinical disorders based on enzyme deficiency will be recognized. Alkaline phosphatase is perhaps the one most likely to be shown to be involved.

Non-specific abnormalities

Jejunal histology is abnormal in a number of conditions such as coeliac disease, tropical sprue, dermatitis herpetiformis and Crohn's disease. Two grades of severity are seen, the most serious being that in which the villi become so completely fused together that they virtually disappear and the mucosal surface becomes an almost continuous sheet (Fig. 4.3b). There is an increase in the number of round cells in the lamina propria and hyperplasia of the crypts of Lieberkuhn. In the lesser degree of damage the villi are still discreet but show great variation in size and shape, being broad, stunted, branched and fused at the tips.

When there is atrophy and fusion of villi there is a great loss of epithelial cells with a corresponding reduction in all enzyme activity.

Jejunal biopsy is a key investigation. While interpretation of the findings is often straightforward the correct appraisal of the histology may require consultation by the clinician and pathologist.

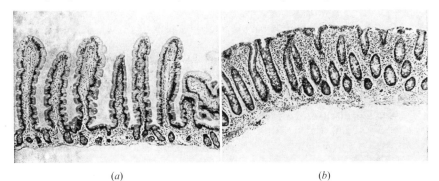

(a)   (b)

Fig. 4.3 (a) Normal jejunal mucosa. (b) Severe abnormality or subtotal villus atrophy.

Pancreatic function tests

Two kinds of pancreatic function tests are currently in use. Both require duodenal intubation. In the Lundh test, pancreatic secretion is indirectly stimulated by by the oral administration of a formula diet. Lipase levels are estimated in the duodenal aspirate. This is the simpler of the two methods. In the second, pancreatic secretion is directly stimulated by the intravenous injection of a highly purified preparation of secretin. The bicarbonate content of the duodenal aspirate is estimated. Mean, normal, hourly bicarbonate secretion is about 15 mM in men and 12 mM in women. For this test a rather thick, double lumen tube is used which requires more experience to pass and position. Its main advantage is that it allows sampling of 'pure' pancreatic secretion, some of which can also be sent for cytological examination.

Miscellaneous investigations

Special tests which may be required for the diagnosis of some of the less common causes of malabsorption are listed below:

Investigation	Diagnosis
Faecal bacteriology for *Mycobacterium tuberculosis*	Intestinal tuberculosis
Faecal examination for ova and cysts	Intestinal infestation
Thyroid function tests	Thyrotoxicosis
Urinary ketosteroids, plasma cortisol	Addison's disease
Measurement of sweat electrolytes	Cystic fibrosis of pancreas
Liver biopsy; mitochondrial antibodies	Biliary cirrhosis
Gland biopsy	Reticulosis
Maximum acid output; gastrin assay	Zollinger-Ellison syndrome

The diagnosis may ultimately rest on the response to specific therapy. Some of the distinct clinical disorders will now be discussed.

Coeliac disease

This congenital disorder, with a hereditary basis, may present for the first time in infancy or adult life. It should not be too readily assumed, however, that an adult presentation is the first manifestation of the disease. Although the patient may have no memory or knowledge of childhood disease, older relatives, especially the mother, may recall abdominal troubles in childhood. More important, perhaps, is the information that the adult patient is significantly smaller than his or her siblings. Moreover, if the patient has evidence of childhood rickets and the siblings do not, this increases the possibility of the childhood disease; social rickets is an environmental disease.

In *infancy* symptoms do not appear until the child is first given food containing gluten. Gluten is the protein in wheat flour which makes dough doughy. It is digested without difficulty by the normal intestine, but not so readily by that of the patient with coeliac disease. Incompletely digested gluten further damages the intestinal epithelium so that what began as a specific derangement of the small bowel goes on to severe generalized disorganization of the villus structure of the mucosae. Such a bowel not only suffers from a reduction in absorbing surface area, but also substantial impairment of its enzyme activity. The severity of disease depends to some extent on the length of bowel involved.

Following the introduction of gluten to the diet the infant fails to thrive, begins to pass typical foul, steatorrhoea stools and suffers painful abdominal distension. Iron-deficiency anaemia develops, and, if hypo-proteinaemia becomes severe enough, oedema appears. Wasting of the buttocks associated with a typical pot belly is highly suspicious in a child not exposed to malnutrition.

While the whole clinical spectrum of severe malnutrition may be seen, the diagnosis does not depend on the recognition of itemized details. Foul diarrhoea, failure to thrive and abdominal distension strongly suggest coeliac disease. Radiology is a useful screening test. As well as the non-specific appearances described earlier it is helpful to compare the maximum width of the small bowel lumen with the transverse diameter of the lumbar vertebrae. In normal children the ratio is not more than 50 per cent.

Jejunal biopsy can be performed even in small infants, but there is some risk of bowel perforation and the examination should be carried out by an experienced investigator. If biopsy cannot be performed the diagnosis may rest upon the response to a gluten-free diet.

In *adults* coeliac disease is diagnosed when malabsorption is found in conjunction with a flat jejunal biopsy, not due to some other specific cause, and gluten is shown to be of aetiological significance. Familial incidence is a valuable clue.

Coeliac disease may present, apparently for the first time, up to the sixth decade. There is no typical presentation. To insist on a 'classical' picture may lead to missing the diagnosis. The clinician's responsibility is to remember that a great variety of symptoms, such as weight loss, anaemia, bone pain, paraesthesia, oedema and skin disorders may be deficiency states. If there is also overt alimentary symptomatology such as diarrhoea, or abdominal discomfort and distension, the real diagnosis is unlikely to be missed. Failing these direct clues malabsorption may not be suspected.

ROLE OF GLUTEN

Gluten is a key substance in the pathogenesis of coeliac disease. It is not the cause of the condition, but it is an essential, specific aggravating factor. Not all patients with the 'coeliac syndrome' respond to gluten withdrawal, perhaps because they have reached a stage of irreversible bowel pathology or because some other as yet unidentified substance is the noxious agent. It is common practice, therefore, to refer to the syndrome which does respond to gluten withdrawal as gluten-induced enteropathy.

The relationship between gluten and coeliac disease was first observed in Holland. Dicke and his colleagues noticed that coeliac children seemed to improve during the wartime period of bread rationing. They followed up what was no more than an inspired guess with a series of clinical experiments which convinced them that gluten was the important substance. It is not yet settled how gluten acts, whether it is a local or systemic effect of gluten itself, a digestion product such as a gliadin, or a metabolite like glutamine.

Gluten exclusion must be strict. The ingestion of even small amounts may either prevent remission or induce relapse. Some patients can, however, tolerate the reintroduction of gluten into their diet. It is difficult to be certain whether this means that there are extremely mild cases of gluten enteropathy who can achieve complete remission, or whether in these cases gluten toxicity has been a non-specific effect on a mucosa damaged by some other primary mechanism, such as acute infection.

One of the practical problems in maintaining strict gluten withdrawal is the wide range of food products, other than the obvious ones of bread and baking, which contain wheat flour. Ice cream and sauces are important examples.

PROGNOSIS OF COELIAC DISEASE

While gluten withdrawal has transformed the prognosis for coeliac children, and substantially improved it for adults, there is still a definite mortality from the disease, particularly among adults whose condition is severe from the beginning, and perhaps especially among those with evidence of childhood involvement. Much has still to be learned about the natural history of the disease, and much new knowledge is likely to accrue as the survivors of proven childhood disease progress into adult life. All of the deaths in our own moderately large series of patients have been individuals with associated lympho-reticular disorder. There is a strong feeling at present that this is the appropriate pathological progression of a tissue which manifests some of the properties of premalignancy. This is a risk which, in contrast with ulcerative colitis, cannot be reduced by total small bowel resection. It remains to be seen whether the early control of the disease by dietary means will improve this aspect of the prognosis.

Sprue

This condition occurs in the tropics and is distinct from coeliac disease. The conditions are similar, however, in so far as they share virtually all of the manifestations of malabsorption, although the bone involvement in sprue may be less of a problem. Jejunal biopsy appearances can be indistinguishable, but are usually less severe in sprue.

Sprue is probably an acquired disease related in some way to environmental and nutritional conditions. It occurs chiefly in the Caribbean, south India, and in countries of south-east Asia. It may affect either the indigenous population or incomers. During the early 1950s the incidence of sprue in British army personnel in Hong Kong reached that of a minor epidemic. In many of the soldiers its onset seemed to follow an acute intestinal infection which had apparently been cured by antibacterial agents. Some of the suggested causes of sprue are infection (bacterial or viral), infestation, vitamin deficiency or a food toxin, such as might occur in rancid fats. It is a curable disease which responds to vitamins, broad-spectrum antibacterials, and other non-specific measures. Occasionally, Europeans will recover only if they leave the tropical environment. Presumably this is the only way they can remove themselves from an unidentified noxious factor peculiar to their tropical environment.

A common presentation of the disease is the triad of sore tongue, weight loss and diarrhoea. Haematological examination reveals a megaloblastic anaemia which is due to folic acid deficiency. The vitamin deficiency is due to malabsorption secondary to intestinal disease, and is not the cause of malabsorption. Experimental folic acid deficiency in rats does not cause malabsorption of fat. Faecal fat analysis, when carried out, usually shows steatorrhoea.

Because of limitations in the medical services in the areas where sprue is endemic, early or mild forms of the disease are not often diagnosed, and it is therefore difficult to build up a complete picture of its natural history. For example, in what percentage of the population is it a mild disorder which undergoes spontaneous recovery? Jejunal biopsy has shown that what would be regarded as mild abnormality in the intestinal mucosa of Europeans is 'normal' in areas of India, south-east Asia and parts of Africa. It is not clear yet whether this is a racial or genetic difference, or whether it represents an effect of chronic environmental factors such as infection or infestation.

Recent preliminary work has shown that an extract of calf jejunum will correct the malabsorption of folic acid in patients with sprue. It has been established that the substance responsible is a heat-stable factor. On the assumption that a similar factor exists in normal human jejunum it is clearly important to discover whether deficiency of such a substance is of primary or secondary importance in the pathogenesis of sprue.

Infection and infestation

Acute bacterial and viral infections may cause transient malabsorption. In most cases this is probably due to temporary, superficial damage to the villi or microvilli. Chronic bacterial infections of the small bowel are uncommon apart from such anatomical abnormalities as blind loops and diverticula. Intestinal bacteria may utilize dietary vitamin B_{12}, perhaps interfere with enzyme systems and cause areas of superficial inflammation of the bowel.

Cholera exerts a different action on the bowel. The vibrio produces a toxin which causes an acute and massive 'exsorption' of fluid and electrolyte associated with almost total concurrent failure of the absorptive capacity of the bowel. The term 'exsorption' denotes the movement of substances from the epithelial cell into the lumen of the bowel, and insorption is the reverse. Nett absorption for any single substance is the algebraic sum of these two processes. These terms have their principal use in considerations of intestinal fluid and electrolyte balance.

Giardia intestinalis (synonym, lamblia), being a protozoal organism by definition, causes infection of the bowel, and not infestation. Although occasionally asymptomatic it is usually pathogenic. The clinical disorder is lambliasis. The thick layer of lamblia on the mucosa interteres mainly with fat absorption.

There are three kinds of infestation known to be associated with malabsorption. *Diphyllobothrium latum*, the fish tapeworm, causes malabsorption of vitamin B_{12} because of utilization of the vitamin by the worm. The condition is often asymptomatic and occurs around the Baltic and the Great Lake regions of North America. *Ascaris lumbricoides*, or roundworm, can cause malabsorption either by blocking the bile and pancreatic ducts or by damaging the mucosa of the small bowel. Occasionally a very heavy infestation may cause intestinal obstruction.

Hookworm infestation by any of the three forms, *Ancylostoma duodenale, A. braziliense* or *Necator americanus*, may cause malabsorption either through mucosal damage or because the secondary anaemia may be severe enough to cause ischaemic dysfunction of the bowel.

Whipple's disease

This rare disease is of interest out of proportion to its incidence. It involves a variety of tissues: joints, lymph nodes, liver, brain, pericardium and pleura as well as the intestine. The typical presentation is malabsorption in a male with additional features of polyarthritis, lymphadenopathy and pigmentation. Symptoms of cardiac, hepatic and cerebral disease may also be present.

Diagnosis is established by lymph node or intestinal biopsy, in which are present foamy macrophages filled with a glycoprotein which stains with the periodic acid-Schiff reagent. The jejunal tissue may be otherwise normal or show clubbing of the villi, dilated lymphatics or even partial villus atrophy. The condition which used to be regarded as fatal can now be 'cured' by antibiotics. At least patients go into long or even indefinite remissions.

The cause of the disease is unknown, but there is evidence which suggests that it may be related to an atypical reactivity between bacteria and abnormal host lymphocytes. Since the latter precondition may be a permanent host feature this may explain the tendency to relapse which some patients have.

GRANULOMATOUS DISORDERS

Ileocaecal tuberculosis

This is now a rare disease in Britain. The presentation is that of lower abdominal pain, perhaps colicky, with fever, intermittent diarrhoea, and sometimes a mass in the right iliac fossa. The demonstration of *Mycobacterium tuberculosis* in stools or ascitic fluid will confirm the diagnosis, but may be difficult to find even in a positive case. Malabsorption need not occur, but if present is likely to be mild steatorrhoea and impaired vitamin B_{12} absorption. The latter is rarely if ever a clinical problem. Sometimes in the absence of positive proof of the diagnosis, it may be necessary to observe the response to chemotherapy.

Crohn's disease

Crohn's disease may cause malabsorption by either of two mechanisms. There may be fistulous blind loops, arising spontaneously or as a sequel to surgery, or there may be generalized mucosal abnormality which tends to be roughly proportional to the severity of the disease. Steatorrhoea and malabsorption of the fat-soluble vitamins may occur in as many as 60 per cent or more of patients with Crohn's disease. Malabsorption of vitamin B_{12} may be severe enough to cause macrocytic anaemia, particularly when there is extensive ileal disease or there have been numerous surgical resections.

Diagnosis of Crohn's disease may present difficulty and, in the absence of the characteristic radiological findings, may remain undiagnosed for many years. It should always be suspected in patients with a provisional diagnosis of adult coeliac disease who are not showing a characteristically good response to the gluten-free diet.

The condition is considered in greater detail on page 201.

DISACCHARIDE INTOLERANCE

Of the intestinal disaccharidases, the enzymes responsible for the final hydrolysis or digestion of the disaccharides, the one most commonly absent or deficient is lactase. Congenital absence of this enzyme, alactasia, has only recently been recognized as the cause of a syndrome of abdominal pain, distension and diarrhoea related to the ingestion of milk. This condition may present for the first time in children or adults. Although in the first instance only lactose absorption is impaired by deficiency of the enzyme, this can give rise to a diarrhoea severe enough to purge out other dietary substances before they are absorbed. Malabsorption of other substances is therefore dependent to some extent on whether they are ingested with the milk or not. Two distinct mechanisms may contribute to the diarrhoea: osmotic purgation by unabsorbed lactose in the small bowel, and irritant purgation in the large bowel by lactic acid derived from the fermentation of the undigested lactose.

The syndrome is easily recognized when there is a clear history of explosive diarrhoea following the ingestion of milk, but sometimes the

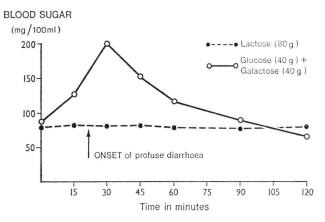

Fig. 4.4 Blood sugar curves in a case of hereditary alactasia. Symptoms were completely relieved by withdrawal of lactose-containing items of diet.

diarrhoea is delayed and the symptoms caused by the milk drinking may be the less flagrant ones of abdominal discomfort and distension. The diagnosis is proved when the typical symptomatology and a flat blood sugar curve follow the ingestion of a test dose of lactose; in addition no symptoms will accompany the normal blood sugar curves which follow equivalent doses of the components of lactose, namely glucose and galactose (Fig. 4.4).

The finding of alactasia by enzyme estimation of intestinal homogenates supports, but as an isolated finding does not warrant a clinical diagnosis of lactose intolerance. Milk intolerance may be related to some constituent of milk other than lactose, e.g. protein.

Sucrase-isomaltase deficiency is a very rare cause of disaccharide intolerance.

These conditions are genetically determined deficiencies of selected enzymes. But when the intestinal mucosa is diseased, as in coeliac disease, there is a generalized and proportionate deficiency of all the enzymes.

INTESTINAL ISCHAEMIA

Vascular conditions causing intestinal ischaemia may be acute or chronic.

Acute intestinal ischaemia

This is usually due to sudden occlusion of the superior mesenteric artery by thrombosis or embolism. When the artery is occluded at or near its origin and restoration of the circulation cannot be achieved by direct arterial surgery, there is infarction of the bowel from a few inches beyond the ligament of Treitz to midtransverse colon, which necessitates resection and jejuno-colic anastomosis. If the patient recovers from the initial catastrophe it may still be possible to achieve caloric and metabolic equilibrium if the duodenum is healthy and there are a few inches of intact jejunum. The problems which this situation presents tax the skills and experience of those handling the case, and every aspect of absorption physiology has to be taken into account. Detailed discussion of management of such cases is outwith the scope of this book. There is, however, a growing number of patients who are maintaining good health after massive bowel resection. This includes young people who have coped with the special demands of adolescent growth.

Chronic intestinal ischaemia

While acute ischaemia of the bowel produces a surgical emergency, the special hazard of chronic intestinal ischaemia is the indsidious and often obscure nature of its presentation. The patients are generally elderly people who have overt arteriosclerosis and may be already the victims of a vascular disorder such as intermittent claudication, cerebral or coronary thrombosis, or angina of effort. They complain of weight loss and vague abdominal pain. If asked, they may agree that the pain comes on after food and is relieved by fasting. This postprandial pain—or abdominal angina, as it is sometimes called—is by no means a constant symptom. Occasionally the abdominal pain comes on with exercise, such as walking. In this case there will probably be severe and extensive calcification or atherosclerosis of the abdominal aorta, with involvement of the iliac arteries as well.

The patients may be suspected of having ulcer dyspepsia and a suspiciously positive barium meal examination will then only delay diagnosis of the true pathology. This is a condition which the clinician has to force himself to think of in any elderly person with obscure abdominal pain. The principal clues which warrant going on to the definitive investigation of lateral abdominal aortography are evidence of malabsorption, flatulence and abdominal distension, other evidence of established arterial disease, and an abdominal bruit.

Although occlusion of the superior mesenteric artery is primarily responsible for the small bowel ischaemia, there is usually also involvement of either the coeliac axis or the inferior mesenteric artery by the time symptoms appear. When the coeliac axis is affected there may be evidence of liver or pancreatic dysfunction also. The superior mesenteric artery is almost invariably occluded internally by atheroma or thrombus. The coeliac axis, on the other hand, is sometimes compressed externally by the arcuate ligaments of the diaphragm.

Reconstructive vascular operations can often restore good circulation to the bowel, but this does not always relieve the symptoms. Moreover, these patients are still at risk from vascular disease in other vital organs and even after good results from surgery they may die a few months later from another remote event. For these reasons, and bearing in mind the technical problems involved in this kind of surgery, operation is not automatically indicated. Some patients are helped by advice to eat small meals and rest after them. Glyceryl trinitrate and other vasodilator drugs are valueless.

PANCREATIC DISEASE

Pancreatic causes of malabsorption may arise from *intrinsic* or *extrinsic* disorders.

Intrinsic causes

Acute pancreatitis (see p. 118)

In this country acute pancreatitis is usually secondary to disease of the biliary tract or to a generalized infection such as mumps. It rarely produces significant malabsorption. In severe cases the pancreas may become haemorrhagic or even necrotic. The latter may result in pancreatic insufficiency, but usually the patient fails to survive such a severe attack; hence the rarity of malabsorption from this cause. Minor cases subside and the gland recovers sufficiently to avoid the occurrence of malabsorption.

Chronic pancreatitis (see p. 125)

True chronic pancreatitis (Fig. 4.5) as distinguished from the entity,

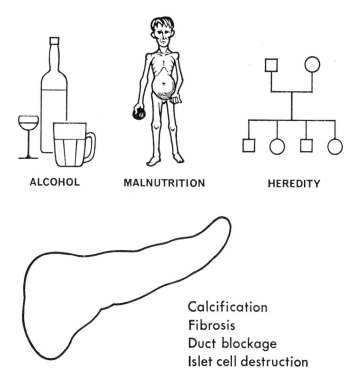

ALCOHOL   **MALNUTRITION**   **HEREDITY**

Calcification
Fibrosis
Duct blockage
Islet cell destruction

Fig. 4.5 The causes of chronic pancreatitis.

chronic relapsing pancreatitis, is better named chronic pancreatic fibrosis. It is rarely a sequel to acute pancreatitis, but is commonly associated with alcoholism, malnutrition and deficiency diseases such as kwashiorkor. Fibrosis of the pancreas occurs first, is followed by parenchymal and duct calcification, and then by duct obstruction which is due partly to the intraductal calcification and partly to the strangulation of ducts and acini by increasing fibrosis.

In the group associated with alcoholism and malnutrition some reversal of pathological changes can occur with treatment of the deficiency state.

Only about 8 per cent of cases of chronic pancreatic fibrosis have steatorrhoea, and only 20 per cent have any form of diarrhoea.

Tumours of the pancreas

Malabsorption is not a common presentation of pancreatic tumours. Since they usually block the common bile duct, jaundice is the main presenting symptom. Tumours of the body of the pancreas usually leave sufficient secreting tissue in the head to prevent malabsorption. Only about 10 per cent of pancreatic tumours have steatorrhoea as a symptom.

Resection of the pancreas for the treatment of tumour, whether gastric or pancreatic, may produce malabsorption, depending on the extent of the resection. Total pancreatectomy always requires replacement therapy with pancreatic enzymes.

Congenital cystic fibrosis

This disease is probably transmitted by a recessive gene. The basic abnormality is an increase in the viscosity of the mucus; hence the alternative name of mucoviscidosis.

In the newborn it may present as meconium ileus. The pultaceous meconium acts as an obstruction which sometimes leads to meconium peritonitis from perforation of grossly dilated gut. In later infancy the presentation is that of inanition despite an apparently adequate diet. Often it is not until early childhood that the large, pale stools appear, which indicate steatorrhoea.

The pathology is generalized cystic change. Similar abnormalities may also be present in the lungs causing persistent cough, recurrent attacks of pneumonia, bronchiectasis and chronic respiratory insufficiency.

Extrinsic causes

This group of causes of pancreatic insufficiency is wholly iatrogenic, arising from the consequences of surgery. The pancreas itself remains normal and capable of normal secretion were it only adequately stimulated.

Diminished gastric acid secretion

There is evidence that operations which reduce gastric acid secretion produce a reduction of 40 to 60 per cent in the volume, bicarbonate and amylase response of the pancreas after a meal. It is possible that in a marginal situation this reduction may be sufficient to precipitate malabsorption from pancreatic insufficiency.

Effect of bypassing the duodenal loop

In operations which bypass the duodenal loop, such as gastrojejunostomy, food passes directly into the jejunum and is then followed by bile and pancreatic juice rather than mixed with them.

Vagotomy

Experimental evidence does not support the suggestion that pancreatic vagotomy might reduce the amount of glandular secretion, but pancreatic stimulation may be reduced as a result of the lowered gastric acid secretion and therefore reduced secretin and pancreozymin stimulation.

MISCELLANEOUS DISORDERS

Antimitotic drugs, such as nitrogen mustard, and pelvic irradiation may cause transient damage to the intestinal epithelium. Malabsorption is not a clinical problem in these patients and will only be detected if specially looked for during the brief period of cellular damage. Neomycin and phenindione are rare causes of malabsorption.

Steatorrhoea can be a symptom of thyrotoxicosis or Addison's disease. Considering the enormous incidence of diabetes mellitus, it is a a very rare feature of this disease. In hyperthyroidism the steatorrhoea is due to intestinal hypermotility. In Addison's disease it may be due to deficiency in cellular alkaline phosphatase. Treatment of these two conditions will improve the steatorrhoea. The mechanism of diabetic steatorrhoea, on the other hand, is not understood and it is not improved by better control of the diabetes.

Liver disease is not as common a cause of malabsorption as one would suspect it might be. In biliary cirrhosis there is usually chronic mild steatorrhoea due to failure of bile to reach the bowel, and in parenchymal cirrhosis there is some failure of bile salt production. But since the bowel is normal and pancreatic function unimpaired, absorption of everything except fat is unaffected.

Mesenteric reticulosis, if it blocks the lymphatics, will cause steatorrhoea. Lymphosarcoma is probably the variety of reticulosis which most commonly involves the bowel in this way.

Minor abnormalities of small bowel epithelium are not infrequent in severe ulcerative colitis, but they are seldom a cause of malabsorption.

TREATMENT

The treatment of malabsorption will be considered in three sections: symptomatic, curative, and maintenance. Apart from the occasional use of steroids, treatment follows strict physiological and pharmacological principles. There is evidence from recent experimental work that the improvement obtained by steroids also has a rational basis.

Symptomatic treatment

The problems most commonly requiring attention are the correction of vitamin and mineral deficiencies and the treatment of anaemia.

VITAMINS

If there is evidence of any vitamin deficiency it is correct to assume there is some degree of deficiency of them all and to give a multivitamin preparation. If the deficiency state is florid and diarrhoea is severe they should be administered parenterally, otherwise the oral route is adequate. Vitamin K need only be given when a coagulation defect has been demonstrated by the appropriate technique.

CALCIUM AND VITAMIN D

It is wise to think of these together. If there is calcium deficiency secondary to malabsorption there is also likely to be hypovitaminosis D. Since the vitamin is essential for calcium absorption, administration of calcium alone will be ineffective.

The dose of calcium should be about 1 to 2g per day, and of vitamin D about 3000 to 5000 i.u. per day. This can either be prescribed as a tablet combining the two substances, namely as tablets of calcium with vitamin D, B.P.C. (each containing 600 mg of calcium and 500 i.u. of vitamin D activity) or separately. Tablets of calcium gluconate contain only 134 mg of calcium so that large numbers have to be taken. The effervescent tablet produced by Sandoz contains 380 mg of calcium. There are several preparations which combine vitamins D and A. If vitamin D is prescribed as calciferol it must be remembered that the standard tablet contains 50,000 i.u. of activity. This is too much for routine use, and can lead to toxicity. Radiostol is a solution of calciferol produced in two strengths, 3000 or 100,000 i.u. per ml.

When it does not conflict with other aspects of management calcium intake can be enhanced in the diet. Parenteral adminstration of calcium and vitamin D may occasionally be necessary during the early management of severe deficiency states.

HAEMATINICS

The anaemia in coeliac children is usually due to iron deficiency. It should be treated by oral administration of ferrous sulphate in appropriate dosage related to age. In adult coeliacs and in sprue, anaemia is usually due to folic acid deficiency. Customary doses are 10 to 30 mg per day, but this is grossly in excess of need. In young adults the anaemias are sometimes dimorphic and both iron and folic acid may be required.

In sprue, folic acid is the primary haematinic deficiency and it is safe to give this alone. In blind loop syndromes, infestations and ileal disease vitamin B_{12} is the required haematinic. If there is ever any doubt about the cause of a megaloblastic anaemia, and pernicious anaemia has not been excluded, folic acid should not be prescribed without vitamin B_{12}. An empirical situation like this should seldom arise.

WATER AND ELECTROLYTES

In severe malabsorption, whatever the cause, if diarrhoea is profuse, water and electrolyte depletion constitutes a serious problem. The situations in which this is most likely to occur are either a relapse of coeliac disease or immediately after bowel resection following acute superior mesenteric artery occlusion. Sodium, chloride, potassium and bicarbonate are all involved and intravenous therapy is essential. Chronic potassium supplementation may be necessary for some patients with massive bowel resections.

PROTEIN

Hypoproteinaemia may be profound and delay recovery as well as cause oedema. Intravenous whole plasma or protein hydrolysates are not often indicated but can sometimes accelerate recovery.

CALORIES

In severe cases a positive calorie balance may only be maintained by parenteral administration of glucose and fat emulsions.

DIARRHOEA

This is usually controlled most satisfactorily by the appropriate specific therapy, such as milk withdrawal, gluten-free diet, anthelmintics, or antibacterials. The most intractable diarrhoeas are usually those produced by surgery in the treatment of peptic ulcer. Postvagotomy diarrhoea can defy such customary remedies as codeine and kaolin-containing mixtures.

ADRENOCORTICAL STEROIDS

Patients who are not responding to rational therapy can improve significantly if given steroids. It is possible that steroids increase the enzyme content of the mucosal cells.

The above medications are usually required only until deficiencies are corrected. But if control of the primary pathology is poor, some of them, especially the haematinics, calcium, vitamin D and potassium, may need to be continued.

Curative treatment

Some of the malabsorptive disorders can be cured by treatment of the primary cause. Offending drugs can be stopped. Surgical blind loops can sometimes be undone. Infestations and infections can be eradicated. Thyrotoxicosis and Addison's disease can be controlled. The gastric hypersecretion of the Zollinger-Ellison syndrome is sometimes amenable to removal of gastrin-secreting adenomas and/or total gastrectomy. Antibiotics may not cure Whipple's disease, but some patients are in prolonged remission after antibiotic therapy and therefore this issue is still *sub judice*. Folic acid and antibiotics may 'cure' sprue, but final judgement awaits certainty about the cause and natural history of this condition.

Maintenance therapy

The most important instructions to patients about long-term therapy relate to **diet**.

GLUTEN

The role of gluten in coeliac disease has already been discussed. If exclusion of gluten from the diet is to be most effective it must be absolute; there are difficulties in ensuring this. First, there may be ignorance of the wide range of foodstuffs which contain gluten. In consultation with a dietician, the physician should issue to the patient a list of all known foods which contain gluten. Secondly, there are the difficulties and embarrassments of social eating which are a real problem for certain patients. Not wishing to be seen to be different, the patient may eat what is available. This happens in school and work canteens, and at holiday resorts. Thirdly, children sometimes chafe at the restrictions imposed on them, and since they do not always appreciate their importance, evade them. Finally, the financial strains of the diet occasionally create difficulties. This has ceased to be a serious problem since gluten-free flour and bread became prescribable.

As yet there is no consensus as to how long a gluten-free regimen should continue. Some patients need to stay on it indefinitely; these constitute the indisputable gluten-induced enteropathies. But a few others, whose initial response to gluten was so good as to seem diagnostic, may remain in good health if gluten is restored to the diet. It is not clear what this means. Perhaps these patients would enjoy even better health if they stayed on the regimen. On balance, if the patients are well and have accommodated themselves to the gluten-free diet, and bearing in mind that there are uncertainties about the natural history of a disease which can be fatal, it would seem wise to continue to regimen.

MILK

The indications for milk restrictions are threefold: first, lactose intolerance due to primary alactasia; secondly, lactose intolerance due to deficiency of the enzyme secondary to the bowel abnormality; and, thirdly, in other milk intolerance syndromes. In the first example the deficiency is permanent and milk withdrawal should be for an indefinite period. In the second, improvement can occur with treatment of the primary condition and milk may be restored to the diet. In the third example, although the precise reason for the milk intolerance may not be known, it is also likely to be permanent.

In the first two instances it is the milk sugar or lactose which is the problem and a list of lactose-containing foods should be prepared. Since milk fat and protein are not important in this respect, the patients can eat butter and cheese. In the last example it is probably milk protein which is responsible.

Food allergy as a cause of alimentary disturbance receives less attention in Britain than in North America. It is always worth while asking patients with bowel troubles if they have any suspicion of pathogenetic food factors.

FAT

Steatorrhoea is not of itself an indication for reducing or withdrawing dietary fat. It is better for a patient to absorb 75 per cent of a daily fat intake of 100 g than one of 20 g or less. Fat-free diets are intolerable and simply add to the problems of maintaining good nutrition. Fat is an important source of calories. In any case, the conditions which cause the worst degrees of steatorrhoea, namely coeliac and pancreatic disease, usually respond to therapy which coincidentally improves the steatorrhoea.

Sometimes, though, fat malabsorption is a serious problem, especially in children and young adults. Recently synthetic triglycerides containing fatty acids of medium-chain length (medium-chain triglycerides), which are largely water-soluble, have been of some success in augmenting fat calorie intake in such patients.

PANCREATIC ENZYMES

Preparations containing the exocrine pancreatic enzymes are of value in conditions of pancreatic insufficiency, particularly fibrocystic disease and chronic pancreatitis. Since these enzymes are inactivated or destroyed by low pH they must be administered as enteric-coated tablets or capsules. So that the enzymes will arrive with food in the duodenum the tablets or capsules are taken during the course of the meal. One preparation is sprinkled over the food before it is eaten.

Replacement pancreatic therapy has transformed the short-term prognosis for children with fibrocystic disease.

VITAMIN B$_{12}$

Pernicious anaemia is a chronic malabsorptive disorder. Patients are kept in good health by the regular parenteral administration of vitamin B$_{12}$ (cyanocobalamin). Dosage schedules vary from 1000 µg per month to 250 µg every two weeks. Patients who have chronic disease of the terminal ileum, or who have had this part of the bowel resected, also have malabsorption of the vitamin and require chronic replacement therapy.

ADRENOCORTICAL STEROIDS

In our experience a few patients have received steroids for short periods with benefit, but none has required maintenance treatment.

SOME CLINICAL PROBLEMS AWAITING SOLUTION

Is coeliac disease pre-malignant?

How does gluten damage the small bowel?

Why does Addison's disease cause steatorrhoea? Is it due to mucosal alkaline phosphatase deficiency?

Are childhood and adult coeliac disease different conditions?

Why does vagotomy cause severe diarrhoea in some patients and not in others?

What is the cause of sprue?

Is there a syndrome of pancreatic insufficiency due to congenital or acquired secretin/pancreozymin deficiency? Is this the cause of the steatorrhoea in the Zollinger-Ellison syndrome?

FURTHER READING

Losowsky, M. S., Walker, B. E. & Kelleher, J. (1974) *Malabsorption in Clinical Practice.* Edinburgh: Churchill Livingstone.

Olsen, W. A. (1971) A practical approach to diagnosis of disorders of intestinal absorption. *New England Journal of Medicine,* **285,** 1358.

Stewart. J. S., Pollock. D. T. Hoffbrand, A. V., Mollin. D. L. & Booth, C. C. (1967) A study of proximal and distal intestinal structure and absorptive function in ideopathic steatorrhea. *Quarterly Journal of Medicine,* **36,** 425.

Watson, W. C. (1968) Assessment of absorption from the small bowel. *Scottish Medical Journal,* **13,** 116.

Young, W. F. & Pringle, E. M. (1971) Children with coeliac disease. *Archives of Disease in Childhood,* **46,** 421.

5. The Biliary System and the Pancreas

Douglas H. Clark, William Manderson and Colin Mackay

THE BILIARY SYSTEM

The biliary tract develops as an offshoot from the foetal foregut. During development, abnormalities may occur not only of the ducts and gallbladder but also of the supplying blood vessels. These are of more concern to the surgeon than to the physician.

BILE

Bile is secreted continuously by the liver and its main constituents are:

> Water
> Inorganic salts
> Bile salts
> Bile pigments
> Cholesterol
> Phospholipids
> Calcium.

Bile salts in the intestine assist in both the emulsification and absorption of fat. The body appears to recognize the need for economy in bile salts, which are conserved by the reabsorption of the greater proportion in the small intestine, the enterohepatic circulation. The other constituents are carried to the intestine for disposal. However, they assume great importance when, for reasons which will be discussed, they precipitate as gallstones (p. 108).

During the interdigestive phases bile, which is continuously secreted by the liver, is stored and concentrated in the gallbladder, the factor of concentration being between 5 and 10 times. The mucosa of the gallbladder achieves this by the absorption of water and inorganic salts, and in this way the concentrations of bile salts, cholesterol, lipids, bilirubin and calcium are greatly increased. In spite of this, gallbladder bile remains iso-osmotic with serum, although the ionic concentration is nearly double. This is achieved by the aggregation of molecules as macromolecular complexes or micelles of large molecular weight (11,000 to 75,000). This complicated physicochemical process is also responsible for maintaining in solution large quantities of cholesterol, which is virtually insoluble in water. Hitherto, it has always been claimed that the maintenance of cholesterol in solution was entirely due to the detergent effect of the bile salts. It has now become apparent that lecithin (one of the phospholipids in bile) in micelle configuration is an even more potent vehicle for the transport of cholesterol. Bile pigments which are also insoluble in water are made soluble by conjugation with glucuronic acid in the liver.

The gallbladder empties as food entering the duodenum stimulates the production of the hormone cholecystokinin, which causes both the contraction of the gallbladder and relaxation of the sphincter of Oddi; bile is thus delivered to the duodenum for admixture with food. The gallbladder and sphincter are also supplied by vagal nerve branches, but there is uncertainty regarding their role in the regulation of gallbladder function. There is some evidence which suggests that after truncal vagotomy the gallbladder dilates and stasis may occur.

Gallstones

The incidence in current clinical practice varies from country to country, being greatest in those with diets containing large quantities of calories with high proportions of meat and fat, and where there is a higher standard of medical awareness. Dietary factors are generally believed to be important. For example, men of British stock in Australia have a higher incidence of gallstones than their counterparts in Britain, those in Australia having a higher meat and fat intake. Patients with hypercholesterolaemia, though prone to vascular degeneration, are not especially liable to gallstones, and hypercholesterolaemia produced experimentally in some animals does not produce gallstones although the vascular system is damaged. Moreover, a relationship between gallstones and serum cholesterol levels in man cannot be established. The high content of carbohydrate in the diet is now coming under suspicion.

Although gallstones are commoner in obese middle-aged females, they are not confined to this group. Patients with gallstones are often not overweight, some are young, and many are lean and frail elderly men and women. A family history is often obtained, but the relative parts played by common environment and genetic factors are uncertain.

GALLSTONE FORMATION

Gallstones are almost invariably formed in the gallbladder; rarely they may arise in other parts of the biliary tree. The three chief factors concerned are:

1. Stasis
2. Infection
3. Alterations in the composition of bile.

1. *Stasis* has long been considered an important factor. During the second and third trimesters of pregnancy atony of the gallbladder can be demonstrated radiologically, and this usually returns to normal after confinement. This is presumably due to the general reduced activity in unstriped muscle during pregnancy, well recognized in the case of the ureters. This stasis may be a factor in the increased incidence of gallstones which is said to occur in women who have had multiple pregnancies.

2. The importance of *infection* in the causation of gallstones has long been upheld, but more recently it has been suggested that infection is probably a secondary phenomenon and not primarily concerned with the genesis of the stones. In the presence of obstruction, infection may determine the deposition of layers and the increase in the size of the gallstones by altering the physicochemical balance of bile and promoting precipitation.

3. *Alterations in the composition of bile* are important. After concentration in the gallbladder, bile is almost completely saturated with cholesterol and slight changes in the factors maintaining this state of equilibrium may result in the precipitation of this substance, and hence the origin of stones.

Recent work suggests that the proclivity to stone formation may be inherent in the quality of bile secreted by gallstone patients. One study comparing hepatic duct bile and gallbladder bile of such patients with samples similarly obtained from patients with normal biliary systems undergoing abdominal operations for other reasons (e.g. peptic ulcer) suggests that the hepatic cell in gallstone patients may produce bile with subnormal concentrations of bile salts and phospholipids, thus reducing micellar attraction holding cholesterol in solution. It has also been noted that the cholesterol and calcium contents of bile are increased in patients with gallstones. Bilirubin, which is held in solution in its conjugated form, may become unconjugated by the effect of β-glucuronidase which has been shown to be present in bile of patients with gallstones. Excessive mucus secretion by the gallbladder mucosa may increase the viscosity of bile and encourage precipitation. Given a bile which, because of the above-mentioned factors, is less stable the final precipitating factors may be stasis, as in pregnancy, obesity, intercurrent infection or a marginal impairment of liver function. Such physicochemical abnormalities in bile might show a familial tendency, or might arise in other diseases, e.g. hepatic cirrhosis, in which an increased incidence of gallstones has been reported. Depletion of the bile salt pool by disease affecting the ileum, e.g. Crohn's disease, by diarrhoea, e.g. post-vagotomy, and by ileal resection predisposes to the formation of gallstones.

TYPES OF GALLSTONE

There are three main types of gallstone:

1. Bile pigment
2. Cholesterol
3. Mixed.

Bile pigment stones are the least common. They are usually multiple and black, and occur when there is a prolonged and excessive load of bilirubin for excretion, as in chronic and well-compensated congenital spherocytosis. The occurrence of these stones in children and young adults should raise the question of haemolysis, especially if there is a family history.

The *cholesterol* stone usually presents as a large single 'solitaire' (Fig. 5.1*a*); characteristically the cut surface shows lines radiating from the centre, a feature which may even show on X-ray. The constituents of mixed stones include cholesterol monohydrate, calcium carbonate and calcium bilirubinate, the concentrations of these substances varying in different stones.

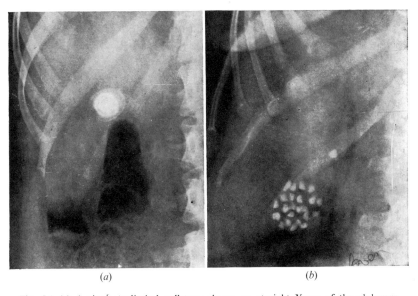

(*a*)   (*b*)

Fig. 5.1 (*a*) A single 'solitaire' gallstone shown on straight X-ray of the abdomen. Concentric rings of calcium have been precipitated at intervals of time. This stone does not show the characteristic radiating spiculation pattern of the typical pure cholesterol stone. (*b*) Multiple gallstones 'faceted' by mutual pressure one against another.

Mixed stones are the commonest, are always multiple and are often present in great numbers. Their size varies from 'sand' to stones more than one centimetre in diameter and they frequently become faceted by mutual pressure (Fig. 5.1*b*). Their cut surface reveals concentric rings, the paler ones being cholesterol and the darker ones bile pigment, both containing salts of calcium. Sometimes these stones are found in large numbers distal to a large 'solitaire' blocking the cystic duct. This arrangement encouraged the view that mixed stones were of inflammatory origin and appeared because of infection superimposed upon obstruction. While this may be correct in these circumstances, mixed stones are found frequently free in apparently normal functioning gallbladders.

CLINICAL PRESENTATION OF GALLSTONES

The presentation of gallstones can be conveniently classified under the headings of silent gallstones, acute cholecystitis and chronic cholecystitis.

Silent gallstones

These give rise to no symptoms. When opaque they may be discovered incidentally on X-ray of the abdomen. Stones may be revealed in the current vogue for regular physical examinations including cholecystography. They may be found during an abdominal operation for another condition. In such circumstances, if it is convenient and appropriate, the stones should be removed.

Several extensive surveys of the natural history of silent gallstones indicate that if the patients live for at least ten years after the discovery of the stones, they have an even chance of developing symptoms, and these are liable to be more severe and associated with complications in elderly patients. The management of patients with silent gallstones is still a subject for debate. Some surgeons, stressing the eventual risk of symptoms and complications advise operation. Others, recognising the small, but appreciable, morbidity and mortality associated with operation, advocate a conservative policy. Recently it has been shown that the administration of chenodeoxycholic acid not only reduces the lithogenic potential of bile, but may cause gallstones to diminish in size and disappear. Further developments in this field may reinforce the conservative approach.

Acute cholecystitis

Typically there is acute severe pain, deeply seated in the epigastrium, radiating to the right hypochondrium, or less commonly, to the left hypochondrium or both. The term 'biliary colic', which is commonly given to this type of pain, is a misnomer because it rarely fluctuates in the fashion of small bowel colic. Usually the pain comes on suddenly, rapidly reaches great intensity and persists without remission for two to three hours or longer, until relieved by the injection of a potent analgesic. The face is usually pale; there is tachycardia and the hands are cold and moist. Vomiting of bile-stained fluid often occurs, and jaundice may be present if the bile ducts are occluded by stone or inflammation. There is marked tenderness and guarding of muscles over the gallbladder, and when acute infection is a major factor there may be systemic toxaemia and pyrexia.

With distension of the gallbladder, irritation of somatic nerves may give rise to more localized pain and tenderness over the gallbladder, backache, and referral of pain to the right shoulder along the phrenic nerve.

Conservative management including rest in bed, suitable analgesics preferably pethidine, and the administration of a suitable antibiotic such as ampicillin or tetracycline, usually results in resolution of the symptoms. Interval cholecystectomy is usually advised, i.e. operation is performed several months after the acute attack has subsided. At the time of cholecystectomy the effect of previous acute episodes may be seen in the form of omental attachment, local fibrosis and adhesions. Some surgeons recommend operation within a few days, especially if a firm diagnosis has been made on clinical and radiological evidence. They claim that this policy is safe and prevents the patient having a further acute episode during the waiting period.

Especially in the elderly, resolution may not occur with conservative measures, and the condition may proceed to empyema of the gallbladder, perforation, abscess formation or generalized peritonitis. Persistent pain, pyrexia, increasing local signs, tachycardia and toxaemia will indicate the need for immediate operation, e.g. cholecystectomy or cholecystostomy.

Chronic cholecystitis

Chronic cholecystitis comprises the clinical syndrome of recurrent bouts of ill-defined dyspepsia with periodic discomfort in the right hypochondrial region. It may take the form of repeated minor attacks such as are described under 'acute cholecystitis' above, or persisting vague dyspepsia, flatulence, heartburn, upper abdominal discomfort and/or fat intolerance over a prolonged period. The symptoms may simulate chronic peptic ulcer, pancreatitis, or hiatal hernia.

Occasionally with obstruction, when the infection is very mild and the gallbladder still distensible, it may enlarge to quite a considerable size due to excessive mucus secretion—the so-called mucocoele of the gallbladder. This mucocoele contains clear or slightly purulent mucus, the other bile constituents having been reabsorbed through the mucosa. On the other hand, repeated damage from infection may cause the gallbladder to become a shrivelled, fibrotic organ contracted firmly around the gallstones. All degrees are encountered at operation, from the apparently normal to the fibrosed remnant.

Treatment of chronic cholecystitis includes advice to take a diet with a low content of fat, and reduction of weight when obesity is present. When symptoms attributable to cholecystitis are found in the presence of gallstones, cholecystectomy should be performed.

RADIOLOGICAL DIAGNOSIS OF GALLSTONES

Straight X-ray

Gallstones contain a variable amount of calcium, but in about 20 per cent of cases it is present in sufficient concentration to allow the stones to be detected on straight X-ray examination.

Oral cholecystogram

This depends on the absorption of an iodine-containing compound from the small intestine, its excretion through the liver into the bile, and its concentration in the gallbladder. It does not give satisfactory results in the presence of jaundice. Seventy per cent of gallstones are positively identified, and presumptive evidence is obtained in a further 25 per cent from non-filling of the gallbladder due to obstruction of the cystic duct.

The 'poorly-functioning gallbladder', i.e. where there is some filling and less than adequate concentration and contraction, is of less significance since more than half of this group are found to be normal after a repeat examination with perhaps a larger dose of contrast medium.

Intravenous cholangiography also has a role in the radiological diagnosis of gallstones. Biligrafin is given intravenously and is excreted rapidly in the bile in high concentration thereby outlining the duct system. Best results are obtained where liver function is normal, though the ducts may be seen in the presence of mild degrees of liver dysfunction. This procedure is indicated where the gallbladder is not visualized by the oral method, where oral cholecystography is not possible because of gastroduodenal disorders, e.g. pyloric stenosis, and where stones in the common duct are suspected. It is less accurate at demonstrating the gallbladder than the oral method. However, if after administration of biligrafin the ducts are adequately visualized but the gallbladder is not seen, this is strong evidence of a stone blocking the cystic duct. Radiologists frequently use it as a complementary measure in those cases where the oral method has failed to show the gallbladder. Absence of the gallbladder shadow by both methods with the ducts visualized is almost 100 per cent diagnostic of an obstructed cystic duct.

Ultrasonography

This new technique has been applied to the biliary system and is effective in determining the size of the gallbladder, especially if it is dilated. Further refinement of the method by grey scaling holds great promise in the diagnosis of gallstones.

Obstructive jaundice

Obstructive jaundice may arise from:
1. A gallstone or gallstones dislodged from the gallbladder and impacted in the common bile duct.

2. Carcinoma arising from the head of the pancreas, hepatic or bile ducts, or ampulla of Vater.

3. Benign stricture of extrahepatic bile duct.

In this section it is convenient to consider these causes together, as the clinical problem presents as one of obstructive jaundice, the cause being unknown.

Obstruction of the common bile duct by a stone or stones migrating from the gallbladder is a fairly common complication of gallstones. Typically this obstruction is painful and intermittent and the jaundice variable. In 10 per cent of the cases, however, the stone is firmly impacted at the lower end of the duct, jaundice is progressive and pain is absent. When the obstruction is complete there is pallor of the bowel motions due to the exclusion of bile pigment from the intestine, and the urine is darker than normal on account of the increased renal loss of water-soluble conjugated bile pigment. Although those biochemical liver function tests which reflect parenchymal damage are usually normal or only slightly disturbed, the serum alkaline phosphatase concentration is usually markedly elevated in the presence of bile duct obstruction from any cause.

Differentiation of gallstone obstruction from that due to carcinoma may be impossible on clinical evidence. Some patients with carcinoma of the head of the pancreas complain of deep-seated epigastric pain and backache. Furthermore, a small carcinoma at the ampulla may occasionally necrose sufficiently to relieve the obstruction, resulting in variation in the depth of jaundice. Benign stricture of the extrahepatic bile ducts almost invariably results from damage at a previous operation. The damaged area is replaced by fibrous tissue, which, as it matures, may contract sufficiently to obstruct the outflow of bile. There is therefore the history of the previous operation to raise the suspicion of the diagnosis. There is much to be said for grouping those cases under the heading 'surgical jaundice'. In this way tedious, expensive, uninformative and delaying investigation may be avoided and earlier treatment instituted.

If a grossly distended gallbladder is clearly palpable below the liver margin in the presence of obstructive jaundice, this is suggestive of carcinoma, but absence of a palpably distended gallbladder has no diagnostic significance.

In the presence of intermittent obstruction ascending infection of the biliary tract may occur, producing intermittent jaundice, pain and fever (Charcot's triad, or intermittent biliary fever). This is a serious complication requiring urgent operation.

Occasionally great difficulty is experienced in differentiating between a 'surgical' and a 'medical' cause of jaundice; e.g. the obstructive phase of viral hepatitis, or the biliary canalicular stasis which may follow the administration of certain drugs (p. 136). It is essential to obtain an accurate history in relation to drugs, injections or infective contacts. The empirical liver function tests are helpful especially when they are repeated at intervals of a few days. The urine should be examined daily for the presence of urobilinogen, which would indicate relief of the obstruction.

Doubt regarding the presence or absence of bile duct obstruction can sometimes be resolved by the radiological procedure of percutaneous transhepatic cholangiography, which comprises directing a long needle into the liver substance and the gradual withdrawal of the needle probing for enlarged ducts. The free aspiration of bile from the needle indicates that the tip is in the lumen of such a distended duct, which can then be outlined by the injection of contrast material (Fig. 5.2).

Endoscopic Retrograde Choledocho-Pancreatography (E.R.C.P.). In certain cases of jaundice this method is invaluable. The ampulla of Vater can be inspected and cannulated. A radio-opaque medium is injected through the cannula, outlining the biliary tree and allowing detection of stones, strictures or other lesions causing jaundice. This technique has also been used for defining the pancreatic ductal system.

When there is strong evidence of obstruction to the extrahepatic bile duct system surgical exploration is required, after prophylactic administration of vitamin K. Stones are removed either through an incision in the supraduodenal portion of the common bile duct or via a direct transduodenal exploration of the ampulla of Vater. It is rarely possible to resect tumours of the head of pancreas, but when these or tumours arising in the lower bile ducts are operable the radical excision usually includes the duodenum, head of pancreas, pyloric antrum, and common bile duct, and therefore requires multiple anastomoses to restore continuity of the upper gastrointestinal tract. Even when the tumour cannot be resected, jaundice may be relieved by diverting bile to the upper small intestine by making an anastomosis between the gall-bladder and either the duodenum or jejunum. Such a procedure gives useful palliation and often significantly prolongs life.

Surgical treatment of benign stricture may prove very difficult. Those in the common bile duct may be excised, with reimplantation of the proximal end of the duct into the upper small intestine. Those at higher levels of the biliary tree may require considerable dangerous exploration, and some ingenuity to achieve drainage of the bile to the intestine.

Gallstone ileus

Gallstone ileus is a rare occurrence. A stone may ulcerate through the wall of the gallbladder, usually from Hartmann's pouch, into the adherent duodenum, and if the stone is large enough it may obstruct the ileum, where the lumen of the bowel is most narrow. Surgical removal of the stone is required.

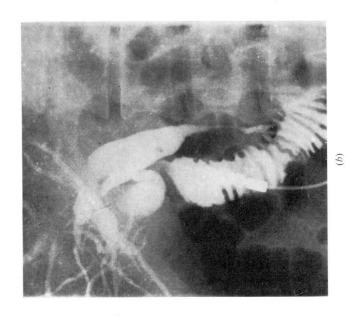

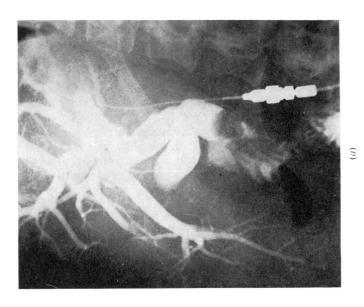

Fig. 5.2 (a) Percutaneous cholangiogram in a 62-year-old woman with a one month history of jaundice and right hypochondrial pain. The common bile duct is dilated and a large non-opaque calculus is present at the lower end. Dye can be seen entering the duodenum. (b) Percutaneous cholangiogram in a 45-year-old man with a two month history of obstructive jaundice. The common bile duct is dilated and a 'rat tail' appearance is seen at the lower end. Dye can be seen entering the duodenum. At laparotomy a large tumour was found arising from the region of the head of the pancreas.

(a)

(b)

Carcinoma of the gallbladder

Carcinoma of the gallbladder is relatively rare and when it occurs gallstones are invariably present. Either recurrent mechanical irritation or exposure to cholic acid derivatives in the stones are possible aetiological factors. However, in view of the rarity of carcinoma of the gallbladder and the prevalence of gallstones, it must be concluded that the gallbladder is rather unsusceptible to such possible carcinogenic agents. In most cases the growth is an adenocarcinoma, but squamous carcinoma arising secondarily to metaplasia of the lining epithelium also occurs. The condition may present with localized pain or with a mass in the right subcostal region, or in the late stages, with jaundice. Because of spread into the adjacent liver, to the biliary ducts or the associated lymph nodes, surgical removal is rarely possible, although occasionally excision of the gallbladder along with a wedge of liver proves successful.

THE PANCREAS

The pancreas is inaccessible to clinical examination. Disease of the organ may declare itself by involvement of surrounding organs, e.g. occlusion of the common bile duct, erosion of a vertebra, or disturbance of gastric or colonic function. Pathological conditions of the pancreas may occur without local physical signs, and the diagnosis in such cases depends upon knowledge of the clinical and biochemical disturbances which may signify pancreatic disease.

ANATOMY

The exocrine portion of the pancreas consists of lobules bound together by loose connective tissue. The lobules are collections of tubular-shaped acini which contain at least two types of cells. The majority are zymogen-containing cells which produce the precursors of the digestive enzymes. There are also cells situated near the centre of the acini, which probably secrete water and bicarbonate. The acinar ducts in turn open into interlobular ducts which join to form the main ducts of the gland. The main pancreatic duct enters the second part of the duodenum at the ampulla of Vater.

PHYSIOLOGY

The daily volume of pancreatic juice in man is between 1000 and 2000 ml. The juice is watery, colourless and odourless. Its pH is 8 to 8·3, due to the presence of bicarbonate, the characteristic anion of the juice. The pancreas has a high turnover of protein in the form of enzymes; the juice contains 1 to 2 g per cent of protein, equivalent to 10 to 40 g of protein daily.

There are three main groups of enzymes.

Proteolytic enzymes. These are secreted in inactive forms. Trypsinogen and chymotrypsinogen are endopeptidases which are stored in the zymogen granules at the apex of acinar cells and discharged on demand into the pancreatic ducts. They are activated by trypsin or chymotrypsin, or by contact with the intestinal mucosa and its activating enzyme, enterokinase, and are most active at pH 8 to 9. Proteolytic enzymes do not reach the cytoplasm of normal cells; the presence of trace amounts of trypsin would provoke proteolysis in the living cell.

Lipase. Unlike trypsin, lipase is secreted in active form, its activity also being highest at an alkaline pH. It splits fat which has been subjected to the emulsifying action of bile salts. The enzyme requires the presence of calcium ions.

Amylase. Amylase is present both in the zymogen granule and in the cytoplasm of the acinar cells and like lipase is secreted in the active form, chloride being a co-factor. The enzyme acts optimally at pH 6·5 to 7·2. It digests starch and maltose, the end product being glucose. Maltase, sucrase and lactase may also be present in pancreatic juice.

Amylase, trypsin and lipase appear in small amounts in the serum of normal people. The pathways by which small amounts of such enzymes find their way into the serum are poorly understood. It is well established, however, from experimental studies in animals, that death of the acinar cells or rupture of ductules from any cause releases pancreatic enzymes into the pancreas and circulating blood.

These observations led to the development of biochemical tests for pancreatic disease which depend upon the demonstration of an increase in serum enzyme concentrations. Under routine laboratory conditions the level of amylase in the serum can be measured rapidly and accurately; for this reason it is the most frequently used diagnostic measurement in clinical practice for the detection of pancreatic cell necrosis.

ENDOCRINE FUNCTION

The islets of Langerhans, which are nests of specialized cells interspersed among the acinar tissue, produce at least two important hormones, insulin and glucagon.

Insulin, from the β-cells of the islets, exerts its well-known hypoglycaemic influence via several effects on carbohydrate metabolism. Glucagon originates in the α-cells, and although it has an action in general antagonistic to that of insulin, its physiological role is uncertain.

Acute pancreatitis

The annual incidence of acute pancreatitis is approximately 5 per 100,000 of the population.

Pathology

In mild cases the only macroscopic change may be oedema of the pancreas. In severe cases, at autopsy or operation, the pancreas is greatly swollen, dark in colour and friable with varying degrees of haemorrhage within its substance. There is oedema of the pancreas and of the retroperitoneal tissues and often a serous ascitic fluid stained with bile or blood. This first collects in the lesser sac forming a pseudocyst, but may later become generalized. White opaque areas are commonly seen scattered over the surface of the pancreas, the mesentery and peritoneum. These are areas of fat necrosis resulting from the action of pancreatic enzymes on tissue fat with the production of glycerol and fatty acids, the latter combining with calcium to form insoluble soaps. A fall in serum calcium may result from extensive fat necrosis and is a reliable sign of severe disease. Infection of the gland may supervene with the later production of local abscesses or general peritonitis. The ileum or transverse colon may be involved in the inflammatory process with disturbance of peristalsis and subsequent distension. Paralytic ileus is a common early sign in the disease. A left-sided pleural effusion or collapse of the lower lobe of the lung may develop and be a source of diagnostic error. Transient glycosuria may be observed during a severe attack due to involvement of the islets of Langerhans.

These events are caused by the release of pancreatic enzymes, particularly trypsin, into the gland. Acute acinar necrosis is accompanied by interstitial oedema and in severe attacks the loss of fluid into the pancreas and retroperitoneal tissues may amount to 20 to 30 per cent of the total blood volume. Haemorrhage into the pancreas or peripancreatic tissues is a sign of severe autodigestion; tryptic digestion of the extravasated blood results in the appearance of an abnormal pigment, methaemalbumin in the serum. The detection of methaemalbuminaemia has been shown to be a reliable indicator of haemorrhagic pancreatitis and of severe disease. Severe attacks of acute pancreatis give rise to shock. Loss of fluid is clearly contributory, but there is also evidence that pancreatic enzymes may precipitate the release into the circulation of vasoactive kinins like bradykinin, which causes vasodilatation and increased capillary permeability. These vasoactive kinins may produce a state of shock not reversed by fluid or replacement of blood. Severe shock is the most common cause of early death in acute pancreatitis. If hypotension is prolonged, acute renal failure may supervene due to acute necrosis of the renal tubules.

Aetiology

The precise pathogenesis of the disease is unknown; it is probable that more than one factor is involved in many cases. The various factors which have been credited with aetiological importance are as follows.

(*a*) Activation of pancreatic enzymes by the reflux of bile into the pancreatic duct. For many years it was believed that acute pancreatitis developed in patients in whom there existed a common termination of the common bile and main pancreatic ducts, the 'common channel' theory. It was postulated that obstruction at the sphincter of Oddi, by an impacted stone or by oedema or spasm of the sphincter, might lead to reflux of bile into the pancreatic duct with activation of pancreatic enzymes. This theory is no longer widely held because it is now known that a common channel is not always present in patients suffering from acute pancreatitis. If bile after incubation for 12 hours with pancreatic juice of high enzyme content or with trypsin is introduced into the pancreatic ducts of animals at pressures sufficiently low not to cause rupture of the ducts, fatal pancreatic necrosis results. Thus, while the common channel theory is no longer tenable, it is possible that reflux of bile, modified in some way, may still be an important factor in the pathogenesis of acute pancreatitis.

(b) Activation of pancreatic enzymes by reflux of duodenal juice. This theory of pathogenesis is perhaps more soundly based since pancreatic enzymes are normally activated by enterokinase from the duodenal mucosa. Such reflux may occur in patients with gallstones because of relaxation of the sphincter of Oddi even in the presence of a normal intraduodenal pressure. This mechanism may account for the close association of gallstones with acute pancreatitis. Acute pancreatitis may also result from an increase in intraduodenal pressure without abnormality of the sphincter of Oddi and the disease has been produced experimentally in dogs by surgically-induced duodenal obstruction.

(c) Obstruction of the pancreatic ducts. The experimental evidence of the importance of pancreatic duct obstruction in the pathogenesis of acute pancreatis is conflicting, but clinical observations strongly suggest that obstruction within the main pancreatic duct, or at the ampulla of Vater, or even in the smaller ductules due to epithelial metaplasia may occasionally be an important factor in the development of the disease.

(d) Vascular factors. Ligation of the major vessels supplying the pancreas rarely causes acute pancreatitis since the pancreas has a very rich collateral circulation. Ischaemia of the tissue can be produced only by interrupting the flow in the smallest blood vessels. Experimental work supports the concept of disease of the capillaries or venules of the pancreas as a factor in acute pancreatitis but it is unlikely that the disease is frequently the result of vascular injury alone. A combination of factors such as ductal obstruction and damage of small vessels due to trypsin is usually present.

ASSOCIATED CONDITIONS

It is important that the clinician be aware of the conditions that are known to be associated with acute pancreatitis since such knowledge may permit him to prevent recurrence or relapse.

Biliary tract disease

In this country gallstones are found in 55 to 60 per cent of cases of acute pancreatitis. This association accounts for the predominance of the female sex in most series reported in Great Britain.

In the remaining 40 to 45 per cent of cases the cause of an attack of acute pancreatitis usually remains unknown but the following conditions may *rarely* be found associated with the disease.

Duodenal ulcer may cause obstruction at the ampulla of Vater and carcinoma of the pancreas and ductal calculi may cause obstruction of the ducts and present with an attack of acute pancreatitis. Chronic alcoholism also tends to predispose to acute pancreatitis, and in the United States of America it is considered to be of major aetiological importance in 25 per cent of cases. In Great Britain this association appears to be less frequent.

Infection

Acute pancreatitis may complicate mumps or viral hepatitis but the disease is usually mild and of brief duration. It may rarely complicate septicaemia.

Trauma

Direct injury to the gland, e.g. by a heavy blow in the epigastrium, can cause acute pancreatitis. Postoperative pancreatitis is a well recognized complication of gastric surgery and is usually attributed to accidental injury to the pancreatic ducts. However, the condition may follow any surgical procedure and, in the absence of evidence of injury to the pancreatic duct, reflux of duodenal juice through an atonic sphincter of Oddi is the probable cause.

Hyperparathyroidism

An attack of acute pancreatitis may be the first sign of hyperparathyroidism. Surgical removal of a parathyroid adenoma lessens the chance of recurrence of acute pancreatitis. It is probable that the acute pancreatic changes are secondary to ductal obstruction by stone formation in the pancreatic ducts due to hyperparathyroidism.

CLINICAL FEATURES

Abdominal pain, sudden in onset, severe and continuous, is the most constant symptom. Although the pain is generalized it is characteristically most severe in the upper abdomen often on the left side. Radiation of the pain through to the back is common, due to extravasation of blood and enzymes into the retroperitioneal tissues. The pain is usually followed by repeated vomiting of small amounts of bile-stained fluid or retching. Vomiting of intestinal contents may occur later in the disease when paralytic ileus and peritonitis develop.

In severe attacks the pain is very intense and tachycardia, hypotension, cold sweating extremities, pallor and cyanosis may be observed, indicating profound peripheral circulatory failure. There may be high fever and in some cases signs of basal collapse of a lung or a pleural effusion may be detected. After several days extravasation of blood near the tail of the pancreas or falciform ligament may lead to bruising in the flanks or umbilicus and these are signs of severe disease.

Physical signs may be few since the pancreas is situated in the retroperitoneal space. Tenderness is usual but rigidity and other evidence of peritonitis only occur when the inflammation involves the peritoneum. Rigidity of the abdominal muscles sometimes develops but it is not of the degree that one usually associates with a perforated viscus. Later in the disease, jaundice may develop due to oedema of the head of the pancreas. A mass palpable in the epigastrium suggests the formation of a pseudocyst in the lesser sac. Abscess formation usually declares itself with continuing fever and leucocytosis and a tender mass may be felt in the abdomen or on rectal examination. Rarely the pancreatic islets are involved in the pathological process to such a degree that diabetes mellitus develops.

DIAGNOSTIC AIDS

The differential diagnosis of acute pancreatitis may be very difficult since the clinical picture closely resembles that of acute myocardial infarction, perforated peptic ulcer and gallstone colic. Intestinal obstruction, mesenteric artery occlusion, ruptured or dissecting abdominal aneurysm may require differentiation.

The following tests may greatly assist in the diagnosis.

1. *Serum and urinary amylase.* The amylase content in the serum may be measured by Somogyi's method. The upper limit of normal is usually about 150 units/100 ml of serum. The level of serum amylase begins to rise within an hour or two of the onset of acute pancreatitis and reaches its maximum in about 24 hours. It remains elevated for about 72 hours, or even longer if morphine has been given. The level may be over 1000 units/100 ml. The transient increase in serum amylase concentration may be missed, and the test has the further disadvantage of not being specific for acute pancreatitis. Levels above normal may occur in other abdominal diseases such as perforated peptic ulcer, cholecystitis and intestinal obstruction, although the increases in these conditions rarely approach those found in pancreatitis. In cases where it is suspected that the increase in serum amylase may have been missed, it is helpful to estimate the urinary excretion of amylase which often shows an increase above normal for some days after the serum level has returned to normal. Urine amylase estimations should be performed on 6 hour or 24 hour collections of urine.

2. *Radiology*. In the early stages of acute pancreatitis straight X-rays of the abdomen are of great assistance in excluding the presence of other conditions, particularly perforated peptic ulcer. If peritonitis and paralytic ileus develop later, fluid levels may be seen. Pancreatic calcification occasionally indicates previous disease. The development of a pseudocyst can often be demonstrated by barium meal examination, particularly by a study of lateral views, when the stomach is seen to be displaced forwards by the collection of fluid in the lesser sac. Radio-opaque gallstones may be seen.

3. *Bilirubin and alkaline phosphatase*. The serum level of bilirubin and alkaline phosphatase may be slightly increased.

4. *Serum calcium*. This may be decreased, and hypocalcaemia is indicative of severe disease, levels below 7 mg per 100 ml being associated with an almost hopeless prognosis. The test is of no diagnostic value in the early stages of the disease. Hypercalcaemia due to hyperparathyroidism is rarely seen during the acute attack and investigation of this disease should be postponed until recovery from the acute attack.

5. *Methaemalbuminaemia*. The detection of methaemalbumin in the serum is an indication of severe disease.

6. *Electrocardiogram*. Changes usually consist of depression of the S–T interval in the limb or praecordial leads with diphasic or inverted T waves. Changes typical of subendocardial infarction have been observed without subsequent autopsy evidence of infarction. These electrocardiographic changes may lead to the mistaken diagnosis of acute myocardial infarction and serum amylase estimations are of great importance in this clinical situation.

Treatment

When the diagnosis can be confidently made treatment should be conservative. However, in cases where there is doubt, laparotomy may be required. If obstruction of the bile duct is found, the appropriate procedure, e.g. removal of stone, should be undertaken. In the absence of obvious associated disease the abdomen should be closed, and medical treatment started.

The first requisite of treatment is the relief of pain. Pethidine is given intramuscularly in a dose of 100 mg and repeated as often as is necessary. Both pethidine and morphine tend to cause spasm of the sphincter of Oddi with resulting increase in intraductal pressure. For this reason atropine sulphate, 0·6 mg, is often given with the analgesic.

Hormonal stimulation of pancreatic secretion is avoided by stopping oral feeding and instituting continuous gastric suction through a nasogastric tube.

Two drugs are possibly of clinical value in lessening the severity of the damage caused by this disorder. These are the trypsin inactivator, aprotinin (Trasylol), and the peptide hormone glucagon. Both are undergoing critical evaluation in clinical trials.

Attention has already been drawn to the gross depletion of circulating blood volume which may develop in this disease. Depending on the severity of the attack 1 to 8 litres of fluid may need replacement. Normal saline should be given initially and plasma substituted in the presence of hypotension. Whole blood is seldom required in the early stages of a severe attack but may be required later when the patient is rehydrated. If, after adequate replacement therapy, oliguria or anuria is noted, acute renal failure should be suspected. This dangerous complication requires special treatment.

A course of antibiotic therapy such as ampicillin is usually given in the hope of preventing or controlling secondary infection.

The signs and symptoms of tetany require the parenteral administration of calcium salts for their relief and a watch must be kept for the development of diabetes mellitus, which is usually transient and mild but which may require insulin therapy. The persistence of paralytic ileus beyond four or five days is a serious complication, and intestinal decompression and intravenous therapy must be continued until bowel motility is restored.

Complications requiring surgical correction may arise in severe attacks. Obstructive jaundice occasionally develops. It is usually transient and due to the oedema of the head of the pancreas. If it persists, then the common bile duct should be explored for gallstones. A collection of fluid localized in the lesser sac, a pancreatic pseudocyst, may uncommonly be felt in the epigastrium and may occasionally reach a large size. If not infected, pseudocysts may be reabsorbed over a period of four to six weeks. If operation is eventually required, internal drainage by anastomosis of the cyst wall to stomach, duodenum or jejunum is followed by disappearance of the cyst.

Prognosis

The mortality rate of acute pancreatitis has declined in the last 20 years but remains in the region of 25 to 30 per cent. Profound shock accounts for most of the deaths occurring early in the illness and is always an indication of severe disease. The presence of flank discoloration, persistent paralytic ileus, hypocalcaemia, methaemalbuminaemia and of surgical complications are later signs of severe disease. Unfortunately neither the severity of the pain nor the height of enzyme levels is a reliable guide to the severity of the attack. Laparotomy without other surgical procedure seems to have no adverse effect on the prognosis.

The mortality rate rises which increasing age and is high in traumatic, postoperative cases, in the presence of established cardiovascular disease, and in patients previously known to be diabetic.

Fortunately about 50 per cent of attacks of acute pancreatitis are relatively mild.

Recurrent acute pancreatitis

The patient may recover completely from the initial attack of acute pancreatitis but develop a second attack some months or years later. Full investigation for possible causal factors during convalescence from the initial attack is essential if recurrent episodes are to be avoided.

If biliary tract disease is present and is successfully treated, the chance of recurrent episodes should be reduced. Hyperparathyroidism or chronic alcoholism may lead to recurrent episodes, but in these conditions full recovery between attacks is unusual and chronic pancreatitis may develop. In the remainder no obvious cause is discovered. Follow-up reveals the occasional case of cancer in the head of the pancreas or ampulla of Vater.

The treatment of recurrent acute pancreatitis is the same as that of acute pancreatitis.

Chronic pancreatitis

Pain is often absent in chronic pancreatitis. Exocrine and endocrine insufficiency are the main problems and the disease may present as obstructive jaundice.

Clinical and pathological features

The condition is characterized pathologically by progressive fibrosis and atrophy of the pancreas. Marked weight loss due to steatorrhoea of pancreatic origin may result and occasionally diabetes mellitus develops. Because of the relative absence of pain the disease may remain unrecognized clinically until obstructive jaundice develops due to fibrotic obstruction of the common bile duct. The jaundice is often mistakenly ascribed to carcinoma of the head of the pancreas, which is a much commoner cause.

Although recognized as a clinical entity for many years, the cause of chronic pancreatitis remains unknown. It has been described in chronic alcoholism. It seems probable that chronic deficiency of protein in the diet may be linked with the disorder since it has been described in kwashiorkor and shown to be the common cause of malabsorption syndrome in East Africa. Other possibilities, the significance of which remain uncertain, are the roles of viral infections and disturbances of autoimmunity.

Diagnosis

In the early stage of chronic pancreatitis, before much pancreatic damage has occurred, confirmation of the diagnosis may be obtained by finding raised levels of serum amylase following an attack of pain, if this is experienced. More commonly the patient is seen in a period of remission, and if there is a history of upper abdominal pain investigation of the biliary tract may reveal evidence of gallstones which should be removed surgically. Hyperparathyroidism should be excluded by measurement of serum concentrations of calcium, inorganic phosphate and protein.

In chronic pancreatitis presenting with jaundice differentiation from carcinoma of the head of the pancreas and other causes of obstructive jaundice is the main diagnostic problem.

In cases of chronic pancreatitis without jaundice the following screening tests may prove helpful in reaching a diagnosis:

(a) *Straight X-ray of abdomen.* Calcification of the pancreas may indicate chronic pancreatic damage, but it is not a common finding.

(b) *Glucose tolerance test.* This may show the changes characteristic of diabetes mellitus, but these are only observed when the pancreas is extensively damaged. The association of diabetes mellitus and steatorrhoea is very suggestive of chronic pancreatic disease.

(c) *Investigation of steatorrhoea.* Investigation for steatorrhoea as described in Chapter 4 may reveal reduced fat absorption due to defective pancreatic secretion.

(d) *Liver function tests.* In the presence of bile duct obstruction these may show raised serum bilirubin and alkaline phosphatase levels.

In many cases, the history and the results of these preliminary screening tests are sufficient for the diagnosis, but in a substantial proportion of cases the diagnosis of chronic pancreatic disease cannot be established without recourse to more complicated tests of pancreatic function. These include tests involving duodenal aspiration which are disturbing and tedious to the patient. They require an experienced operator since vomiting or retching may vitiate the test.

Tests requiring intubation

The secretin test. This involves the fluoroscopic positioning in the duodenum of the distal tip of a double-lumen gastroduodenal tube, so that the gastric and duodenal contents are obtained simultaneously. The pancreas is stimulated by the intravenous administration of secretin (1 clinical unit of secretin per kg body weight) and the duodenal aspirate is collected for 80 minutes into cooled containers. The volume, pH and bicarbonate concentration of the juice are measured. A normal response should give a volume of not less than 2 ml per kg body weight, with a bicarbonate concentration of at least 90 mEq per litre. Complete obstruction of the pancreatic ducts is suggested by a decrease in both volume and bicarbonate concentration. A low volume with normal bicarbonate concentration suggests partial obstruction of the pancreatic duct.

The secretin-pancreozymin test. Many workers believe that combined stimulation of pancreatic secreton by secretin and pancreozymin is more useful than stimulation by secretin alone. High levels of diagnostic accuracy have been reported with the combined test, but it should be noted that experience with this test is more limited than with the secretin test. After duodenal intubation an intravenous infusion of secretin and of pancreozymin is given over a period of 90 minutes, with the object of achieving maximal stimulation of the pancreas while avoiding the unpleasant vasomotor reactions that not uncommonly follow the administration of these enzymes as a single intravenous bolus.

The Lundh test. This uses a standard test meal as the stimulus of pancreatic secretion. In this test a single lumen tube is passed into the duodenum under fluoroscopic control. The tryptic activity in the duodenal aspirate is measured, and in a two-hour collection is normally greater than $9\mu Eq/min/ml$. Slightly lower values may be found in non-pancreatic steatorrhoea.

Cytology of duodenal aspirate. Papanicolaou stained smears of aliquots of duodenal aspirate, or fluid obtained at endoscopic retrograde choledocho-pancreatography may reveal the presence of neoplastic cells, and such a finding is of critical diagnostic value in suspected pancreatic carcinoma. The percentage of positive results varies widely from centre to centre (30 per cent to 90 per cent), and clearly this test is very dependent on the skill and experience of the pathologist.

Scanning of pancreas. Use has been made of the avidity of the pancreas for amino acids, required for the synthesis of enzymes. Radioactive selenomethionine, which is concentrated by the pancreas is given, and the radioactivity from the pancreas is measured by scintillation counter. This is at present the only technique for the direct demonstration of pancreatic morphology without laparotomy, and although still in the experimental stage the diagnosis of pancreatic carcinoma by the demonstration of a filling defect, and of chronic pancreatic disease by the demonstration of a diffuse reduction of uptake of radioactive material, has been possible. There are many technical difficulties to overcome before this test becomes a routine procedure, but it may prove a useful screening test in the diagnosis of pancreatic disease.

Scanning of the pancreas by ultra-sound techniques has not yet established itself in clinical practice, but promises to be of special value in detecting pseudocysts of the organ.

With the increasing incidence of pancreatic disease a reappraisal of tests of pancreatic function is needed, and we await the results of multi-centre trials for a pronouncement on the comparative value of the tests now available, and on the best ways of performing them. The Lundh test has certain advantages over the secretin and pancreozymin test. It is simpler to perform, is cheaper and has no unpleasant side-effects. It has the disadvantage that the stimulus to pancreatic secretion cannot be exactly measured and cannot be guaranteed as precisely as in the hormone tests which claim to differentiate between pancreatic carcinoma and chronic pancreatitis.

Medical treatment

In chronic pancreatitis the attacks of pain, when these occur, are often precipitated by the ingestion of alcohol. Alcohol should therefore be avoided by such patients. All patients should be advised to avoid large meals as these may cause excessive stimulation of the damaged pancreas.

When signs of pancreatic insufficiency appear, treatment consists of the oral administration of a proprietary preparation of pancreatic enzymes, e.g. Cotazym B, Nutrizym and Pancrex-V. They should be thoroughly mixed into the patient's food, and alkalis should be given to buffer gastric acidity. There is no evidence that any one of these preparations is superior to the others. The only guide to their effectiveness is correction of steatorrhoea. Diabetes mellitus may require specific therapy with oral hypoglycaemic agents or insulin.

Surgical treatment

In our experience operation is rarely required. However, the following procedures have been used.

Surgery is indicated for the treatment of pseudocysts or abscesses, but these complications are rare. Surgical treatment is also employed in an attempt to relieve pain on the occasions when medical efforts have failed.

Sphincterotomy, i.e. transduodenal division of the sphincter of Oddi, performed to ensure free drainage from the bile and pancreatic ducts, has failed to fulfil its promise of relieving pain in all cases. It carries a low mortality and is technically easier to perform than other operations and for these reasons is usually the first choice. Other procedures have been devised with the aim of draining the pancreatic secretion from the tail of the pancreas to the jejunum. However, the only operation that gives predictable relief is complete pancreatectomy. In this country one seldom encounters chronic pancreatitis of sufficient severity to require this operation, which carries a high mortality rate and a high incidence of postoperative morbidity. At laparotomy the differentiation of areas involved with chronic pancreatitis from carcinoma of the head of the pancreas may be impossible if no secondary deposits of tumour are detected.

Biopsy in chronic pancreatitis is seldom helpful. It carries the risk of fistula formation and histological interpretation of the tissue changes is very difficult since chronic pancreatitis and carcinoma may co-exist.

Carcinoma of the pancreas

The commonest type of tumour to occur in the pancreas is an adenocarcinoma arising either from the acini or probably more often from the ducts. The tumour is usually scirrhous, but rarely cystadenocarcinoma. It is commoner in men than in women, and the peak incidence is in the 50 to 70 years age group. Fortunately it is much less common than carcinoma of other alimentary organs such as the stomach or large bowel, for it is often difficult to diagnose, even at a relatively late stage, and curative treatment is rarely possible.

The tumour occurs mainly in the head or body of the pancreas, and if it arises in the head of the organ it may soon obstruct the lower end of the common bile duct, thus presenting clinically as steadily increasing obstructive jaundice. Certainly the onset of painless obstructive jaundice in someone in this age group should raise the serious suspicion of this disease. Apart from this fairly dramatic mode of presentation other clinical features are usually caused by extension of tumour beyond the pancreas itself into other intra-abdominal organs, or to the posterior abdominal wall; or manifestations of blood-borne or lymphatic metastases. The first abnormal sign may be hepatic enlargement, ascites, subcutaneous secondary deposits in the region of the umbilicus, or some other clear sign of advanced intra-abdominal malignant disease.

Any of the following should give rise to suspicion of the disease:

Unexplained weight loss, possibly accompanied by a vague history of mild dyspepsia.

Upper abdominal pain mainly in the left subcostal region and extending into the back, especially if this is partly relieved by the patient sitting up and leaning forward.

Melaena, or repeated loss of small quantities of blood in the bowel motions, explained by ulceration of the growing tumour into the duodenum.

Chronic diarrhoea possibly associated with steatorrhea.

The onset of mild diabetes with no previous history of such a disorder.

Episodes of either superficial or deep venous thrombosis in the legs without any obvious local precipitating factors.

Unexplained continuous or intermittent pyrexia.

Change in abdominal contour, the appearance of subcutaneous nodules or lymph node enlargement.

The diagnosis is easiest to establish in the presence of the characteristic progressive obstructive jaundice; confirmation of the absence of bile pigment from the stools, an increase in the bile pigments in urine, but corresponding lack of urobilinogen, and a marked elevation of the serum alkaline phosphatase will usually give sufficient grounds for an exploratory laparotomy. Where other less suggestive symptoms and signs are present the following further aids to diagnosis may be of value. First, barium meal examination may demonstrate some distortion of the contour of the duodenum, the result of invasion by tumour in the head of the pancreas. Widening of the normal C-shaped outline of the duodenum has been stressed as an important sign, but considerable enlargement of the head of the pancreas is required to cause this abnormality. The radiologist can also help on occasions by selective angiography in which he injects contrast medium directly into the coeliac and/or superior mesenteric arteries, to search for an abnormal vascular pattern within the pancreas.

Scintiscanning of the pancreas after the intravenous injection of selenomethionine may show a failure of areas occupied by tumour to take up the amino acid.

Pancreatic function tests as described on page 126 may show a failure of exocrine pancreatic secretion response following stimulation to the gland by secretin and/or pancreozymin.

Sometimes, however, the results of all these investigations are equivocal, and the diagnosis is only established at exploratory laparotomy. If there is a strong suspicion of the disease in spite of apparently negative investigations, laparotomy should be advised. If the tumour is encountered early enough, it is sometimes possible to excise it radically. For tumours in the body and tail of the organ this involves excision of the distal portion of the pancreas along with the spleen. Removal of tumours in the head of the pancreas requires excision of the lower end of the stomach, the entire duodenum, the distal portion of the common bile duct, and several inches of jejunum, along with the head of the pancreas; the severed common bile duct, the stomach, and the stump of pancreas each requires to be anastomosed separately into the remaining jejunum. This operation (Whipple's procedure) is a major operation with a high mortality and morbidity risk. Unfortunately the great majority of tumours are found to be inoperable by the time they come to surgery, and any radical procedure is usually out of the question. If obstructive jaundice is present, or imminent, very worthwhile palliation can be achieved by anastomosing the distended gallbladder to the duodenum or jejunum, and this is usually followed by the prompt disappearance of the jaundice. Attempts have been made to relieve the sometimes distressing pain of the disease by division of the splanchnic nerves, but this is unreliable, and often brings about little or no benefit.

Itch is sometimes a considerable problem as the disease advances, and on occasions some slight relief can be obtained by the oral administration of cholestyramine, but once the obstruction to bile flow becomes complete this medication loses its effect. Ascitic fluid can be aspirated, repeatedly if necessary, and this may relieve some symptoms. Increasingly strong analgesics and sedatives are often required during terminal care.

Insulin-secreting islet-cell tumours

These are rare, usually benign solitary adenomas. Malignant change, characterized either by local extension, or by distant spread, occurs in 10 per cent. The tumours have an equal sex incidence and may occur at any age, although symptoms usually appear in middle age.

The typical solitary adenoma which may arise in any part of the pancreas is usually a distinctive reddish brown, but may be difficult to distinguish from normal pancreatic tissue. It is usually small and well-circumscribed from the surrounding tissue and so easily 'shelled out' by the surgeon. It may be accompanied by similar adenomata of other endocrine glands, particularly of the parathyroid and pituitary glands —the so-called polyglandular syndrome. Microscopically the adenoma cells closely resemble normal islet cells, the β-cell usually predominating.

Clinical features

Attacks of hypoglycaemia are characteristic of insulinoma. They are due to the excessive or inappropriate secretion of insulin by the tumour. Hypoglycaemia produces symptoms due to release of adrenaline, e.g. shaking, anxiety, sweating, hunger, weakness and palpitations, and to neuroglycopenia, e.g. headache, paraesthesia, visual disturbance, changes in mood and behaviour, convulsions, drowsiness and coma. The presence of an insulin-secreting tumour should be strongly suspected when such symptoms recur, especially if they develop in the fasting state or are provoked by exertion.

Diagnosis

Insulin-secreting islet-cell tumour is easily diagnosed once the condition has been suspected. In 90 per cent of cases fasting hypoglycaemia can be demonstrated following an overnight fast, providing the test is performed on three or more occasions and a reliable method for the estimation of blood glucose is used. Measurement of plasma insulin levels at the time of hypoglycaemia may reveal absolute or relative hyperinsulinaemia, a finding strongly suggestive of the diagnosis of insulin-secreting tumour.

In the remaining 10 per cent of cases these simple tests yield inconclusive results. In this group, special tests designed to provoke hypoglycaemia are employed. Fasting for 72 hours or stimulation of insulin secretion by substances like glucagon, leucine or tolbutamide may reveal hypoglycaemia with inappropriate insulin secretion. The glucagon test is most commonly used. The tolbutamide test can be dangerous and should be reserved for those cases in which the diagnosis seems unlikely. Coeliac axis arteriography may locate the tumour in about one-third of cases. Co-existing parathyroid or pituitary adenomata should be excluded before operation is advised.

Treatment

In all cases surgical exploration of the pancreas should be carried out without delay since surgery offers the prospect of permanent cure. For several days before operation the patient should eat liberal amounts of those foods which he has found effective in controlling his attacks. Intravenous glucose supplements should be available before and during operation.

The surgeon should mobilize the pancreas so that careful examination of the whole gland is possible, to exclude the presence of multiple tumours. Once identified, the tumour is usually easily enucleated. If the capsule is not well-defined the growth should be resected with a small margin of pancreatic tissue. If, after a careful search, no tumour can be found, it is usually recommended that the distal part of the body and tail of the pancreas be resected in hope that the tissue removed will contain the adenoma.

In the rare cases of malignant tumour total resection of the pancreas is performed, if the operation is technically possible.

FURTHER READING

Bouchier, I.A.D. (Ed.) (1973) *Clinics in Gastroenterology—Diseases of the Biliary Tract.* London: Saunders.

Carey, C. (Ed.) (1973) *The Pancreas,* St. Louis: C.V. Mosby.

Howat, H.T. (Ed.) (1972) *Clinics in Gastroenterology—The Exocrine Pancreas.* London: Saunders.

Kune, G.A. (1972) *Current Practice of Biliary Surgery.* Edinburgh: Churchill Livingstone.

6. The Liver

I. W. Dymock

The presenting symptoms and signs of liver disease may vary widely: secondary involvement of the central nervous system is often as important as the alimentary findings. Laboratory data and special radiological, isotopic and biopsy techniques are frequently employed in reaching a diagnosis and in measuring the progress of the illness.

NORMAL BILE PIGMENT METABOLISM

Bilirubin is the bile pigment responsible for the characteristic yellow colour of jaundiced serum and tissues: each day some 300 mg of this pigment is produced and exreted by the healthy adult. About 85 per cent of this bilirubin is derived from the haemoglobin liberated from the circulating red cells at the end of their life span. Most of the remaining bilirubin is derived from bone marrow haems released during ineffective erythropoiesis, and the smallest part originates from haem pigments contained in liver cells. The exact chemical reactions involved in the production of bilirubin have not been determined, but they are known to involve the conversion of the ring protoporphyrin haem to the linear tetrapyrrole biliverdin which in turn is converted to bilirubin.

Under normal conditions bilirubin is soluble in fat but insoluble in water, and its transport in the serum is made possible by firm binding to the serum albumin. As under normal circumstances the albumin content of 100 ml of blood is sufficient to bind 40 mg of bilirubin, this ability to transport is rarely saturated. This protein binding usually prevents bilirubin excretion via the kidney. Under certain circumstances other substances with a strong protein binding ability, such as the sulphonamide sulphafurazole (Gantrisin), may displace bilirubin with release of the pigment into the tissues producing jaundice.

The subsequent metabolism of bilirubin involves its transport into the liver cell, but the mechanism by which it is separated from albumin is not understood. Inside the liver cell it is bound to an as yet unidentified macromolecule, which is immunologically distinct from albumin. The bilirubin now reacts with uridine diphosphoglucuronic acid (UDPGA) under the influence of the enzyme glucuronyl transferase to form bilirubin diglucuronide. This enzyme is located in the microsomal fraction of liver cells and is deficient or absent in certain congenital unconjugated hyperbilirubinaemias. Bilirubin diglucuronide is water soluble.

After glucuronidation, bilirubin is transferred across the liver cell to the bile canaliculus into which it is secreted against a concentration gradient. The bilirubin then passes along the bile radicles to the common bile duct and to the intestine where, under the influence of the intestinal bacteria, it undergoes deconjugation and hydrogenation to 'stercobilinogen' and unconjugated bilirubin. Most of these are excreted in the stool, but some stercobilinogen may be reabsorbed from the colon to re-enter the liver and be excreted via the kidney as urobilinogen.

BILIRUBIN DETERMINATIONS

For many years it has been known that the bilirubin in bile was water-soluble whilst the bilirubin in serum was not. However, in jaundiced patients both water-soluble (conjugated), and the non-water-soluble (unconjugated) forms may be present. The chemical determination of the serum bilirubin is done with van den Bergh's diazo reagent, which normally reacts with the water-soluble or conjugated form giving a 'direct' reaction. The addition of alcohol renders the water-insoluble unconjugated bilirubin soluble in water, and measurement by van den Bergh's method then gives a 'total' bilirubin representing the combination of unconjugated and conjugated bilirubin. The difference between these two represents the 'indirect', or unconjugated, form. Under normal circumstances the total bilirubin does not exceed 0·8 mg per 100 ml and the 'direct' reacting conjugated bilirubin is not more than 0·2 mg per cent.

JAUNDICE

Jaundice is an increase in the amount of the bilirubin in the blood and other body tissues. In the patient this is seen as a yellow discoloration of sclera, skin and mucosae. The increase in bilirubin levels may result from either increased production due to the excessive breakdown of red corpuscles (haemolytic jaundice) or because of failure of the mechanism for removal of bilirubin from the circulating blood as it passes through the liver. This failure of excretion may be due to either dysfunction of the liver cells so that they cannot remove the bilirubin from the circulating blood (hepatocellular jaundice) or from obstruction to the flow of bile from the liver (obstructive jaundice) resulting in diffusion of bilirubin compounds from the liver back into the blood.

Haemolytic jaundice

This is the least common of the three types of jaundice and is usually the least noticeable. The haemolysis may arise on account of abnormalities in the red blood cells, or the action of various lysins. The elevation in the serum bilirubin level is usually slight (up to 5 mg per cent) and other features of the haemolytic process are usually dominant. The urine contains increased quantities of urobilinogen but does not contain bilirubin, hence the previous name for the condition, namely 'acholuric jaundice'. The stools usually retain their normal colour but on chemical analysis excess urobilinogen may be detected.

Hepatocellular jaundice

Hepatic, or hepatocellular, jaundice is the term used to describe the type of jaundice due to liver cell damage, when the ability of the diseased liver cells to remove bilirubin from the blood and excrete it into the biliary system is impaired. The commoner causes of this type of jaundice are virus hepatitis and hepatic cirrhosis, but it may also occur in other parenchymal disorders of the liver, including severe congestive cardiac failure. Other clinical evidence of hepatic dysfunction is usually present (pp. 144–148). The stools are usually normal in colour; the urine contains urobilinogen and sometimes bilirubin. The bilirubin which is present in the blood is partly of the conjugated and partly of the unconjugated variety, and the total bilirubin concentration may occasionally reach 40 mg per cent, although more commonly it is less than 20 mg per cent. Other biochemical features in the serum include markedly elevated transaminase levels and a moderate increase in the alkaline phosphatase.

Obstructive jaundice

In this type of jaundice the flow of bile is obstructed by a lesion in either the biliary tract or the surrounding structures. Most commonly this occurs in the extrahepatic portion of the biliary tree, and the commonest causes are impaction of a gallstone usually at the lower end of the common bile duct, a carincoma of the head of pancreas producing extrinsic pressure on the bile duct or a carcinoma of the ampulla of Vater (see p. 128). Less common causes are strictures resulting from previous inflammation or surgery, and lymph nodes in the porta hepatis. Intrahepatic lesions, such as a hepatoma, may sometimes produce this type of jaundice, but these lesions usually obstruct either the right or the left hepatic duct, rarely both ducts.

In this situation the bilirubin level often reaches very high levels of 30 to 40 mg per 100 ml, and is associated with a marked increase in the serum alkaline phosphatase concentration. In addition the serum transaminases may be moderately elevated, due to secondary hepatic damage. The urine contains large quantities of bilirubin but no urobilinogen, and the stools are pale. Bile salts, which are produced by the liver, may accumulate in the blood and are responsible for the pruritus and bradycardia which are often found in these patients.

Differential diagnosis

Although in most patients with jaundice it is usually possible to place them in one of these three categories, in some instances this may be difficult due to overlap in the clinical features and in the biochemical tests. However, all patients with jaundice merit detailed investigation and this may include laparotomy.

In the interrogation of the patient with jaundice it is particularly important to enquire regarding jaundice in the relatives or contacts, the presence of other symptoms such as abdominal pain, whether any drugs have been taken recently, and if there have been any similar episodes in the past. The laboratory investigations which may be required are many, but it is particularly important to measure the serum total and conjugated bilirubin, alkaline phosphatase and transaminase levels. In addition all these patients should have urine examined for the presence of bilirubin and urobilinogen, and the colour and character of the stools should be inspected. A plain radiograph of the abdomen should be included in the investigations as this may demonstrate a radio-opaque gallstone. In every instance laboratory tests should be performed to detect a coagulation defect. If the prothrombin time is abnormal vitamin K therapy should be commenced.

In most patients with obstructive jaundice it is due to an extrahepatic biliary obstruction originating from cholelithiasis or a carcinoma in either the head of the pancreas or the ampulla of Vater. In these patients surgical management is imperative. However, in some the jaundice is due to a lesion for which surgery is contra-indicated. This may occur in some patients with virus hepatitis who enter a phase of the illness in which the jaundice is obstructive in nature. Other conditions in which surgery is contraindicated are those in which the obstruction is at the canalicular level as with some drugs such as chlorpromazine and methyl testosterone. In primary biliary cirrhosis severe obstructive jaundice may develop in a manner which is similar to that described above, and in these patients and in those with drug jaundice or virus hepatitis a laparotomy may be associated with a rapid deterioration. Wherever possible these less common causes of obstructive jaundice should be excluded prior to surgery, by the newer techniques including liver scanning and E.R.C.P., with radiological demonstration of the biliary and pancreatic ducts. In some patients liver biopsy may be indicated.

VIRAL LIVER INFECTIONS

Viral hepatitis

Although many viral diseases can produce a hepatitis, this term usually refers to infectious hepatitis (type A), and serum hepatitis (type B).

Infectious hepatitis (Type A). This form of virus hepatitis is usually transmitted by the faecal–oral route and is often associated with poor hygiene. Food and water appear to become contaminated from the excreta of an infected individual. Less commonly, it may be transmitted by the parenteral route. Infectious hepatitis tends to occur sporadically and usually only isolated cases are encountered. From time to time, however, explosive epidemics arise and these tend to occur in institutions, hospitals, schools and communities where large numbers of people, particularly children, are in close proximity. Major epidemics occur during wars and there have been large numbers of reported cases in the past 30 years from North Africa, Korea and Vietnam.

The incubation period is from one to eight weeks, and the patient probably remains infective up to two weeks after the onset of the disease. During the same period blood and serum are also infective and parenteral transmission may occur.

Other possible sources of infection which have been incriminated include sea food, milk, orange juice and water supplies. Virtually any foodstuff may become a carrier source for the virus.

Serum hepatitis (Type B). The virus of serum hepatitis (homologous serum jaundice) is usually transmitted by the parenteral route but it can be acquired orally, and by sexual contact. The main source of infection is from needles, syringes, tubing, serum, blood and blood products. The risk from the transfusion of a single unit of blood was formerly about 1 per cent, but in some areas where there are professional blood donors the risk is much higher. Human dried plasma is a potential source of virus hepatitis, although this risk has been minimized with the use of small-pool plasma from perhaps 8 to 12 donors instead of the 100 or so used formerly. Routine testing of donor blood for the hepatitis antigen (see page 140) has, however, reduced this risk substantially. Staff and patients in renal dialysis units are particularly at risk. Patients undergoing open-heart surgery with cardiopulmonary bypass also have an increased risk of developing serum hepatitis, as do 'main-line' drug addicts who frequently share syringes and needles. In addition there is a high incidence of serum hepatitis in persons who have been recently tattooed, individuals in malarial areas where the mosquito is a vector, and amongst homosexuals.

The incubation of serum hepatitis is from six weeks to six months and the period of infectivity may be up to one week after the onset of jaundice. The patient may be infective for up to three months prior to the onset of symptoms.

Pathology

Macroscopically and microscopically the lesions of infectious hepatitis and serum hepatitis are identical.

If the patient dies after a very short course, then the liver will show the classical appearance of acute yellow atrophy. The liver is usually small and the cut surface shows patchy or total yellow atrophy. For some reason, the left lobe appears to be more severely affected. Early regeneration nodules may be obvious if the patient has died in the recovery phase.

Histological examination of the hepatitic liver will show a well-preserved reticulin network if death has been early. Later, the reticulin network will collapse. Necrosis and autolysis of the liver cells is the main feature, with polymorphonuclear infiltration of the portal tracts. Eosinophil bodies may be present and their frequency is related to the prognosis; when they are more frequent the prognosis is poor. Centrilobular cholestasis may occur and is associated with more severe jaundice.

Clinical features

Not all patients with virus hepatitis develop jaundice. In fact, the anicteric form of the disease may be about ten times more common than the classical disease state.

Prodromal symptoms occur in all patients and may be present for up to a week before the onset of jaundice. The main features at this time are malaise, anorexia, headache and the loss of the desire to smoke or to drink alcohol. In addition, there may be discomfort in the right hypochondrium, usually attributed to stretching of the liver capsule. Two to eight days after developing these symptoms jaundice appears; this frequently coincides with some improvement in appetitie. Many patients have pruritus for a few days as the jaundice appears. The liver is usually just palpable in the right midclavicular line and is smooth and tender. One in five patients has palpable splenomegaly. With jaundice there is darkening of the urine and there may be some pallor of the faeces; this latter sign becomes marked should there develop a phase of biliary obstruction.

In the uncomplicated case, recovery begins one to two weeks from the onset of jaundice. The stools rapidly regain their normal colour, the jaundice lessens and the urine colour lightens. Splenomegaly, if present, subsides rapidly, but the hepatomegaly may return to normal only some weeks later.

Clinical investigations

Urine examination at the onset will reveal the presence of bilirubin and an excess of urobilinogen. The bilirubinuria persists throughout the illness, but the urobilinogen may disappear temporarily should there be an obstructive phase due to cholestasis; this clears during the recovery phase and urobilinogen returns to the urine.

The serum total bilirubin level rises rapidly but rarely exceeds 25 mg per cent. With this, the alkaline phosphatase is also elevated, but it seldom rises above 40 King-Armstrong units per cent. The levels of serum transaminases are markedly elevated in all patients; the alanine amino-transferase (G.P.T.) may reach particularly high levels, as this enzyme is more specific for liver damage than the aspartate (G.O.T.).

A mild leucocytosis is usually found in viral hepatitis and the pro-thrombin time may be prolonged. The E.S.R. is usually elevated.

Complications

Not every patient with viral hepatitis pursues an uneventful course. The commonest complication which occurs is for the disease to have a more prolonged course with persistent jaundice. The jaundice in these patients is almost always obstructive and is associated with intra-hepatic cholestasis. In this situation, the possibility that the lesion is due to obstruction to the bile ducts must be considered. The giving of ad-renal corticosteroids to such patients will, in the cholestatic jaundice of viral hepatitis, produce a rapid reduction in the level of serum bilirubin. There is no beneficial effect if the obstruction is extrahepatic. The use of corticosteroids does not affect the course of the hepatitis nor does it produce a permanent improvement.

About 5 per cent of patients show rapid clinical deterioration with the onset of acute liver failure. Following the onset of jaundice these patients soon become deeply comatose, and there is frequently an associated acute renal failure. Clinical examination usually reveals a small shrunken liver which cannot be detected on percussion. Death is almost invariable, despite full supportive measures (see page 154) which are aimed at providing sufficient time for liver regeneration to occur.

Almost 5 per cent of patients will have a relapse following recovery from an attack of viral hepatitis. This is usually associated with inges-tion of alcohol or undue physical exertion. Commonly, the jaundice is not so marked as during the initial episode and the liver function tests do not show the same degree of abnormality. Further bed-rest is usually followed by an uneventful recovery.

Some patients may have a clinical course marked by persistence of jaundice with consistently abnormal liver function tests. Fortunately, this type of chronic persistent hepatitis is uncommon, and it requires to be differentiated by liver biopsy from chronic active hepatitis which has presented acutely. In this situation, corticosteroids or azathioprine may be of value.

Treatment

There is no specific treatment for viral hepatitis. The patient should be in bed until the pyrexia settles and general well-being has returned. Various non-specific regimens may help the patient and reduce the incidence of complications, although there is no real evidence for this. It is usual to give the patients a diet with a content low in fat and high in carbohydrate and protein. Probably the giving of an adequate number of calories, regardless of the form, is the most important measure.

Should liver failure develop, the general measures for this condition should be instituted together with more specific measures, such as exchange blood transfusions.

Prophylaxis. If individuals have been in contact with, or are liable to be exposed to, cases of viral hepatitis, the use of human gamma globulin is recommended. There is evidence that this preparation, obtained from the serum of immune subjects, will reduce the incidence of frank hepatitis and may abort the more severe attacks. The usual dose is 750 mg by intramuscular injection and the effect lasts for about three months. Recently a new type of hyper-immune globulin against type B hepatitis has become available also.

Hepatitis-associated antigen (synonyms: Australia antigen; SH-antigen). This antigen was originally detected in the serum of an Australian aborigine but has since been reported as being present in the serum of patients with viral hepatitis. The position is by no means clear but it has been found in the serum of over 75 per cent of patients with serum hepatitis, but in less than 15 per cent of patients with infectious hepatitis. It may be detected in blood taken for transfusion and, if subsequently administered, serum hepatitis is likely to occur.

The antigen has also been demonstrated in patients with chronic liver disease such as cirrhosis, chronic active hepatitis and hepatoma, and it has been postulated that these conditions are produced following a Type B infection. The incidence of antigenaemia varies in different countries, being low in Britain (about 1:750 persons) and high in Mediterranean, African and Asian countries. The virus has been identified by electron microscopy of serum, and consists of small round forms, tubular particles and the larger Dane particles which are probably the virus itself (Fig. 6.1). The antigen may be detectable in the serum of patients developing hepatitis for up to three months prior to jaundice, but it usually is eliminated within a week or two of the onset of the acute illness. There is a high incidence of carriage of the antigen in drug addicts.

CIRRHOSIS

Hepatic cirrhosis

Cirrhosis can be defined as a late result of liver injury producing a diffuse process in the liver, characterized by fibrosis, regeneration nodules formed from the normal lobular structure, and intrahepatic portasystemic vascular shunts. As the aetiological factors and mechanism of production are unknown in most cirrhotic patients, it is customary to classify cirrhosis according to its pathological characteristics (Table 6.1).

In a micronodular cirrhosis there is an involvement of every lobule and the nodules are of lobule size (about 1 mm) and are surrounded by fine bands of fibrous tissue which contain both portal tracts and centrilobular areas (Fig. 6.2*a*), although as a rule neither these portal tracts

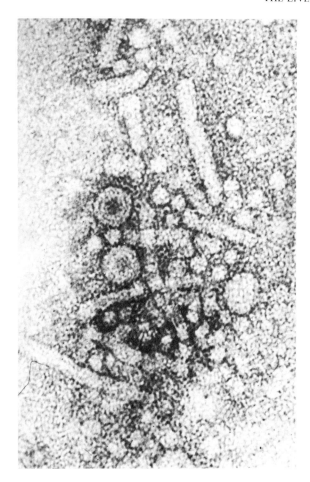

Fig. 6.1 Electronmicrograph of the serum of a carrier of the Hepatitis B antigen. The predominant particle is the small round form (20 nm size) with in addition some tubular forms and a few of the large (42 nm) Dane particles with an inner core and outer coat.

nor the central veins can be identified. This absence of central veins is an important differentiating feature from hepatic fibrosis. In time these micronodular types of cirrhosis progress to the macronodular type. When the histological features are in the intermediate stage they are classed as mixed cirrhosis. In the macronodular cirrhosis, the nodules are usually at least 1 cm in size. Within these larger nodules the central veins and portal tracts can usually be identified giving a semblance of a lobular structure (Fig. 6.2b). This type of cirrhosis is usually found in end-stage cirrhosis, regardless of its aetiology. Biopsy diagnosis of macronodular cirrhosis may prove difficult, as the sample produced by

Table 6.1 Classification of the cirrhoses

New classification	Old classification
Macronodular	Postnecrotic Posthepatic

Micronodular	Portal
	Laennec's
	  Alcoholic
	  Nutritional
	  Diffuse septal

Mixed (a combination of micro- and macronodular)	

Fibrotic conditions
  with progression to cirrhosis, e.g.
    Biliary cirrhosis
    Haemochromatosis
    Cardiac cirrhosis	

the needle biopsy may not be altogether representative. Biopsy diagnosis of a mixed or micronodular cirrhosis is, on the other hand, much easier; the main features to be looked for are fibrosis with loss of lobular structure, nodule formation and liver cell regeneration. Fragmentation of the biopsy is frequent.

Liver biopsy

A sample of the liver substance can be obtained by using a special needle introduced directly into the liver under local anaesthesia. The indications for liver biopsy, in addition to the diagnosis and assessment of cirrhosis, include:

Unexplained hepatomegaly or splenomegaly
Jaundice of unknown cause
Assessment of treatment in haemochromatosis (p. 159)
Diagnosis of storage disorders, e.g. glycogen storage disease and amyloidosis
Diagnosis of reticulosis
Determination of cell-type in hepatic tumours (p. 161)
Granulomatous disease with hepatomegaly.

Certain precautions must be observed prior to liver biopsy. These are:

1. The patient must be co-operative.
2. There must be no bleeding tendency.
3. The prothrombin time must be no more than two seconds prolonged over the control.
4. The platelet count should exceed 100,000 per mm^3.

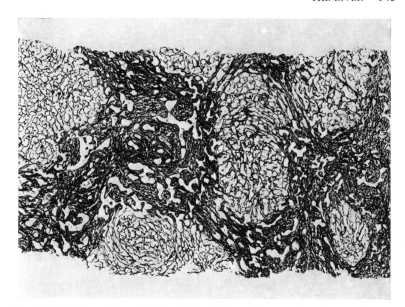

Fig. 6.2 (*a*) Micronodular cirrhosis. Marked fibrous tissue condensation can be seen surrounding almost uniformly-sized nodules of liver cells. The central hepatic veins cannot be identified. (Reticulin stain; × 70.)

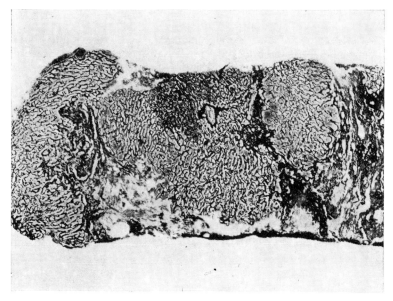

Fig. 6.2(*b*) Macronodular cirrhosis. Fibrous tissue condensation is again evident but the nodules are larger and of varied size and shape. A central hepatic vein can be identified in the central nodule. (Reticulin stain; × 70.)

5. Blood group should be known and one litre of blood cross-matched prior to the biopsy.
6. Hydatid disease must *not* be suspected (p. 156).

In most of the patients with macronodular cirrhosis the aetiology is unknown (cryptogenic cirrhosis). Factors which have been suggested as causative in these patients have included anicteric and asymptomatic viral hepatitis, food toxins, malnutrition, drugs and disordered immunological mechanisms.

The clinical features of hepatic cirrhosis are those of chronic liver disease, though in some instances the patient may have no symptoms, physical signs or biochemical abnormalities. General non-specific features are common and include malaise and lethargy, as well as the more specific features of portal hypertension or liver cell failure. Specific points to be looked for on examination are hepatomegaly, splenomegaly, ascites, oedema, jaundice and the neurological and the psychiatric features of a portasystemic encephalopathy (p. 153). Other physical features include palmar erythema, cutaneous telangiectasis and pigmentation, spider naevi, finger clubbing, white nails and a hyperdynamic circulation. Weight loss is common though it may be masked by fluid retention.

There are no specific biochemical tests for cirrhosis and most patients will have a moderately raised alkaline phosphatase level, mild hyperbilirubinaemia and, if there is cellular damage, elevated transaminase levels. The serum albumin level is usually low and the gamma globulin increased. A low total body potassium level is commonly found, though the plasma potassium may remain normal. A useful test of liver function is the bromsulphthalein retention test. The dye is injected intravenously in a dose of 5 mg per kg body weight. Blood samples are taken before injection and at intervals from 5 to 45 min. Normally by 45 min less than 6 per cent of the dye is present in the blood. If liver function is impaired the dye is not excreted into the bile and high levels are detectable in the serum. The test is only valid if the patient is not jaundiced. Occasionally, anaphylactic reactions occur on using bromsulphthalein. A mild normochromic anaemia is common, but if there has been intestinal haemorrhage, the anaemia may be hypochromic. Occasional patients have macrocytes in the peripheral blood film but the anaemia does not respond to either vitamin B_{12} or folic acid. The prothrombin time is usually mildly prolonged and in some instances responds to vitamin K. An intravascular coagulation state may be present, particularly in liver cell failure and there may be increased fibrinolysis. The liver scan (p. 162) shows a small irregular liver with an increased splenic uptake.

Whenever possible, liver biopsy (p. 142) should be performed in patients with suspected cirrhosis, to establish the diagnosis, identify the type of cirrhosis and its stage of development.

Alcoholic liver disease

The precise relationship between ingestion of alcohol and the development of cirrhosis is not known. Some alcoholics do not develop cirrhosis and although it is possible that associated protein malnutrition may play a role, some cirrhotic patients have been known to have had a high protein intake for many years. Alcoholic cirrhosis is more common in men. The liver is usually enlarged and the cirrhosis is of the micronodular type, though it may later progress to become a mixed or a macronodular cirrhosis.

The clinical presentation is often that of end-stage cirrhosis with portal hypertension, ascites or liver cell failure. In addition, after particularly heavy drinking, jaundice, anorexia, abdominal pain and the pathological features of an alcoholic hepatitis may be the presenting features. Delirium tremens, peripheral neuritis, Wernick's encephalopathy and vitamin B deficiency may all occur. Management is based on withdrawal of alcohol and the treatment of specific complications. The former may precipitate delirium tremens; chlorpromazine, chlordiazepoxide and diazepam are all useful in treating alcohol withdrawal symptoms. Supplements of vitamin B should be given to all patients and a high protein and calorie intake encouraged. Total abstention from alcohol should be maintained. This usually demands skilled psychiatric advice. Valuable support can be obtained from Alcoholics Anonymous.

Macronodular cirrhosis

A macronodular cirrhosis is the commonest variety in the United Kingdom. In almost half of the patients a history of an attack of viral hepatitis can be elicited, but in the remainder no specific aetiology can be demonstrated. Most patients are middle-aged, females being affected three times as commonly as males. The liver is usually reduced in size and is nodular with large coarse irregular nodules.

Portal hypertension (p. 147) is frequently found in these patients and bleeding from oesophageal varices is often the presenting feature. Any other complications of a cirrhosis may develop. Diagnosis is based on clinical features and is established by liver biopsy. The specific complications of portal hypertension, liver cell failure or neuropsychiatric disturbances (p. 153) are treated as appropriate.

Primary biliary cirrhosis
(Hanot's cirrhosis; xanthomatous biliary cirrhosis; chronic non-suppurative cholangitis)

The aetiology of primary biliary cirrhosis is unknown, but recent work suggests that it may be due to an immunological disturbance which may have a familial basis. It is almost entirely confined to females over the age of 45 and is characterized by chronic jaundice, severe pruritus, cutaneous xanthomata and bone changes.

The basic pathological lesion involves the bile ducts which in the early stage show necrotic, swollen and hyperplastic epithelial cells, a surrounding granuloma and a dense lymphocytic infiltrate. Later, the bile ducts can no longer be recognized but the portal tract infiltrate increases, eventually becoming fibrotic with associated cholestasis (Fig. 6.3). The liver is usually enlarged with, in the later stages, a macronodular cirrhosis.

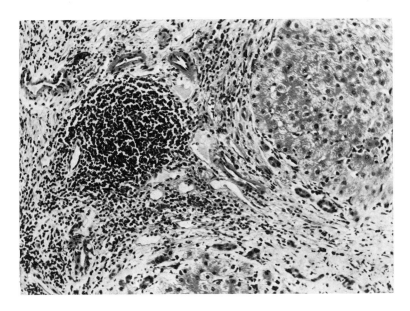

Fig. 6.3 Primary biliary cirrhosis. There is a marked round cell infiltrate in the portal tract area and sheets of fibrous tissue surround the liver nodule. Small bile ductules are present with swollen epithelial cells. The liver cells contain pigment due to cholestasis. (H and E; × 250.)

Patients usually present with cholestatic jaundice and pruritus. The bilirubin level is usually from 5 to 10 mg per cent with a markedly elevated level of alkaline phosphatase. Hepatomegaly is usual and any of the complications of cirrhosis may occur. Cutaneous xanthomata are frequent particularly around the eyes, and steatorrhoea due to chronic bile-salt deficiency is common. Bone changes occur including osteo-porosis, secondary hyperparathyroidism and osteomalacia. The osteo-malacia is due to vitamin D deficiency as a result of the steatorrhoea. A bleeding tendency due to both chronic liver disease and deficiency of vitamin K occurs.

The diagnosis can often be made on the basis of abnormal liver function tests and the demonstration of a raised level of IgM and mitochondrial antibodies which are found in over 95 per cent of patients. The liver biopsy changes are characteristic. The main differential diagnosis is from a cholestatic jaundice due to drugs or an obstruction of the common bile duct. Treatment is mainly symptomatic. Phenobarbitone may relieve the itch and lower the bilirubin level, while cholestyramine will also relieve itch. Vitamin D and vitamin K should be given for the osteomalacia and bleeding diathesis respectively. Portal hypertension (p. 148), ascites (p. 151) and liver failure (p. 153) should be treated as appropriate. The use of the immunosuppressive drug azathioprine has been suggested recently and may prove beneficial. The prognosis is poor, most patients dying within five years of diagnosis.

Chronic hepatitis

It has recently become possible to separate different forms of chronic hepatitis depending on the main histological features, and there is some evidence to support subdivision into the two groups, chronic active hepatitis and chronic persistent hepatitis. Each tends to occur more frequently in a different type of population and the outcome may vary depending on the individual type. Chronic active hepatitis, usually a disease of young females, almost invariably leads to cirrhosis and is almost certainly an immune disease. Corticosteroids produce both symptomatic and biochemical improvement and prolong life. The chronic persistent pattern, which is more common in males of Mediterranean origin, has, as a rule, a more favourable outcome.

Portal hypertension

In portal hypertension there is increased pressure in the portal venous system due to obstruction to the flow of portal venous blood. This obstruction may be either within the liver (intrahepatic) or within the portal or splenic veins (extrahepatic). Portal hypertension is usually classified as presinusoidal or postsinusoidal, depending on the relationship of the obstruction to the hepatic sinusoid (Table 6.2).

Table 6.2 Classification of portal hypertension

Presinusoidal	Postsinusoidal
Intrahepatic	Intrahepatic
Cirrhosis	Veno-occlusive disease
Hepatic fibrosis	Cirrhosis
Schistosomiasis	
Tropical splenomegaly?	
Extrahepatic	Extrahepatic
Portal vein block	Budd-Chiari syndrome
Tropical splenomegaly?	Cardiac failure

In the investigation of portal hypertension and in the preparation of the patient for portacaval shunt operations, radiology of the portal venous system is essential. This can be simply achieved by the technique of percutaneous trans-splenic portal venography. Precautions similar to those for liver biopsy (p. 142) are required. It is possible to outline the splenic vein and other tributaries of the portal vein by injecting contrast medium directly into the splenic pulp through a needle introduced under local anaesthesia.

In portal hypertension a collateral circulation develops between the veins of the portal and systemic circulations. The main sites of these collateral vessels are:

1. At the oesophagogastric junction between the left gastric vein and the intercostal, diaphragmatic and minor azygos veins.
2. Between the haemorrhoidal veins of the portal circulation and the inferior haemorrhoidal veins draining to the inferior vena cava.
3. Between the umbilical veins and the veins of the abdominal wall draining to the systemic circulation.
4. At any point where the abdominal viscera meet the retroperitoneal tissues as in the splenorenal ligament and in the diaphragmatic area.
5. In abdominal wound scars.

The main clinical feature of portal hypertension is alimentary bleeding which may be of variable severity. In about 4 per cent of patients with alimentary bleeding it is due to portal hypertension and in those the immediate mortality is 40 per cent. The bleeding is usually from oesophageal varices (Fig. 6.4) or from varices in the gastric fundus, but occasionally it can be from an associated peptic ulcer. Variceal haemorrhage is usually massive with large volumes of fresh or only minimally altered blood being vomited. Early diagnosis is essential and the stigmata of liver disease should be looked for in every patient with a haematemesis or melaena. Early and adequate blood transfusions should be given and the pulse, blood pressure and central venous pressure should be recorded half-hourly. Specific measures to control the haemorrhage include:

(a) The passage of a Sengstaken trilumen tube with balloons in the oesophagus and stomach to occlude both the oesophageal and gastric varices. Once this tube has been passed the pharynx must be aspirated regularly as the patient cannot swallow. Continuous nursing care is essential to avoid inhalation of regurgitated material.
(b) Posterior pituitary extract (pitressin) lowers portal venous pressure and may stop bleeding. It is usually accompanied by rapid evacuation of the bowel and urinary bladder. It is given intravenously as an infusion of 20 units every 30 minutes. It should be used with care in elderly patients as it may precipitate coronary artery occlusion.

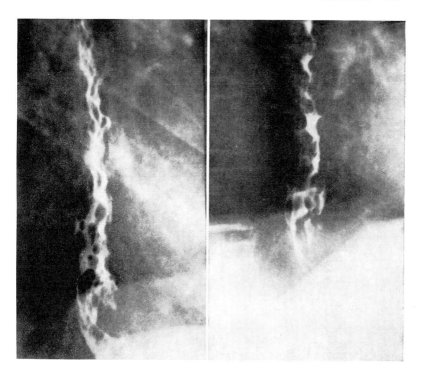

Fig. 6.4 Oesophageal varices. Barium swallow in a 40-year-old man with an alcoholic cirrhosis who was admitted following a haematemesis. The oesophagus is slightly dilated and the large varices can be seen as multiple filling defects.

If these medical measures fail to control bleeding, then arrangements should be made for emergency surgery. The various possibilities include an oesophageal or gastric transection in which the submucosal area of the oesophagus or stomach is transected and resutured, thus obliterating the venous channels. Any such operation should be followed within two months by a definitive shunt operation. Emergency portacaval anastomosis is practised in some centres, but carries a high (40 per cent) mortality. More recently it has been possible to inject, via an oesophagoscope, a sclerosing solution directly into the veins.

In considering a patient for an elective portasystemic shunt operation, several criteria are necessary:

   (i) Liver function must be adequate. In practice this means a bilirubin of less than 2 mg per cent and a serum albumin of more than 3 g per cent.

 (ii) There should be no ascites.

(iii) There should be no history of portasystemic encephalopathy (p. 153).

(iv) There should be a patent portal or splenic vein (Fig. 6.5) and if a splenorenal shunt is to be considered, the renal vein should be normal.

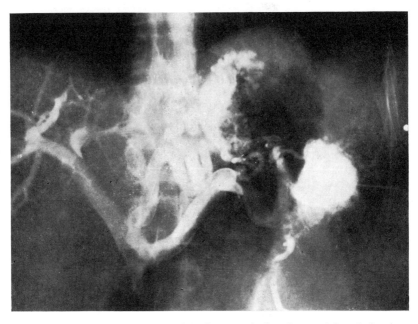

Fig. 6.5 Splenic venogram. A pool of dye is present in the spleen, and the splenic vein, portal vein and intrahepatic portal veins have been filled. The portal vein is patent. The dilated left gastric vein can be seen to be filled and dye is passing along this to collaterals at the cardia.

Two types of portacaval anastomosis are used. In the side-to-side anastomosis, the portal vein and the inferior vena cava are anastomosed without the portal vein being divided. It has the disadvantage that there is a higher postoperative incidence of portasystemic encephalopathy. In the end-to-side operation, the portal vein is ligated and divided in the hilum of the liver and the free end is anastomosed to the vena cava. This produces a more dramatic fall in portal venous pressure and the incidence of encephalopathy is less.

If neither of these operations is practical, an anastomosis of the splenic vein to the renal vein, or the insertion of a dacron tube prosthesis between the superior mesenteric vein and the inferior vena cava, may be carried out.

After portasystemic shunt operations, certain complications may occur. These include:

Portasystemic encephalopathy
(in almost 20 per cent of patients)

Persistent ankle oedema
Hepatocellular damage
Gastric hypersecretion
Repeated infections
Myopathy with paraplegia
Haemosiderosis.

Portal vein block

Portal vein block accounts for about 10 per cent of patients with portal hypertension. It is usually due to portal vein thrombosis. Although in most instances no cause can be found for the portal vein thrombosis, it may arise as a late sequel to umbilical sepsis or catheterization of the umbilical vein. Occasionally it is due to a cavernous transformation of the portal vein, which is thought to be congenital. Liver function and liver histology are both normal. The prognosis is good provided that the portal pressure can be lowered. Portacaval shunt operations are usually impractical and splenorenal or superior mesenteric-inferior vena caval anastomoses have to be considered.

Ascites

One of the common complications of portal cirrhosis is the development of ascites. The mechanism of production of ascites is still incompletely understood, but a number of factors are known to play a part. These are:

1. Increased portal venous pressure (p. 147). In extrahepatic portal vein obstruction ascites is rare, so that elevation of portal venous pressure alone is rarely causative in producing ascites. Intrahepatic portal hypertension, on the other hand, increases hepatic lymph production, which may play a role in the development of ascites.
2. Hypoalbuminaemia. In chronic liver disease circulating levels of albumin are decreased due to reduced hepatic albumin synthesis and dilution in the expanded extracellular fluid volume which is associated with cirrhosis. Reduction in the circulating albumin levels in turn lowers the effective colloid osmotic pressure. Hypoalbuminaemia alone rarely produces ascites, but will do so in association with increased portal venous pressure.
3. Increased lymphatic lymph production. In portal hypertension, hepatic lymph production is increased. This normally drains to the thoracic duct but the lymphatic system may not be able to cope with the expanded flow resulting in congestion and dilatation of the hepatic lymph channels. This in turn results in 'weeping' of lymph from the liver surface and is probably the major source of ascitic fluid.
4. Increased secretion of aldosterone. In chronic liver disease the level of aldosterone may be increased due to increased secretion by the

adrenal and impaired detoxication by the liver. This results in increased retention of sodium and fluid.

5. Increased intra-abdominal pressure from ascites already produced may lead to reduced cardiac output, lowered renal blood flow and glomerular filtration, resulting in increased fluid retention. This may stimulate the renin-angiotensin mechanism which further increases aldosterone secretion.

6. Antidiuretic hormonal activity may also be increased.

The clinical symptoms of ascites are those of abdominal distension and discomfort, anorexia, dyspnoea and peripheral fluid retention. Pleural effusions are frequent and umbilical and inguinal herniae may be produced. The abdominal skin is tense and shiny, and abdominal and leg veins may be prominent. In the abdomen, the free fluid can be demonstrated by shifting dullness and a fluid thrill. Palpation of the liver is difficult. The biochemical features are those of chronic liver disease. The serum electrolytes may show hypokalaemia and hyponatraemia, a low level of serum sodium (130 mmol/l) being associated with a poor prognosis. If patients with ascites develop pyrexia, infection of the ascitic fluid should be considered. A diagnostic aspiration should always be done to exclude infection, for cytology and for protein estimation.

The treatment of ascites should be directed towards a slow and steady removal of the ascitic fluid. Body weight and the serum electrolytes should be measured daily. Rapid fluid removal may precipitate portasystemic encephalopathy which is probably due to the development of hypokalaemic alkalosis. The main features of treatment are:

(*a*) Bed rest.

(*b*) Restriction of dietary sodium. Normally it is sufficient to stop adding salt to food, but in ascites resistant to treatment severe salt restriction to less than 20 mEq per day should be commenced.

(*c*) Diuretic therapy. Bendrofluazide 5 to 10 mg per day should be tried at first. If unsuccessful, frusemide 40 to 240 mg per day or ethacrynic acid 50 to 150 mg per day can be used. The more powerful the diuretic the more liable the patient is to develop portasystemic encephalopathy.

(*d*) An aldosterone antagonist such as spironolactone should be added to the regime if the ascites proves resistant; suitable dose is 50 mg four times a day.

(*e*) Ascitic fluid reinfusion. More recently it has been possible to treat ascites by its withdrawal and subsequent re-infusion intravenously. Prior to re-infusion the fluid passes through an ultra-filter which removes both salt and water, producing a fluid of high protein concentration. This procedure is usually associated with a spontaneous diuresis, and the patient can then be treated by maintenance diuretics and/or a low salt diet.

Portasystemic encephalopathy

Portasystemic encephalopathy may occur as an episode during the course of a chronic disease of the liver or it may be a terminal feature of acute fulminant hepatitis. Patients with severe parenchymal disease of the liver may experience episodic stupor or frank coma from time to time. A number of factors appear to be important in the development of this complication. They are:

Severe damage to the liver parenchyma.

Free communication between the portal venous system and systemic venous system with access of portal blood to the cerebral circulation.

A susceptible brain.

In patients with chronic liver disease there is frequently a precipitating factor. The following may be contributory:

1. Intestinal haemorrhage. This will provide an abundant source of nitrogenous products which can be absorbed into the portal system. Most patients with chronic liver disease who have intestinal bleeding experience some degree of portasystemic encephalopathy.
2. Hypokalaemia. Patients with liver disease have a low level of whole-body potassium. Enthusiastic diuretic therapy for ascites may precipitate an episode of hepatic failure.
3. Unduly rapid removal of ascitic fluid may cause loss of potassium, or hypotension.
4. Sedation. Sedative drugs, particularly morphine, may precipitate coma in patients with liver disease and should be avoided in such circumstances.
5. Infection and surgical trauma have also been incriminated, as has hypotension.

Aetiology

The precise biochemical mechanisms leading to hepatic coma are unknown. Ammonia has been blamed in the past and there is no doubt that most of the above precipitating factors will produce a rise in the level of blood ammonia. However, this is not the whole answer and the correlation between ammonia levels and depth of coma is not good. Other nitrogenous products may produce intoxication of the susceptible brain. Whatever the cause of the encephalopathy, it seems likely to be multifactorial.

Clinical features

The principal clinical feature is stupor or coma with a varying level of consciousness. This may range from mild drowsiness or disordered sleep-pattern to a deep coma with no response to external stimuli. The minor degrees of portasystemic encephalopathy are usually associated with somnolence, apathy, lethargy and a lack of spontaneity. The personality of the individual may change dramatically, quiet introspective individuals becoming aggressive, irritable and childish. A whole spectrum of personality change is seen. The intelligence of the individual may deteriorate markedly and inability to perform mental arithmetic is seen at an early stage. The speech may become slow and slurred and the voice monotonous. A characteristic foetor may be detected on the breath.

The neurological signs which may be detected at this stage include hyperreflexia, constructional apraxia and a characteristic flapping tremor, best seen with the arms extended and the hands in full dorsiflexion. The physical signs and symptoms can usually be reversed with appropriate therapy, but in some individuals a permanent neuropsychiatric disorder may develop. This is associated with poor mental function and personality change as well as the other signs listed above. It is believed that in these individuals there is organic brain damage.

The diagnosis of portasystemic encephalopathy may be confirmed by finding a raised level of blood ammonia. Characteristic changes are seen on the electroencephalograph with a generalized slowing of the normal α-rhythm activity (8 to 13 c.p.s.) and its replacement by a slow δ - activity of about 4 c.p.s. Serial tracings can be of assistance in assessing the success of therapy.

Treatment

It is most important at the outset to look for any precipitating factor such as intestinal haemorrhage or over-enthusiastic diuretic therapy, and give corrective treatment.

General measures. (1) If the patient is comatose then routine nursing care of such a patient should be instituted. (2) If there has been recent alimentary bleeding it is worth while to purge the patient with magnesium sulphate, orally or by an enema. (3) Intestinal bacteria have an important role in portasystemic encephalopathy, being responsible for the breakdown of protein substances in the gut to nitrogenous products including ammonia. The use of non-absorbable antibiotics such as neomycin sulphate or framycetin sulphate is recommended. The usual dose of neomycin is 4 to 8 g per day in divided doses. (4) It is usual to exclude protein from the diet. At a later date, when the patient is fully conscious and alert, protein may be reintroduced gradually in increments of 10 g per day at weekly intervals. (5) Potassium supplements in the order of 3 to 4 g per day should be given.

Management of the resistant case. In some patients with severe liver damage and with a large portacaval shunt, liver failure may prove resistant to the therapy outlined above. In these patients the use of the synthetic disaccharide lactulose may be considered. It alters the pH of the faeces and decreases the intestinal transit time. Alternatively, *Lactobacillus acidophilus* is worthy of trial. This acts by altering the bowel flora. If the patient's general condition is sufficiently good, an ileorectal anastomosis with colonic exclusion can be considered, but the results of this operation are far from encouraging.

Exchange blood transfusion. In the management of the patient with acute fulminant hepatitis the above measures have little to offer. In this special situation exchange blood transfusion may be tried.

Fresh whole blood is given intravenously while blood is being removed through an intra-arterial cannula. It is usual to exchange up to 12 units of blood over three or four hours and the procedure may require to be repeated within 24 hours.

Pig liver perfusion. Recently, a number of workers have described the use of isolated pig liver perfusion chambers to treat hepatic failure. Blood from the patient is passed through a fresh pig liver and then returned to the patient's circulation by another vessel. The pig liver is able to act for up to six hours and effectively removes toxic metabolic products from the perfused blood.

Heparin therapy. The suggestion that intravascular coagulation occurs in acute liver failure has led to the use of heparin therapy. The results of treatment are disappointing and its use should be reserved for patients with gross disseminated intravascular coagulation.

Charcoal column haemoperfusion. Recently resin-coated activated charcoal columns have been used to remove toxins from the patient's circulation. The early results are encouraging.

Prognosis

The prognosis of the patient with chronic liver disease and porta-systemic encephalopathy is moderately good, provided that coma is not deep. The presence of coma or precoma is a contraindication to any subsequent portal-systemic shunt for portal hypertension. Coma developing during acute fulminant hepatitis is almost always fatal.

Leptospirosis

Leptospiral infections are frequently encountered in man. The most frequently seen is Weil's disease, due to *Leptospira icterohaemorrhagia*. This organism is transmitted from the rat, which when infected carries it in its renal tubules. Human infection occurs from contact with infected rat urine. The disease occurs principally among farm-workers, miners, sewage workers and people in the fish-cutting industry.

The incubation period in man is 7 to 15 days and most infections are seen in summer and autumn. The early symptoms are those of fever, prostration, abdominal pain, vomiting, headache and confusion, and these may be accompanied by bronchitis and conjunctivitis. Jaundice appears after about one week and is associated with a haemorrhagic tendency and haematuria, bleeding from mucous membranes and into the skin. Severe renal damage occurs in many patients, who show oliguria and a rising level of blood urea; the urine contains bilirubin and protein. Meningitis is common. The jaundice is often more severe than would be expected from the liver function tests and is aggravated by a failure of excretion of bilirubin in the urine and release of bilirubin from tissue haemorrhages. Cardiac arrhythmias and hypotension occur.

Laboratory examinations reveal polymorph leucocytosis, liver function tests suggesting hepatocellular damage with a disproportionate rise in bilirubin level, and a bleeding diathesis. In the early stages there is a leptospiral bacteraemia which can be seen on thick blood films or demonstrated on blood cultures, and in the later stages the agglutination tests for *L. icterohaemorrhagia* are positive, with rising titres in the second and third weeks. Liver biopsy demonstrates focal necrosis, marked cellular regeneration and polymorph infiltration in the periportal area.

Penicillin in large doses is the treatment of choice, though the efficacy of this is in doubt and almost 15 per cent of patients die, mainly due to renal failure. A few patients have a relapse. Reduction in morbidity and mortality is best directed towards prevention among exposed individuals by the use of protective clothing and the administration of immune serum.

Pyogenic liver abscess

These abscesses usually arise as a complication of another focal infection lying within the portal venous drainage area. The commonest primary infections include appendix abscesses, diverticular disease and gallstones with cholangitis. The causative organism is usually *Escherichia coli*, but a *Pseudomonas* or a *Streptococcus* may be found.

The main clinical features are weight loss, anaemia, hepatomegaly, and fever with associated upper abdominal discomfort, rigors and occasionally jaundice. Laboratory findings include leucocytosis, abnormal liver function tests with an elevated alkaline phosphatase and a low serum albumin, a high erythrocyte sedimentation rate and filling defects on the liver scan (p. 162).

Treatment is by surgical drainage of the abscess. A careful search should be made for any possible primary infection and appropriate antibiotic therapy given.

Hydatid disease

This is due to infection with the tapeworm *Echinococcus granulosus*, which is transmitted to humans from dogs. The disease is uncommon in Britain, though it does occur in sheep farming areas of Wales. Ova liberated from the tapeworm are carried to the liver and other organs where they develop into the adult cyst. This cyst in turn enlarges progressively and daughter cysts within the cyst cavity are usual. The cyst is usually surrounded by a firm fibrous capsule. More than 70 per cent of the cysts occur in the liver, but they may also be found in the lungs, intestine, spleen and brain. Whenever a cyst is found in one of these other organs a liver cyst is usually also present. Multiple cysts are common.

Many cysts are asymptomatic in man, being found only at autopsy. The commonest presenting feature is hepatomegaly which is noticed by the patient. Upward displacement of the diaphragm is common. Some patients have vague upper abdominal discomfort. Eosinophilia may be present.

The diagnosis may be easily made in many cases by the demonstration of a calcified cyst-like mass or masses within the liver or in the lung. The calcification is produced by calcium deposition in the cyst capsule. The diagnosis can be confirmed by the intradermal (Casoni) test, in which sterile cyst fluid is injected, producing a wheal and a flare in positive tests. Complement fixation and haemagglutination tests are also available. Localization of the cyst within the liver is essential prior to treatment and hepatic scanning has proved of value. Hepatic arteriography (p. 162) and portal venography (p. 148) may also help to locate the cyst-likely areas, showing an alteration or compression of the vascular tree.

Surgical treatment is always indicated, as rupture of the cyst may prove fatal due to an anaphylactoid reaction, the cyst protein being strongly antigenic. At laparotomy prior to removing the cyst, formalin or alcohol should be injected into it to sterilize the daughter cysts. Rupture of the cyst during removal can result in severe anaphylaxis or the dissemination of daughter cysts throughout the abdomen.

Hepatic amoebiasis

Amoebic abscess of the liver is the usual form of amoebic infection found in the liver, though multiple small focal lesions may also occur. The infection, due to *Entamoeba histolytica*, reaches the liver from the portal venous system, where it localizes at the level of the hepatic sinusoids, multiplying and forming abscesses which do not have a definite capsule, the limitation being marked with necrotic liver cells, leucocytes and red blood cells. This debris is reddish-brown and thick, being usually described as like anchovy sauce. Although the infection is secondary to colonic infestation, many patients do not give a history of amoebic dysentery and some have never been in a tropical country. Secondary bacterial infection occurs in 20 per cent of patients.

The clinical features are the gradual onset of a pyrexial illness, weight loss, anaemia with upper abdominal or lower chest pain on the right side, which may be pleuritic in nature. An associated pulmonary right lower lobe consolidation, pleurisy or effusion is common. The liver is enlarged and tender and localization of the abscess on clinical examination is occasionally possible. Radiological examination of the chest and abdomen confirms the hepatomegaly with the diaphragm being displaced upwards, and the lower lobe changes in the chest X-ray. Liver function tests are often normal though there is a polymorph leucocytosis but no eosinophilia. Liver scanning reveals the site of the abscess (p. 162). Stool examination may reveal cysts. A haemagglutination test is most valuable, being positive in almost every instance.

Treatment is usually with metronidazole, this drug having largely replaced emetine hydrochloride, and oral chloroquine. The treatment is continued for 10 days, the patient being confined to bed during this period. Needle aspiration of the abscess may be performed after drug treatment has started. Failure to respond to therapy should raise the possibility of a secondary infection and appropriate measures instituted as for pyogenic liver abscesses.

Although other infections with parasites do occur, they are rarely seen in this country and the reader is referred to a textbook of tropical medicine.

Budd-Chiari syndrome (hepatic vein occlusion)

Obstruction of the hepatic veins produces a characteristic syndrome with ascites, tender hepatomegaly and portal hypertension. In most instances it presents in an acute form, the aetiology of which is unknown. It has been suggested recently that the altered coagulation pattern produced by oral contraceptives may precipitate thrombosis in an hepatic vein. The occlusion usually occurs at the junction of the hepatic veins and the inferior vena cava and in some the thrombosis extends into the vena cava, producing venous congestion and oedema in the lower half of the body. Some patients have been found to have an endothelial diaphragm extending across the hepatic vein and this has proved amenable to surgical removal.

In the acute form there is a rapid onset of upper abdominal discomfort and ascites. The liver is enlarged and tender, and splenomegaly is usual. Although in many patients the diagnosis is made only at laparotomy, the liver scintiscan is pathognomonic, showing isotope uptake only in the caudate lobe which has a separate venous drainage into the vena cava. Serial scans will show progressive increase in the size of the caudate lobe as this hypertrophies, taking over the function of the remainder of the liver. Liver biopsy (p. 142) shows characteristic centrilobular venous congestion.

The prognosis in the acute form is poor. Surgical exploration with aspiration of clot from the hepatic veins and vena cava is often unsatisfactory. Anticoagulation has little to offer though an infusion of the fibrinolytic agent streptokinase has proved beneficial. In the chronic form, ascites and peripheral oedema are usual and these may prove resistant to treatment. In this type, progression to cirrhosis is the usual outcome.

Veno-occlusive disease

In this variant of the Budd-Chiari syndrome the centrilobular veins are occluded by thrombus but the main hepatic veins remain patent. The condition is usually seen in the West Indies and is almost confined to children under 10 years of age. The drinking of bush teas has been incriminated as these contain toxins which produce an endophlebitis in the centrilobular area. The clinical features and physical signs are similar to these in the Budd-Chiari syndrome. However, almost 50 per cent of patients make a complete recovery, the remainder dying in the acute phase or developing cirrhosis.

Haemochromatosis

In haemochromatosis the physiological mechanism governing absorption of dietary iron is impaired and excessive accumulation of iron occurs as the storage compounds ferritin and haemosiderin. Over a period of time the normal total body iron of 3 to 4 g may increase to as much as 25 g. This excess iron is stored throughout the body particularly in the tissues of the liver, pancreas, myocardium and the endocrine organs.

It is convenient to classify iron overload states into primary idiopathic haemochromatosis, of which the aetiology is unknown, and those in which the development of haemochromatosis is a secondary phenomenon (Table 6.3). In the patients with secondary iron overload, haemosiderosis usually occurs without tissue damage, whereas in idiopathic haemochromatosis tissue damage is present.

Table 6.3 Classification of iron overload states

1. Primary idiopathic haemochromatosis
2. Secondary haemochromatosis
   (a) Cirrhosis with siderosis
   (b) Sideroblastic anaemia
   (c) Bantu siderosis
   (d) Haemolytic anaemia—
       (i) Thalassaemia major
       (ii) Hereditary spherocytosis

Primary idiopathic haemochromatosis

In idiopathic haemochromatosis the main clinical features are of a cirrhosis with heavy iron deposition in the liver. In addition, cutaneous pigmentation, diabetes mellitus, hypogonadism, cardiac involvement, or an arthritis may be present.

The aetiology of idiopathic haemochromatosis is disputed, though the balance of opinion favours a hereditary basis. Some maintain that this is a variant of nutritional cirrhosis occurring in subjects exposed to a high intake of alcohol and iron. The finding of iron overload in alcoholic cirrhosis supports this hypothesis, and it has been noted that over 30 per cent of patients with idiopathic haemochromatosis have an excessive intake of alcohol.

Most patients are male from 50 to 70 years of age. There is usually clinical evidence of liver damage with hepatomegaly, right hypochondrial discomfort and splenomegaly. More than 60 per cent of patients are diabetic, many requiring insulin therapy. Hypogonadism, with loss of libido, and an arthropathy are common. The latter presents as swelling and tenderness of the metacarpophalangeal and proximal interphalangeal joints of the index and middle fingers; the large joints, particularly the knee and hip joints, may also be affected. Cardiac complications include myocardial infarction, congestive cardiac failure and cardiac arrythmias.

Cutaneous pigmentation is striking in most patients, the pigment being classically described as bronzing, being due to the deposition of iron and melanin in the skin. Testicular atrophy is usually found.

The diagnosis of haemochromatosis can usually be confirmed by the presence of a high serum iron level, together with a high percentage saturation of the iron binding capacity of the serum. Perl's stain of liver cells reveals the iron to be in the hepatocytes, fibrous tissue, and Küpffer cells. Histological examination may reveal either a typical cirrhosis or minor fibrosis. The fibrosis may be reversible with treatment. Another important investigation is to measure chelatable body iron stores. Desferrioxamine, a specific iron-chelating agent, is given intravenously and promotes the excretion of iron in the urine, the quantity excreted being proportional to body stores of iron. The family of the patient should be investigated for evidence of iron overload, as the prognosis appears to be improved if the disease is detected at the asymptomatic stage.

The treatment of choice for haemochromatosis is venesection. It is usual to remove from the patient one pint of blood weekly until he becomes anaemic or until the body stores of iron are depleted. As each 500 ml of blood removes 250 mg of iron, this may take up to 18 months. The complications of idiopathic haemochromatosis should be appropriately treated.

The long-term prognosis of haemochromatosis is moderately good, the main complication in the long term being the development of a hepatoma. Any deterioration in the patient's condition should raise this suspicion.

Venesection therapy may require to be repeated after three or four years.

Secondary haemochromatosis

Haemochromatosis can also occur as a secondary feature in cirrhosis, sideroblastic anaemia and haemolytic states.

The treatment of patients with the secondary variety is more difficult than those with idiopathic haemochromatosis. Venesection is not practised in many of those with haemolysis, due to the co-existing anaemia. Patients with cirrhosis and secondary iron overload tolerate venesection very poorly, and desferrioxamine therapy is also poorly tolerated.

Hepatolenticular degeneration (Wilson's disease)

Hepatolenticular degeneration is a hereditary disorder of young people in which copper is deposited in the liver, basal ganglia, cornea and other tissues. There is increased intestinal absorption of copper in association with reduced level of blood copper and concentration of plasma caeruloplasmin. This latter compound, an α-2-globulin, normally binds most of the blood copper, but in these patients the level is reduced so that the copper is carried in a loose association with the albumin from which it is readily dissociated and transferred to the tissues. The exact pathogenesis is uncertain though it has been suggested that the low caeruloplasmin level is the primary defect.

The pathological changes include hepatic cirrhosis, basal ganglia degeneration, and in the cornea copper deposition may be detected in the so-called Kayser-Fleischer rings seen particularly near the limbus.

The treatment of choice is penicillamine, which binds tissue copper, the chelate being excreted in the urine. The therapeutic dose is 1200 mg q.d.s. by mouth and it should be continued for at least a year. Effective treatment results in improvement in both the neurological and hepatic signs and disappearance of the Kayser-Fleischer rings. Maintenance therapy is subsequently required.

TUMOURS OF THE LIVER

Primary tumours of the liver are rare, but secondary hepatic deposits from a primary carcinoma elsewhere are not uncommon.

Primary liver tumours

The commonly encountered primary liver tumours are the malignant hepatoma and the malignant cholangioma.

Aetiology

There is an association with hepatic cirrhosis and haemochromatosis, both of which appear to increase the risk of development of primary hepatic tumour. There may be some relationship to previous type B virus hepatitis.

Primary hepatic tumours are found throughout life with a peak incidence from 60 to 80 years. They occur four times as commonly in males as in females.

Diagnosis of liver tumours

Malignancy must always be suspected in the patient with unexplained hepatomegaly, and useful support to the diagnosis may be obtained by either liver scanning or selective angiography.

Hepatic scintiscanning. Following the intravenous injection of a gamma-emitting radioisotope the liver can be scanned by a moving scintillation counter producing a typewritten print-out of the isotope concentration, its pattern, and the size of the liver (Fig. 6.6a). In cirrhosis the isotope uptake will be patchy and reduced. Hepatic tumours, either primary lesions or metastases, will be seen as filling defects in the scan (Fig. 6.6b).

Hepatic arteriography. Transfemoral retrograde hepatic arteriography may demonstrate the abnormal vascular pattern of a tumour. Under local anaesthesia an arterial catheter is inserted into the femoral artery in the groin and advanced under radiographic control as far as the coeliac axis. The catheter is then manoeuvred into the hepatic artery and after rapid injection of radio-opaque dye, serial radiographs are taken.

Treatment

Wherever practical, laparotomy is done, and if the tumour is confined to one lobe, part of the liver can be excised. The remaining normal liver tissue will rapidly regenerate, but the presence of cirrhosis (p. 140) is a relative contraindication to a partial hepatectomy as regeneration of liver tissue in cirrhosis is minimal.

As many hepatic tumours are located diffusely throughout the liver most patients are not suitable for partial hepatectomy, and in this situation a number of less radical procedures can be considered. Hepatic artery ligation or the infusion of a suitable cytotoxic agent into the portal venous system or hepatic artery may on occasions be tried.

Secondary tumours of the liver

The management of secondary tumours of the liver is essentially similar to that detailed for primary tumours. If the diagnosis of metastatic liver tumour has been made at laparotomy when the primary growth was resected and local resection of the hepatic metastases was not possible, then cannulation of the portal system can be performed. Postoperatively the patient can then receive an appropriate cytotoxic agent into the liver tissue in a high concentration.

CONGENITAL AND FAMILIAL LIVER DISEASE

Only brief mention of the commoner disorders is made here.

Congenital biliary atresia

Two distinct varieties of biliary atresia are recognized in which the

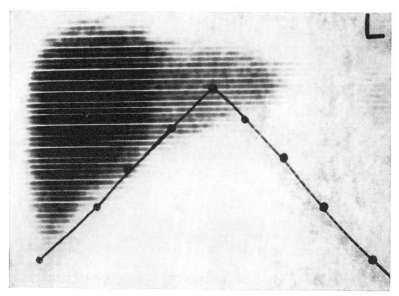

Fig. 6.6(*a*) Technetium⁹⁹ sulphur colloid liver scan. The shape and size of the liver is normal and isotope uptake is uniform. There is minimal isotope uptake by the spleen.

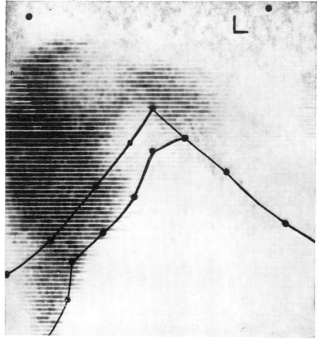

Fig. 6.6(*b*) Technetium⁹⁹ sulphur colloid liver scan. In this patient with a primary hepatocellular carcinoma there are multiple filling defects in this enlarged liver. A selenomethionine scan demonstrated uptake in these filling defects, a finding suggestive of a hepatoma.

atresia may be mainly intrahepatic or extrahepatic. Some overlap between the two types is frequently found.

If untreated, the children with extrahepatic biliary atresia will rarely survive more than three years but those with an intrahepatic obstruction can survive into early adult life. In both groups the outcome is usually fatal unless surgical treatment has been successful.

Clinical features

In both groups of infants jaundice develops during the first week of life and increases progressively. The jaundice is obstructive in type with pale stools, dark urine and pruritus. There is hepatomegaly.

Treatment

Surgery represents the major hope of cure and exploration of the biliary tree is usually undertaken at two to four months. If a lesion is extrahepatic an attempt can be made to anastomose the gallbladder or a dilated upper biliary or hepatic duct to the jejunum.

Should surgery fail to produce a satisfactory result, then supportive treatment is necessary with vitamin K and a low fat diet. Medium-chain triglycerides may be of value in reducing steatorrhoea and improving nutrition. Phenobarbitone may be beneficial in reducing jaundice. In the future, such infants will be candidates for hepatic transplantation.

The hyperbilirubinaemias

These syndromes were formerly thought to be rare, but it is known now that they may be present in up to 5 per cent of the population. In most instances the diagnosis is made incidentally and the patient is symptom-free. The main variants are shown in Table 6.4, the most common by far being Gilbert's syndrome. Some patients with unconjugated hyperbilirubinaemia develop vague upper abdominal discomfort, nausea, anorexia and vague ill-health, and in this situation the use of an enzyme-inducing drug such as glutethimide or phenobarbitone may be indicated.

Polycystic disease of the liver

Polycystic disease of the liver rarely gives rise to symptoms on its own, but is usually diagnosed when the associated polycystic kidneys are detected. The liver cysts vary in size from a few millimetres to over 10 cm and increase in size with the passage of years. There are usually adequate liver cells remaining in these livers and hepatocellular function is good. Portal hypertension is not a feature. Liver scanning (p. 162) will reveal multiple filling defects within the liver. The prognosis is excellent, the only indication for direct treatment being aspiration of a distended cyst which is causing pain.

Table 6.4 The hyperbilirubinaemias

Type	Bilirubin levels	Frequency	Other features
Conjugated			
Dubin-Johnson Syndrome	Up to 8 mg per cent	Uncommon	Chocolate-brown pigmentation of the liver
Roter Syndrome	Up to 8 mg per cent	Uncommon	—
Unconjugated			
Gilbert's Syndrome	Up to 5 mg per cent	Up to 4% of the population	
Crigfer-Najjar Syndrome	5 to 40 mg per cent	Rare	Usually present at birth May cause kernicterus May be fatal in severe cases
Primary Shunt Hyperbilirubinaemia	Up to 8 mg per cent	Very rare	Bilirubin derived from a source other than red cell breakdown

The glycogen storage diseases

Six different glycogen storage diseases have now been described, of which five affect the liver with heavy deposition of glycogen in liver cells. The classification of the various types together with the basic defect is given in Table 6.5.

Table 6.5 The glycogen storage diseases

Type	Synonym	Enzyme deficient
I	Von Gierke's	Glucose-6-phosphatase
II	Pompe's	Lysosomal acid and glucosidase
III	Cori's	Amylo-1,6-glucosidase
IV	Anderson's	Amylo-1,4,1,6-transglucosidase
V	McArdle's	Phosphorylase (muscle)
VI	Her's	Phosphorylase (liver)

Von Gierke's disease is by far the commonest. This usually presents in early childhood with hepatomegaly and symptoms of hypoglycaemia or ketosis. Splenomegaly is never found, providing a valuable differentiating sign from other childhood causes of hepatomegaly. The only other feature on clinical examination is physical retardation. The mental development is normal unless hypoglycaemia has been severe. The basic defect is an absence of hepatic glucose-6-phosphatase resulting in the inability to release glucose from glycogen. The diagnosis is suspected by a negative glucagon test. The administration of glucagon normally produces a rise in blood glucose within one hour. These patients do not achieve an adequate response. The diagnosis can then be confirmed by the finding, on liver biopsy, of glycogen-laden liver cells. Enzyme analysis of the biopsy specimen will yield minimal levels of glucose-6-phosphatase diagnostic of this type.

Treatment is indicated for stunting of growth, recurrent hypoglycaemia or excessive hepatomegaly. Two different approaches have been successful. The corticosteroid triamcinolone induces the enzyme glucose-6-phosphatase resulting in more adequate glycogen breakdown. Should this not be adequate a portacaval shunt operation will result in freshly absorbed glucose being directed to peripheral tissues, bypassing the liver. The surgical approach has proved successful in this condition although it does involve a major operation.

FURTHER READING

Boucher, I. A. D. (Ed.) (1973) Diseases of the biliary tract. *Clinics in Gastroenterology*, **Vol. 2,** No. 1.

Scheuer, P. (1968) *Liver Biopsy Interpretation*. London: Baillière Tindall & Cassell.

Sherlock, S. (1975) *Diseases of the Liver and Biliary System*. Oxford: Blackwell.

Tygstrup, N. (Ed.) (1974) Viral hepatitis. *Clinics in Gastroenterology*. **Vol. 3,** No. 3.

7. The Acute Abdomen (including Intestinal Obstruction)

David C. Miln and Ronald M. Ross

The diagnosis of conditions presenting as acute abdominal emergencies depends mainly on the interpretation of clinical findings; these may be supplemented on occasions by the results of selected X-ray or laboratory investigations.

HISTORY

The sudden onset of symptoms is always a distressing experience, and while taking the history the clinician has the opportunity not only to make a diagnosis, but also to alleviate the patient's anxiety and gain his confidence. It is necessary to phrase questions in a manner which can be understood by the patient. Attention should also be paid to changes in symptoms and signs which may have occurred since the onset of the illness as this may give a vital clue to the diagnosis.

PAIN

Although pain is a feature common to all abdominal emergencies, sufficient differences exist in its site, character and development to indicate its underlying origin.

If the patient complains of upper abdominal pain the source lies in the foregut (stomach/duodenum/gallbladder/liver or pancreas), while pain from lesions of the midgut is referred to the umbilical area, and from those of the hindgut to the lower abdomen. As the lesion progresses, more exact localization occurs as the overlying parietal peritoneum becomes involved.

A valuable additional pointer to the location of the lesion is reference of the pain outwith the abdomen. One example is shoulder tip discomfort caused by an inflamed gallbladder stimulating the sensory nerves of the diaphragm which share the same cervical segments of the spinal cords as those of the shoulder region.

The exact mechanism producing pain has not been fully elucidated. Certainly the gross dilatation of the bowel in paralytic ileus is not accompanied by severe pain, nor does handling, cutting or cauterizing the bowel wall evoke any painful sensation. In general it would appear that the factor common to all painful lesions of the gut is the potential for producing local ischaemia. This may arise from sustained tonic contraction of the gut wall as in intestinal obstruction, from a local inflammatory process in which thrombosis and endarteritis are features, or from an acute vascular occlusion or infarct.

Pain may be colicky or steady in character. Colic refers to pain which recurs in spasms intermitting at regular intervals with periods of freedom. Resulting as it does from strong contraction of smooth muscle it implies an obstructive element. Steady pain on the other hand is more suggestive of irritation or traction involving the visceral or parietal peritoneum.

VOMITING

Vomiting is a common accompaniment of many minor illnesses, but when it is persistent it should suggest that the cause is intra-abdominal. Copious vomiting may lead to signs of dehydration, which, if marked, may be reflected in a dry furred tongue, thin thready pulse and loss of elasticity of skin. It should also be remembered that although thirst is a feature of water deprivation or depletion, it may be absent when there has also been a significant loss of electrolytes as occurs in high intestinal obstruction.

Two other terms used to describe vomiting deserve mention since their significance is not always fully understood.

'Faeculent vomiting' occurs in high small bowel obstruction due to the bacterial decomposition of bile producing a 'faecal' odour. It does not mean that faeces are present in the vomitus.

'Projectile vomiting' is a forcible ejection of the vomitus and the term is now commonly used to describe the characteristic vomiting in congenital pyloric stenosis.

Recurring episodes of vomiting unaccompanied by other alimentary signs may be due to raised intracranial pressure of a brain tumour.

BOWEL HABIT

Since the definition of constipation and the exact meaning of diarrhoea vary according to each individual patient, it is often useful to start by enquiring if there has been any recent alteration in bowel habit. From this starting point one can then enquire in detail about the severity of such changes. When constipation, i.e. a lessened frequency of bowel motions, is present, it is desirable to enquire also regarding any difficulty in the passage of flatus. Diarrhoea implies increased frequency in daily bowel habit and is accompanied by the passage of fluid, mucus or blood.

PAST HISTORY

Full details of previous illness, operations and any current treatment should be recorded since this information may be helpful in reaching a diagnosis. An accurate history of drugs which have been taken recently should be obtained either from the patient or from a close relative; some drugs, e.g. ganglion-blocking agents, may cause signs leading to diagnostic difficulty. Steroid therapy may need to be increased if emergency operation is required.

PHYSICAL EXAMINATION

Acute abdominal disorders give rise to both local and systemic signs.

The discovery of other lesions on general examination can often throw light on the cause of the abdominal symptoms.

The information obtained from a careful history usually suggests a tentative diagnosis, and this awareness leads the examiner to look for specific signs. This is a practical approach as opposed to the 'routine' method of abdominal examination.

Certain basic points of routine must, however, be followed.

Inspection

The abdomen is first observed for distension, asymmetry of contour and evidence of restriction of movement with respiration. It is often useful to ask the patient to cough or attempt to sit up to demonstrate a hernia or haematoma of the rectus sheath, which might be missed by palpation alone.

Palpation

This should begin over the quadrant least likely to be affected, in order to obtain standards on which muscle guarding and rigidity can be judged. Comparisons can then be made between one area and another. Next, an attempt is made to palpate deep structures and feel specifically for any abnormal masses that may be expected from the history. A search for the point of maximum tenderness is best postponed until this stage, otherwise the patient may become apprehensive and find difficulty in relaxing the abdominal muscles.

Percussion can be used not only to determine whether the liver is enlarged, or the urinary bladder distended, but also to detect the shifting dullness characteristic of a peritoneal effusion. The presence of free gas in the peritoneal cavity leads to loss of the normally dull percussion note over the liver.

Since testicular swellings can be associated with abdominal symptoms the scrotum must also be examined.

Auscultation

The silent abdomen in peritonitis, the hollow tinkling sounds of bowel obstruction and the increased frequency of bowel activity in enteritis are all easily recognized. The vascular bruit over the aorta or iliac arteries affected by gross atherosclerosis will not, however, be heard unless the clinician specifically listens for it.

To complete the examination of the acute abdomen, rectal examination must always be done and on occasion vaginal examination is also indicated.

Since many of the conditions to be mentioned under the 'Acute Abdomen' are dealt with in other chapters, only brief reference is made to them in the following pages.

Peritonitis

One has only to observe the change which takes place in the peritoneum during a routine laparotomy to appreciate how actively this glistening membrane can react to any form of irritation. On becoming congested and spongy it is capable of discharging leucocytes rapidly into the peritoneal cavity, or producing fluid rich in antibodies, and by its adherence to surrounding structures it helps to localize infection. This latter function is aided by the subdivision of the peritoneal cavity into compartments by the transverse mesocolon, the pelvic brim, the midline structures and the paracolic gutters.

Peritonitis results from the spread of infection from an inflamed abdominal organ, directly from an abdominal wound, from the female genital tract, or on rare occasions it may be secondary to septicaemia.

Initially the symptoms are those of the causative lesion, but as the infection extends the classical signs of a spreading inflammatory process appear. The abdominal pain becomes more diffuse, fluid balance is disturbed by vomiting, by the loss of electrolyte and protein into the peritoneal cavity, and by sweating.

Treatment is aimed at aiding the peritoneum to fulfil its natural function. The patient's head and trunk are raised in an attempt to localize the pus in the pelvis. Nasogastric suction is employed to relieve vomiting and to facilitate the assessment of intestinal fluid loss. Intravenous fluids are administered to correct electrolyte depletion and restore acid-base balance. A broad spectrum antibiotic, e.g. ampicillin or occasionally lincomycin or clindamycin is given in effective dosage intravenously. Pethidine is prescribed as required for relief of pain and anxiety. In most instances the peritonitis is due to the discharge of infective material into the peritoneal cavity. Operation is therefore necessary to remove the continuing source of infection or to drain the affected compartment and allow localization of the process.

Following recovery from peritonitis the possibility of a subphrenic or pelvic abscess developing in the ensuing weeks must be remembered. In addition, over the longer term the patient remains susceptible to intestinal obstruction due to residual peritoneal bands and adhesions.

Appendicitis

One of every seven people in this country develops appendicitis at some time in his or her life. Obstruction of the lumen by a faecolith or inflammation of the mucosal surface are the common initiating factors.

The presenting features vary, depending on both the pathology of the attack and the anatomical position of the organ.

OBSTRUCTIVE APPENDICITIS

Blockage of the appendicular lumen results in stasis and conditions which favour the multiplication of the commensal bacteria *Escherichia coli* and *Streptococcus faecalis*. Strong contractions by the appendix in its attempt to expel the blockage, and distension of the organ added to by the inflammatory response, cause central colicky abdominal pain. As the inflammation progresses to involve the serosal surface, tenderness can be elicited by palpation over the organ. If the obstruction to this virtually closed loop is relieved the condition may resolve, otherwise further distension of the appendix results in compression and thrombosis of its blood supply leading to gangrene of its wall and perforation.

In the early stages of obstructive appendicitis there may be little or no pyrexia and a normal white cell count.

CATARRHAL APPENDICITIS

As the disorder is inflammatory from the outset there is usually early constitutional upset with a raised temperature and leucocytosis and the patient has a 'toxic' appearance. Also, because of free drainage from the appendix into the caecum the central abdominal discomfort is less acute and of slower onset than in the obstructed case. In some cases the attack may resolve at this stage, but in others secondary obstruction of the lumen occurs due to enlargement of the lymphoid follicles of the submucosa. The symptoms then become those of obstructive appendicitis.

It follows that the distinction between the two types of appendicitis is artificial, but it explains why one patient may look 'toxic' and have a marked leucocytosis while another may have more marked abdominal symptoms with little apparent general upset.

In 60 per cent of cases the inflamed appendix is retrocaecal and the irritation of the psoas muscle may cause the patient to lie with the right hip flexed. If the appendix lies in contact with the ureter the patient may complain of dysuria. A ruptured retrocaecal appendix forms an abscess which may point in the loin or track along the psoas muscle.

Should the inflamed appendix lie in the pelvis it may irritate the rectum to produce diarrhoea, or the bladder to cause an increased frequency of micturition. Rectal examination may detect a pelvic abscess pointing into the rectum, or tenderness caused by the presence of a pelvic appendicitis.

In the child, in whom the appendix is usually relatively longer than in the adult and in whom the omentum is often not sufficiently developed to contain the inflammatory process, the danger of diffuse peritonitis is increased. Mortality and morbidity are also greater in the elderly where symptoms prior to perforation are often mild, and peritonitis is a lethal complication.

Treatment

Within the first 48 hours of an attack, treatment is appendicectomy. In the presence of peritonitis which shows no sign of localizing, laparotomy, drainage and where possible appendicectomy is the treatment of choice. Histological examination of the appendix identifies the rare case of carcinoid tumour, or the presence of worms requiring further treatment.

If first seen in the later stages and there is already evidence of local abscess formation conservative treatment is best. This consists of giving ampicillin 500 mg orally four times daily in addition to analgesics to relieve pain. Nasogastric suction is required if there is associated paralytic ileus; intravenous fluid replacement may be indicated and this route may be used for administration of antibiotic.

Acute salpingitis

This can usually be distinguished from appendicitis on the basis of an accurate history and a pelvic examination.

The pain which is caused by distended Fallopian tubes and inflammation of the overlying peritoneum is usually lower abdominal from the outset. There is an early and marked elevation of both temperature and pulse rate. The usual history includes menstrual irregularity and, in cases of ascending infection, vaginal discharge.

Abdominal findings usually consist of distension, tenderness, and rigidity of the lower abdomen. Vaginal examination demonstrates any purulent discharge and allows palpation of the inflamed and distended Fallopian tubes which prolapse into the pouch of Douglas.

Once a definite diagnosis has been made a conservative routine is begun. While awaiting the result of bacterial culture of a high vaginal swab, penicillin in high dosage is desirable. The patient is confined to bed, pethidine and intravenous fluids are given, and a close watch is kept for resolution of the inflammation on the basis of a fall in pulse rate and temperature. Should a local abscess form in the rectovesical pouch it is best incised and drained through the posterior vaginal wall or rectum.

Acute ileitis

This uncommon condition occurs usually in young adults, and the symptoms are difficult to distinguish from those of appendicitis. At laparotomy, which is often necessary because of the possibility of appendicitis, the last few inches of the terminal ileum are found to be reddened, thickened and congested. The adjacent mesentery, which also tends to be oedematous and inflamed, contains large fleshy lymph nodes. The cause of the condition is unknown.

If the diagnosis can be confidently made no surgical treatment may be necessary, since in 50 per cent of patients with acute symptoms the condition resolves and the patient has no further trouble. In the remainder the disease recurs in subacute or chronic form.

On discovering the condition at laparotomy nothing should be done to the diseased segment of intestine. Removal of the appendix is a matter for the personal preference of the surgeon. The patient should be reviewed as an outpatient in case the condition recurs in a subacute or chronic form as described in Chapter 9.

Meckel's diverticulum

This additional appendage arising from the ileum is found in a small percentage of people. Like the vermiform appendix it is subject to obstruction, inflammation and perforation. There may be bleeding from a peptic ulcer associated with ectopic gastric mucosa in the diverticulum. The clinical presentation is similar to acute appendicits. Excision of the diverticulum or excision of the local bowel segment and end-to-end anastomosis may be necessary.

Small bowel perforation

Abdominal trauma may produce bruising, devitalisation and rupture of the bowel close to its point of fixation at the duodenojejunal flexure.

Rarely, perforation occurs in the ileum from ingested foreign bodies, tumour involvement or damage to the bowel wall by thiazide diuretics. The clinical features resemble suppurative appendicitis.

Mesenteric adenitis

In children, adeno virus infection occurs in the lymph nodes of the mesentery, resulting in central and right iliac fossa pain similar to appendicitis. However, there is commonly also soreness of the throat and cervical adenitis, and vomiting is rare. Laparotomy may be necessary to ensure that serious appendicitis is not missed.

Acute cholecystitis—see Chapter 5.
Perforated peptic ulcer—see Chapter 3.
Diverticular disease—see Chapter 12.
Acute pancreatitis—see Chapter 5.

ACUTE INTESTINAL OBSTRUCTION

The clinician must attempt to answer three vital questions whenever intestinal obstruction is suspected.

1. Is the obstruction due to simple occlusion or is there evidence of strangulation?
2. At what level in the bowel has obstruction developed?
3. Is it possible to diagnose the cause of the obstruction?

The common causes of obstruction of small bowel are incarcerated external herniae, adhesions, and bands which cause kinking or volvulus. Large bowel obstruction occurs most frequently in the elderly where it is due to faecal impaction, carcinoma, diverticular disease or volvulus. The less common causes of obstruction often have other distinct clinical features and will be discussed separately.

CLINICAL FEATURES OF OBSTRUCTION

Colic
In small bowel obstruction the sudden onset of severe colic is often the first symptom. It is experienced all over the abdomen, but is usually maximal at the umbilicus. By contrast, colic in large bowel obstruction is usually experienced after the appearance of other symptoms, is more insidious in onset and is located mainly in the lower abdomen.

Increasing frequency and intensity of abdominal colic is a warning of impending strangulation.

Vomiting
The more proximal the obstruction the more rapidly does vomiting occur and the greater the risk of electrolyte and fluid depletion. In high jejunal obstruction vomiting quickly follows the first episode of pain, whereas in the more common ileal obstruction it may be delayed for a further four to six hours. In colonic obstruction vomiting occurs relatively late and it is exceptional for it to be profuse enough to cause the dehydration and electrolyte depletion.

The normal quantities of fluids and electrolytes passing into and out of the gastrointestinal tract are illustrated in Figure 7.1 and the principal disorders of this balance are outlined in Figure 7.2.

Distension
Since the degree of the distension is dependent on the length of bowel obstructed, there is practically none with a jejunal lesion and a slight amount of central abdominal distension in ileal obstruction. In large bowel obstruction the distension may be gross and more marked in the flanks and upper epigastrium. Generalized abdominal distension without pain suggests a paralytic ileus.

Constipation
Complete obstruction of the distal colon is almost invariably associated with absolute constipation, with passage of neither faeces nor

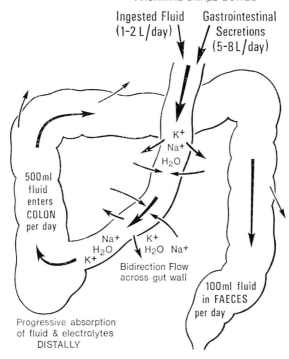

PROXIMAL SMALL BOWEL

Ingested Fluid
(1-2 L/day)

Gastrointestinal
Secretions
(5-8 L/day)

K^+
Na^+
H_2O

500 ml
fluid
enters
COLON
per day

Na^+
H_2O
K^+

K^+
H_2O Na^+

Bidirection Flow
across gut wall

100 ml fluid
in FAECES
per day

Progressive absorption
of fluid & electrolytes
DISTALLY

Fig. 7.1 Normal pattern of salt and water absorption by the bowel.

flatus, even following enemeta. In small bowel obstruction bowel motions may continue for a few days after the onset of the acute attack.

Pulse rate and temperature

These are usually normal initially, but are increased when a significant degree of hypovolaemia, or secondary infection, develops.

Abdominal examination

Since herniae are common causes of intestinal obstruction, careful examination of the inguinal, femoral and umbilical regions is essential; the presence of scars from previous abdominal operations may be relevant. On palpation there is usually tenderness over the site of obstruction. The presence of peritoneal irritation from strangulated bowel may lead to 'rebound tenderness'. Vigorous peristalsis may produce noises which can be heard without a stethoscope. When the obstruction has progressed the bowel becomes distended and less active. Auscultation then reveals periods of silence intermitting with high-pitched tinkling sounds. The rectum must always be digitally examined for impacted

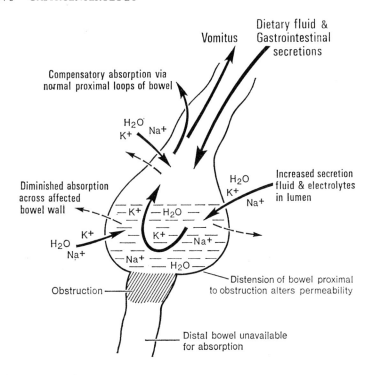

Fig. 7.2 Effect of intestinal obstruction on fluid and electrolyte absorption.

faeces, or tumours in the rectum or in the rectovesical pouch. The rectum may be ballooned distal to a complete obstruction.

The only ancillary investigation of immediate help is the taking of straight X-ray films of the abdomen. Films taken with the patient in the erect position may show fluid levels in the small intestine (Fig. 7.3); this finding usually indicates a lesion in the distal small bowel. With a colonic lesion the caecum is very distended if the ileocaecal valve is competent, and the extent of the gas in the colon will indicate the site of obstruction. In a volvulus of the pelvic colon a single huge loop can be seen extending from the left iliac fossa. (Fig. 7.4). Occasionally the X-ray films may demonstrate a foreign body or gallstone ileus.

Fluid and electrolyte changes in intestinal obstruction

The balance between absorption and secretion of fluid and electrolytes by the bowel is altered, leading to copious loss of fluids from the body. The management of this problem requires an understanding both of the normal mechanisms involved in salt and water absorption, and of the abnormal handling of fluid and electrolytes which occurs after intestinal obstruction.

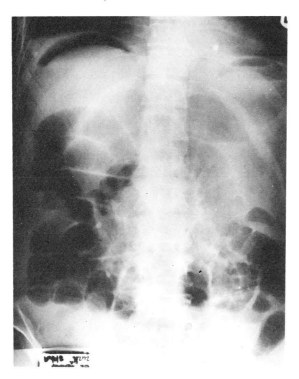

Fig. 7.3 Acute small bowel obstruction due to adhesions following recent operation. Small bowel distended. Fluid levels present. Gas under both domes indicates pneumo-peritoneum from recent laparotomy.

Salt and water absorption by intestinal tract. The intake of fluid and electrolytes in the diet represents only a small proportion of the total load of water and salt presented to the gut for absorption (Fig. 7.1). In the adult, 5 to 8 litres of alimentary secretions (saliva, bile, gastric, pancreatic and intestinal juices) enter the upper intestinal tract each day. Normally, virtually all this large volume of dietary fluid and secretions from the proximal bowel is reabsorbed in the lower small intestine and colon.

Experimental studies have shown that there also is a constant exchange, in both directions, of water and electrolytes across the intestinal mucosa.

As a result of this bidirectional movement of fluids between the gastrointestinal lumen and the body, the composition of the upper small intestinal contents is modified so that it resembles extracellular fluid in tonicity and electrolyte content. Most of this isotonic solution of water and electrolytes is then subsequently absorbed in the distal small bowel so that only about 400 to 500 ml of fluid reaches the colon

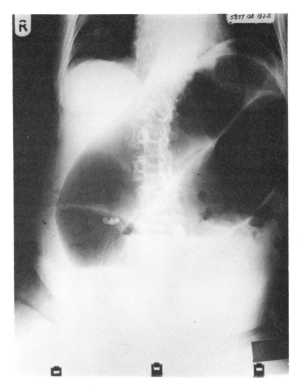

Fig. 7.4 Volvulus of the sigmoid. Gross distension of the sigmoid loop with fluid levels.

each day. In the large bowel, intestinal contents are further modified by removal of water, sodium and chloride, and the addition of potassium, so that normally less than 100 ml of fluid is lost in the faeces each day.

Fluid and electrolyte changes after intestinal obstruction

Following obstruction the accumulation of fluid within the lumen of the gut depends on a combination of factors (Fig. 7.2).

1. The deprivation of the absorbing surface of bowel distal to the obstruction. The intestinal contents, unable to pass the obstruction, accumulate above it, and their volume is progressively augmented by addition of alimentary secretions. The importance of this factor naturally depends on the site of the obstruction—the higher the level of obstruction, the more serious the consequences in terms of fluid loss.

2. A second factor is the progressive impairment in the absorptive capacity of the intestine proximal to the site of obstruction. This part of the gut becomes distended, its motility is altered and its circulation impaired. These changes result in alteration in the

bidirectional movement of fluid and electrolytes across the bowel immediately above the obstruction. The initial effect, occurring within about 12 hours, is a reduction in the flow from the bowel to the bloodstream. This alteration persists, extends proximally, and is accompanied after about 24 to 36 hours by an increased flow in the reverse direction, from the blood back into the bowel lumen. The net result is further accumulation of water and electrolytes in the intestinal lumen. This explains why fluid losses within the obstructed bowel may be considerably greater than the volume calculated simply on the basis of sequestration of alimentary secretions.

3. Accumulation of fluid above an obstruction results in increased intraluminal pressure and some of the intestinal contents may pass proximally into loops of normal bowel still capable of absorption. Ultimately the proximal loops may become affected in turn, but the lower the level of obstruction in the gut the slower the effects will be to develop, and the longer the proximal intestine will continue to absorb. This compensatory mechanism is, of course, less effective where obstruction occurs proximally in the bowel.

Systemic effects of intestinal obstruction are due both to salt and water depletion, and to the accompanying acid-base disturbance.

(*a*) Salt and water deficit. Fluid which accumulates in distended loops of obstructed bowel has a cation composition very similar to that of plasma. As salt and water are lost in isotonic proportions little change in intracellular fluids occurs, but there is reduction of the extracellular fluid space including the intravascular compartment. Progressive contraction of the intravascular compartment is accompanied by haemoconcentration, with little change in the concentration of plasma electrolyte concentrations. Reduction of plasma volume leads to lowering of the cardiac output, and if not corrected, eventually results in oligaemic shock.

(*b*) Acid-base disturbance. Patients with severe fluid depletion following obstruction usually develop a metabolic acidosis due to loss of bicarbonate in the intestinal fluid, the ketoacidosis of starvation, and uraemia resulting from oligaemia.

Management

An intravenous infusion is started immediately, and fluid replacement is guided by biochemical findings in samples of serum. Blood will almost certainly be necessary to combat the hypotension which accompanies strangulation.

Nasogastric suction relieves vomiting and in some cases can decompress the bowel sufficiently to relieve the obstruction. If this correction of fluid balance and bowel decompression fail to relieve symptoms within a few hours, laparotomy becomes mandatory.

At operation the procedure may be simply that of dividing a fibrous band or untwisting a loop of bowel. If, however, non-viable strangulated small bowel is present it must be resected together with its thrombosed section of mesentery and continuity re-established by end-to-end anastomosis. In many cases it is also advisable to decompress the bowel before closing the abdomen. With large bowel obstruction the dangers of primary resection are great. The distended and thinned colonic wall is not suitable for anastomosis, and escape of colonic content leads to a virulent peritonitis. For this reason the safest procedure is to open the bowel proximal to the obstruction in the form of a temporary colostomy. In obstruction of the ascending colon relief can be achieved by side-to-side anastomosis between the ileum and transverse colon. The diseased segment can be resected at a later date when the patient is fit and the bowel adequately prepared by poorly absorbed sulphonamides and/or antibiotics, e.g. neomycin.

Intussusception

Intussusception arises when one part of the bowel is invaginated into the lumen of the adjacent segment and propelled distally. The majority of cases occur in babies under one year of age, and males are affected more often than females. The starting point is thought to be hyperplasia of lymphoid tissue in the terminal ileum which then projects into the lumen and is passed into the caecum like a foreign body. The disorder may, however, begin at other levels of either the small or large bowel. Rarely in adults a polyp or tumour in some part of the bowel initiates the process.

In babies the attack starts with an agonizing cry of pain which quickly passes off to return minutes or hours later. Palpation of the abdomen reveals no tenderness, guarding or rigidity, but the right iliac fossa feels empty, and a small palpable mass may be detected under the right lobe of the liver or in the left hypochrondrium. Blood may be passed per rectum or found on digital examination of the rectum. An X-ray of the abdomen may confirm the obstruction and even outline the intussusception. The presence of these features is sufficient to make the diagnosis.

The treatment is by surgical operation, and in most cases reduction of the intussusceptum by manipulation will be successful. In the irreducible type, resection or bypass anastomosis is necessary.

Volvulus

In this condition a segment of bowel rotates on the axis of its mesentery, occluding first the lumen at either end of the loop and, if unrelieved, the blood supply, producing strangulation. Traction on the apex of the loop and elongation of the mesentery both predispose to volvulus. The following are the commonest sites.

Pelvic colon. In this situation the traction on the mesentery may be a constipated loop of pelvic colon. The condition, which mainly affects elderly men, starts with sudden lower abdominal colic precipitated by straining on defaecation or by a sudden increase in abdominal pressure during exertion. The onset may be accompanied by tenesmus and slight rectal bleeding. Constipation is absolute and within a few hours the distended loop of pelvic colon is obvious on inspection of the abdomen. Later there is generalized abdominal distension and local tenderness over the increasingly ischaemic pelvic colon.

At the earliest opportunity decompression should be attempted by sigmoidoscopy and the passage of a rectal tube into the distended segment. Should this fail laparotomy is required. Simple untwisting of the volvulus and maintenance of its reduction by a rectal tube passed up to the affected area may be all that is required. However, if this treatment fails operative reduction is required. If the volvulus recurs, later elective resection of the pelvic colon is advisable.

Small bowel. At this level the predisposing factor is usually a previous abdominal operation or peritonitis which has produced a peritoneal adhesion to the small bowel. The symptoms are those of small bowel obstruction with tenderness over the distended loop. The latter is often apparent on a straight X-ray. Treatment consists of untwisting the volvulus at operation and dividing the adhesion. If gangrenous bowel is present this must be resected and continuity restored.

Caecum. When the mesentery to the terminal ileum, caecum and ascending colon is lax, and only the caecum is anchored by peritoneum, volvulus can occur. This situation is rare.

NEONATAL VOLVULUS

Neonatal volvulus is a developmental anomaly with incomplete rotation of the midgut. Bile-stained vomiting a few days after birth, and an X-ray showing gas in the stomach and duodenum only, suggest the diagnosis. Immediate operation is required to remedy the situation.

Urinary calculus

Impaction of a urinary calculus in the renal pelvis or ureter is a further common cause of acute abdominal pain, and on occasions the differential diagnosis from other disorders may be difficult. Classically there is a sudden onset of severe pain in the region of the kidney and along the ureter, and also there may be some dysuria. The detection of red blood cells on microscopic examination of the urine usually gives confirmation of the diagnosis.

Rupture of the spleen

In countries where malaria and parasitic diseases are endemic there is often gross splenic enlargement which predisposes to spontaneous rupture. In this country the more usual cause of splenic rupture is trauma by a blow on the left side and there may be associated rib fractures in this area. If the tear has been large the clinical features become immediately apparent, but in a number of instances the initial symptoms are only of vague general discomfort in the left upper abdomen followed a few hours or days later by signs indicating internal haemorrhage. In these cases a haematoma produced at the time of injury has been contained temporarily, but ruptures later into the general peritoneal cavity. Pain referred to the tip of the left shoulder is a fairly common sign of splenic rupture and is due to the irritation of the overlying diaphragm.

In the acute phase these patients are shocked due to blood loss. There is usually rigidity of the abdominal wall muscles and palpation usually demonstrates tenderness all over the abdomen although this is maximal in the left hypochondrium. The referred shoulder tip pain is increased by gentle pressure over the spleen and occasionally more dramatically when the foot of the bed is raised as part of the treatment to combat hypotension.

Straight X-ray of the abdomen may show increased density in the left hypochondrium, elevation of the left dome of the diaphragm, displacement of the gas bubble in the stomach to the right, and possibly fracture of the tenth, eleventh, or twelfth ribs.

Treatment consists of giving morphine to relieve pain and rapid blood replacement to allow laparotomy at the earliest possible moment. Splenectomy is performed and blood clot evacuated from the peritoneal cavity.

Ruptured aneurysm of the abdominal aorta

The patient is often an elderly atherosclerotic subject who initially develops a dull abdominal pain which passes through to the lumbar region. He becomes shocked, pale and sweating, with a subnormal temperature and a thin thready pulse. As the blood from the ruptured aortic aneurysm spreads to fill the retroperitoneal tissues the blood pressure falls, and the pain becomes more severe. Examination shows central abdominal distension with tenderness over the palpable aneurysm, but little or no muscle guarding.

It is at this stage that surgical intervention is most likely to be successful. In the subsequent 24 hours there is a risk of fatal bleeding into the peritoneal cavity.

It should therefore be appreciated that once the diagnosis is made blood transfusion should be started and the patient taken urgently to the operating theatre. Once the aneurysm has been isolated by vascular clamps it is opened and substituted by a synthetic graft.

OTHER CAUSES OF ACUTE ABDOMINAL PAIN

In addition to the acute surgical emergencies there are numerous other causes of abdominal pain which should be kept in mind. In some the abdominal symptoms are mild in comparison to the general condition of the patient, as in diabetes mellitus or epilepsy. In basal pneumonia, common in elderly bedridden patients, there may be referred upper abdominal pain.

A myocardial infarction producing abdominal pain is often difficult to distinguish from cholecystitis or pancreatitis. In other cases an acute episode of vomiting may raise the possibility of gastritis or food-poisoning. Enteritis, although epidemic at certain times of the year, can on occasion be difficult to distinguish from appendicitis. Porphyria because of its rarity is only likely to be diagnosed by its possibility being recalled or noticing that the urine becomes red on being left standing. Other conditions which may uncommonly present with abdominal pain include herpes zoster and epidemic myalgia.

The best guarantee of making the correct diagnosis lies in a careful history and examination, avoiding preconceived ideas, repeating abdominal examinations when required, and where necessary arranging an exploratory laparotomy.

FURTHER READING

Anqell, J. C., Havard, C. W. H. *et al.* (1972) *British Journal of Hospital Medicine*, **7**, 429–472.

Cope, Z. (1963) *The Early Diagnosis of the Acute Abdomen.* 12th Edn. London: Oxford University Press.

Shepherd, J. A. (1975) *A Concise Surgery of the Acute Abdomen.* Edinburgh: Churchill Livingstone.

8. Intestinal Infections

K. A. Buchan and Peter McKenzie

MICROBIAL DISEASES OF THE INTESTINAL TRACT

Since the beginning of the antibiotic era bacterial infections have
assumed a less prominent role in human disease. Bacterial infection
remains, however, the most common of all intestinal diseases. In recent
years there has also been an increasing awareness of the role played by
the microbial flora of the intestine in certain alimentary diseases.

NORMAL FLORA OF THE ALIMENTARY TRACT

Before changes in the intestinal flora associated with disease can be
understood, some knowledge of the nature and the mechanism of
colonization of the bowel is of considerable value.

The stomach is relatively free from micro-organisms when empty.
Many organisms, in saliva, upper respiratory tract secretions and
ingested food, are swallowed but are destroyed by gastric acid. It is
probably for this reason that small numbers of acid-resistant yeasts
(usually *Candida albicans* and *Torulopsis glabrata*) are the only organisms of note to be found in normal individuals.

The jejunum has a sparse microbial flora. The main mechanism preventing a permanent and dense colonization is the forward propulsion
of the intraluminar contents at a rate which exceeds the multiplication
rate of the organisms present. This tends to favour the elimination
rather than the accumulation of a resident flora. The acidity of gastric
juice and the presence of bile in the duodenum are selectively inhibitory
to the majority of ingested bacteria. This disinfectant-like action is
probably important in minimizing the contamination of the small
bowel.

In normal individuals the flora of the jejunum consists of small
numbers (usually $< 10^5$ per ml) of aerobic lactobacilli, streptococci
and yeasts.

In the terminal ileum there is considerable variation in the flora. The
bacterial content most often resembles that of the jejunum. Occasionally it resembles that of the colon, but whether this is a true colonization
or due to reflux through the ileocaecal valve is uncertain.

The colon is the only part of the intestinal tract which supports a rich resident flora. The quality and quantity exhibit little individual variation and there is a considerable similarity amongst all mammalian species. This is indeed remarkable when one considers the multitudinous varieties of bacteria which must pass through the intestine in the lifetime of an individual.

The colon in many respects acts like a sump. Its contents have a slow rate of forward flow in comparison to the remainder of the intestinal tract. The resident flora is therefore in a state of bacterial ecological equilibrium. Whereas in the small intestine organisms must be in a growth phase to maintain a resident flora against the flow rate through the lumen, in the colon they exist in a resting phase. Thus if even half of the contents of the colon were emptied in one day, then only 50 per cent of the remaining organisms would be required to undergo a single division to maintain the bacterial count. Under normal circumstances the caecum is the site at which multiplication takes place: 'foreign' organisms are prevented from multiplying by environmental conditions, which are anaerobic, and by the population pressure of the resident flora.

The flora is mainly anaerobic, consisting of the obligatory anaerobes, bacteroides and anaerobic lactobacilli. These constitute on average 98 per cent of the total flora. The remaining species most often encountered are *Escherichia coli*, *Clostridium welchii*, enterococci, aerobic lactobacilli, *Staphylococcus albus* and yeasts. The total bacterial count is in the order of 10^{10} viable organisms per ml. In summary, the flora of the intestinal tract in a normal individual can be compared to the botanical flora of a lofty Scottish peak: the summit (the stomach) supports little growth; the steep slopes (the small intestine) may precariously support a sparse flora; the glen below (the colon) supports a rich and varied flora.

Diseases of the intestinal tract associated with micro-organisms may be due to specific intestinal pathogenic species or secondary to alterations in the intestinal flora.

Bacillary dysentery

The dysentery organisms belong to the group Shigella, and the commonest epidemic type in this country is *Shigella sonnei*. *Shigella flexneri* occurs less frequently and the other important type, *Shigella shigae*, is found only in the tropics.

Since World War II there has been an increasing high prevalence of dysentery in Great Britain and, indeed, it is now the most widespread of all infections. At one time it was a scourge of prisons and mental institutions, but it is now finally established as a nuisance endemic disease in day nurseries and in the homes of the less well-endowed social classes. Since 1955 the notifications in England and Wales have never been less than 20,000 per year. In 1960 the huge total of 43,285 was reached and these notifications are only the 'tip of the iceberg'. Why it has increased is difficult to understand, but it is certainly associated with defective hygiene and sanitation.

Dysentery can only be acquired by swallowing the organisms. These are excreted by the bowel, and in nursery schools or in the home the spread can be traced from the lavatory seat to hands and thereafter directly or indirectly to the mouth. Spread by water in this country is rare, but food can occasionally be infected by a worker in a canteen who is suffering from dysentery or who is a 'carrier'. This situation can give rise to an explosive outbreak, and if those who have become infected belong to homes where hygiene and sanitation are below accepted standards there is further opportunity for the continued spread of the infection.

Pathology

The incubation period for dysentery is from two to seven days. The pathological changes mainly affect the large bowel. In Sonne infection there are mild inflammatory changes with increased secretion of mucus giving rise to loose stools which may have small flecks of blood. Flexner infections are often mild but on occasion (as with Shiga) can cause intense inflammatory changes resulting in ulcerated areas, especially in the rectum and sigmoid colon.

Clinical manifestations

The predominant symptom is diarrhoea, which is often accompanied by colicky abdominal pain, and there may be ten to twenty loose bowel movements in the first 24 hours. Initially the stools consist of loose faecal material and later may be mainly mucus flecked with blood.

In Sonne and mild cases of Flexner, the illness has mainly subsided by the end of the second day. In this country dysentery is essentially a mild disease mainly because Sonne is the predominant type of infection. However, Flexner and Shiga infections can give rise to a very acute illness. Where the diarrhoea is frequent and severe, the patient is febrile, toxic and rapidly becomes dehydrated. Occasionally in children Flexner infection can cause a profound toxic illness, with prostration often preceding the occurrence of diarrhoea and the diagnosis of dysentery therefore remaining unsuspected. Unless appropriate resuscitative measures are immediately instituted, death can occur.

Diagnosis

In most cases where there are frequent loose stools with blood and mucus the diagnosis of dysentery is easily made. (But in every infant and child the abdomen should be examined carefully for muscle guarding and tenderness.) Retrocaecal appendicitis can be mistaken for dysentery, but in the former the diarrhoea is usually infrequent and there is muscle guarding and tenderness in the right side of the abdomen. In infants the possibility of intussusception must always be considered, and the characteristic stool changes and clinical signs sought (see p. 180).

Treatment

Sonne dysentery is usually a mild illness and the worst is over within 48 hours. It is now generally accepted that in the majority of cases there is no indication for antibiotic therapy. Mist. kaolin et morph. is a time-honoured symptomatic remedy, but a tablet containing diphenoxylate hydrochloride 2·5 mg and atropine sulphate 0·025 mg is an effective intestinal sedative. The adult dose is two tablets six-hourly.

If the illness is severe then specific chemotherapy is indicated. In this country most strains of Shigellae are resistant to sulphonamides but are usually sensitive to streptomycin, nalidixic acid and the tetracyclines. These drugs are given orally for a period of five days. The adult dose is: streptomycin 2 g six-hourly; nalidixic acid, 1 g six-hourly; and tetracycline 250 mg six-hourly. Nalidixic acid has the advantage of not being an antibiotic and has been essentially free of the problems of resistance and 'transferred resistance'.

In cases admitted to hospital it has been the custom to obtain three negative specimens of faeces or rectal swabs prior to dismissal. However, this is not necessary in every case. The period of infectivity is from the beginning of the illness till the organism disappears from the faeces, but the period of greatest infectivity is during the diarrhoeal phase. When the stools become formed the infectivity is low and the carrier state does not last for more than a few weeks. Where the patient is a food handler, a nurse or a child from a day nursery then bacteriological cure is necessary and six successive negative specimens are required. A five-day course of chemotherapy (e.g. nalidixic acid) may be necessary to achieve this.

Prevention

Dysentery has been said to be the most highly preventable disease which is 'unprevented'. In hospital all loose stools should be reported as being due to 'dysentery'. The most important single factor in the prevention of spread is the frequent ritual of 'washing of hands' by nursing and medical staff.

Amoebic dysentery

Amoebic dysentery is a tropical illness and arises following the oral ingestion of the cysts of the protozoon *Entamoeba histolytica*. The primary lesions are in the large bowel but extraintestinal lesions can occur, the commonest being amoebic hepatitis.

The only origin of infection is a 'human carrier'. Amoebic cysts passed in faeces can be ingested following direct contact or indirectly through infection of water or food. These play an important role in the spread.

In the intestines the amoebic cysts dissolve and the resulting vegetative forms penetrate the host's tissues giving rise to ulceration of the colon.

Clinical picture

Following an incubation period which can vary from a few days to several months, the acute dysenteric attack begins with diarrhoea. The patient passes frequent loose stools which are watery and contain blood and mucus. The acute attack usually lasts for a few days but can be prolonged for several weeks. Where inadequately treated, there can be attacks and remissions, eventually resulting in chronic amoebic dysentery with a clinical picture similar to ulcerative colitis.

The commonest extraintestinal complication is acute hepatitis which can result in abscess formation. There is pain and tenderness over the region of the liver and this is accompanied by fever, rigors and sweats. When abscess occurs the liver is enlarged and on X-ray the dome of the diaphragm is seen to be elevated and immobile. Liver abscess can occur up to 20 years after the initial infection.

The diagnosis is made by finding of *Entamoeba histolytica* in the stool. It is essential that the stool should be collected in a warm bedpan and examined microscopically without delay. In patients with the chronic pattern of disease excretion can be irregular, and repeated examination of stools may be necessary. Sigmoidoscopy may be required to establish the diagnosis. Ulceration will be observed and scrapings can be taken for microscopy and histology.

Treatment

Amoebic dysentery should be treated with a combination of direct-acting systemically effective amoebicides (emetine and quinoline derivatives) and broad-spectrum antibiotics.

ACUTE AMOEBIC DYSENTERY

Days 1 to 3   Dehydroemetine hydrochloride 60 mg daily, i.m. injection.

4 to 10   Dehydroemetine bismuth iodide (EBI) 100 mg thrice daily orally, and tetracycline 1 g daily. A satisfactory substitute for EBI is diloxanide furoate (Furamide) 500 mg thrice daily. It has the advantage of being non-toxic.

CHRONIC AMOEBIC DYSENTERY

Days 1 to 2   Chloroquine diphosphate 600 mg daily.

3 to 21   Chloroquine diphosphate 300 mg daily, and di-iodohydroxy quinoline 1 g daily.

As emetine is a cardiac depressant and gastrointestinal irritant, it must be given under strict supervision. The patient must be in bed during the time of administration, and the drug must not be repeated for at least two weeks.

Giardiasis

This is due to infestation with a small protozoal parasite, *Giardia lamblia*, and may give rise to mild but persistent diarrhoea in children. Search should always be made for the parasite or cysts in the stools of children with recurrent diarrhoea where no bacterial pathogens have been cultured.

The stools are quickly cleared of the protozoon by the oral administration of mepacrine 25 mg thrice daily for five days, or metronidazole (Flagyl) 200 mg thrice daily for seven days, which is equally effective and has the advantage of having no toxic side-effects.

Infantile gastroenteritis

Infantile gastroenteritis is a syndrome where the main features are diarrhoea and vomiting. In the early part of this century, each summer and autumn in the industrial areas of our British cities there were large epidemics with great loss of infant life. The disease still occurs where there is overcrowded housing, inadequate sanitary conditions or deficient standards of hygiene. The incidence has fallen steadily but it is still an important cause of morbidity and death in the first six months of life.

In many outbreaks neither bacterial nor viral pathogens have been isolated but certain agglutinable strains of *Escherichia coli* are now regarded as causal pathogens. These strains seldom cause any clinical upset in children over two years. Gastroenteritis seldom occurs in an infant who has been solely breast fed. The stool in the breast-fed infant is markedly acid in reaction and the bowel flora consists almost exclusively of *Lactobacillus bifidus*. The bowel milieu is such that the pathogenic *E. coli* are unable to flourish, in contrast to the ease of colonization in the bottle-fed baby.

Clinical picture

The infant is disinclined for feeds, and soon diarrhoea and vomiting occur. Initially the stools are grass-green, but if the illness continues they become more frequent and watery, containing little faecal material. Very soon there is evidence of dehydration. In the moderately ill case the child is irritable, the skin is pale, the lips are bright red, the tongue is dry and the eyes are slightly sunken.

Where there is more marked dehydration the infant becomes much more irritable and fretful. The eyes, fontanelle and abdomen are obviously sunken, and the skin of the abdomen can be lifted up in folds between the thumb and forefinger. Thirst is present and the child may feed avidly often only to vomit immediately. When loss of weight exceeds 10 per cent of the infant's body weight the condition becomes critical due to oligaemia and peripheral circulatory failure. The infant lies immobile, the skin is cold and waxy, the eys and fontanelle are sunken. The extremities are cold and cyanosed. Recovery requires energetic restoration of body fluids.

The loss of electrolytes in the stools and vomitus usually equals or is greater than the loss of body water and this results in 'hypotonic dehydration'. It is this form of dehydration which has been described above.

However, where the loss of body water exceeds the loss of electrolytes, the dehydration is of the hypertonic or hypernatraemic type. This is a highly dangerous situation because the infant may not appear obviously dehydrated, the skin on palpation feeling 'doughy' or 'velvety'. However, there is evidence of acidosis, the respirations are rapid and convulsions may occur followed by unconsciousness. The diagnosis of hypernatraemic dehydration is confirmed on estimation of serum electrolytes when the sodium concentration is in excess of 150 mmol/l and there is a markedly raised blood urea level. Unless hypernatraemic dehydration is recognized and dealt with expeditiously, permanent brain damage may result. When death occurs there is often evidence of cerebral haemorrhage at autopsy.

The essential causative factor in hypernatraemia is inadequate intake of water. This may be due to:

1. Reluctance to feed
2. Withdrawal of fluids because of vomiting
3. Attempts to thicken feeds
4. Giving of hypertonic glucose solutions.

Diagnosis
The diagnosis of gastroenteritis is normally quite easily made, but it must be remembered that diarrhoea and vomiting can occur when an infant is suffering from pneumonia, otitis media, meningitis or urinary tract infection. It cannot be overstressed that where there is diarrhoea and vomiting in an infant, thorough clinical examination is essential.

Treatment
Where the dehydration is mild, all milk feeds should be withdrawn and half-strength physiological saline or half-strength Hartmann's solution (Compound Injection of Sodium Lactate) 200 ml per kg per day given in small feeds every two hours. After 24 hours, if the vomiting has ceased, dilute milk feeds can be introduced and the 'saline' solution reduced and gradually withdrawn.

Where hypotonic dehydration is severe hospital admission is essential. Attempts at feeding by mouth are discontinued and intravenous therapy instituted. The commonly used fluid is 5 per cent dextrose in half-strength physiological saline, but the authors have found half-strength Hartmann's solution effective. In the first four to six hours the dehydrated infant should receive 45 to 65 ml per kg body weight and thereafter the quantity is 130 to 200 ml per kg per day. After 24 to 48 hours on intravenous therapy the diarrhoea and vomiting have usually abated. Dilute feeds are introduced and the intravenous fluids reduced accordingly.

Severe hypertonic (hypernatraemic) dehydration requires fluids intravenously, and in order to avoid giving excess electrolytes the saline or Hartmann's solution should not be more than one-fifth normal strength. Where acidosis is a marked feature it may be necessary to add bicarbonate to the i.v. solution. However, the whole regime should be regulated by frequent estimations of serum electrolytes.

Where the dehydration is of such severity as to be associated with peripheral circulatory failure the infant should be nursed in an incubator or an oxygen tent.

Antibiotics have little or no place in the treatment of infantile gastroenteritis, but if there is evidence of parenteral infection, for example, otitis media, or pneumonia, then it is important that the appropriate antibiotic should be given.

Typhoid and paratyphoid fevers (the enteric fevers)

Prior to the availability of good water supply and sanitation, typhoid fever was a frequent and deadly disease in Great Britain. At present between 100 and 250 cases are notified each year with a mortality of less than 1 per cent. About half the infections are contracted by people on holiday in Mediterranean countries. *Salmonella typhi* is a purely human pathogen, and most of the cases of typhoid fever occur singly or in small numbers infected by carriers excreting the organism in faeces or urine. Two notable occurrences of widespread outbreaks in recent years have been in 1963 when 68 British visitors to Zermatt, Switzerland, were infected by 'drinking water', and in 1964 in Aberdeen when a most exceptional source, a tin of infected corned beef, gave rise to typhoid in 400 people.

Pathology

After ingestion the organisms pass from the intestine to the mesenteric glands, and then via the thoracic duct and the bloodstream to the liver, gallbladder, spleen and bone marrow, where they proliferate. This occurs during the incubation period. There is then a secondary bacteraemia which gives rise to the signs and symptoms of the period of invasion, and at this time the organism can be grown on blood culture.

Following a secondary invasion of the intestine from the gallbladder the Peyer's patches become swollen and ulceration occurs in the severe cases. Persistent foci may remain in the gallbladder and kidney after clinical recovery. The patient may continue to excrete organisms and become a chronic faecal or urinary carrier.

The incubation period is 7 to 14 days.

Clinical picture

There is frequently a history of the patient having returned from a holiday abroad. The onset of the illness is insidious, with malaise, lethargy, headache, vague abdominal discomfort and often epistaxis. The temperature increases in stepwise fashion, and by the end of the first week reaches 39° or 40°C. The pulse rate does not increase proportionately. Leucopenia is usual.

By the beginning of the second week the patient looks toxic and ill. The cheeks are flushed, the tongue is dry and heavily furred and the lips and teeth are covered with sordes. The spleen is palpable and in most cases about the tenth day of illness 'rose spots' appear on the abdomen and the lower part of the thorax. These rose spots are small maculopapules which fade on pressure. Over a period of a few days the rash comes out in crops but it is usually sparse. There is marked mental dullness and often a low muttering delirium. Diarrhoea can occur at this stage, the stools being loose and green—the classic 'pea soup' stools. However, in many patients constipation is the rule. The illness reaches its peak in the third week and this is when the serious complications of intestinal haemorrhage or perforation can occur. In the majority of cases there is a favourable outcome. The temperature falls by lysis, the general condition improves rapidly, the appetite returns and sometimes becomes voracious.

This description is that of an untreated case of typhoid fever. Where adequate chemotherapy is given, the acute part of the illness is markedly shortened.

Complications

Intestinal haemorrhage. This usually occurs during the third week when there is sloughing of the ulcers of the Peyer's patches. The bleeding can vary from a few streaks of blood in the stool to massive haemorrhage. When severe, the incident is marked by a rapid fall in temperature with a sharp rise in pulse rate.

Perforation of an ulcer is a very serious complication and, as with haemorrhage, usually occurs in the third week. There is usually severe abdominal pain (but this can be absent) associated with rigidity of the abdominal wall.

Osteitis. This late complication is rare and occurs in the ribs, tibiae or vertebrae.

Diagnosis

The diagnosis of typhoid fever may be suggested if there is a palpable spleen and 'rose spots' are present. However, a definitive diagnosis can be made only as the result of laboratory investigation.

Blood culture is positive during the first week of illness.

Faeces and urine culture only become positive at the beginning of the second week.

The Widal reaction (serum agglutination) becomes positive during the second week. There is a steep rise in the H (flagellar) titre and a slower but significant rise in the O (somatic) titre. Vi antibody occurs only in typhoid and is an indication of the presence of 'living bacilli'. During the acute phase it appears in low titre, but persistence is suggestive of the carrier state and indicates need for repeated culture of faeces and urine.

Certain Salmonellae including *Salmonella typhi* can be phage-typed, which is most useful in epidemiological surveys. It allows the strain from a carrier or other source of infection to be typed and linked up with strains from other sources.

Treatment

Chloramphenicol has been found to be extremely effective in the treatment of typhoid fever. The adult dose is 500 mg six-hourly, continued until three days after the temperature has returned to normal, and thereafter 250 mg six-hourly for a further 7 to 10 days.

The usual response to this treatment, therefore, is:
1. The temperature returns to normal with three or four days of commencing treatment.
2. Toxaemia abates within 48 hours.
3. Appetite becomes normal in a few days and at the end of 10 days convalescence begins.

Recent claims have been made for the use of trimethoprim/sulphamethoxazole (Septrin) in typhoid fever. Clinical trials have shown this combination to be as effective as chloramphenicol and it has the advantage of being free of the hazard of blood dyscrasia.

All typhoid patients must have six consecutive culture-negative specimens of faeces and urine before leaving hospital. Because excretion of organisms can be intermittent, repeat specimens should be cultured at intervals till six months after the illness. When the convalescent carrier state arises, ampicillin in large doses over a period of some weeks may be effective in achieving negative cultures.

The gallbladder is a recognized source of continuing infection. If there is evidence of gallstones or cholecystitis then cholecystectomy is justified and this measure is often effective in clearing up the carrier state.

Chronic carriers become the responsibility of the public health authorities who keep them under surveillance.

Prevention

Provision of pure water supplies and adequate surveillance of 'carriers' are fundamental preventive measures.

For those in attendance on cases of enteric fever the ritual of 'washing of hands' is the most important single factor in prevention of the spread of infection.

Typhoid paratyphoid vaccine (TAB)—two doses with one month interval gives protection in average circumstances. Where water supplies are suspect, as in underdeveloped areas, TAB should not be regarded as giving absolute protection and drinking water must be sterilized.

Salmonellosis

In addition to *Salmonella typhi* and *S. paratyphi* the Salmonella group has over 200 types which are intestinal pathogens. Salmonellae have been found in almost every animal species. Indeed, the most widespread zoonosis is Salmonella food-poisoning, and two-thirds of all human infection is due to a single type, *S. typhimurium*. Most human infection with this organism is from meat, but a considerable source is duck eggs and bulk dried egg. The commonest manner by which infection is conveyed is by processed meat preparations such as pies and reheated stews. A hazard which is not usually appreciated is that, in ordinary cooking, the temperature reached at the centre of a joint of meat removed from deep freeze is often quite inadequate to kill off organisms which may be present.

Since World War II there has been a marked increase in the incidence of salmonellosis. The feeding habits of the populace have changed considerably. Almost every member of a family has at least one meal per day away from home—in school or works canteen. This communal feeding increases the opportunity for spread of infection. Most episodes involve single cases or one family, but there can also be widespread outbreaks such as occurred in the west of Scotland between August and October 1968 when there were 472 cases of infection with 12 deaths. *Salmonella typhimurium* phage-type 32 was the offending organism.

Incubation period

This is usually 12 to 48 hours.

Clinical picture

The onset is abrupt with vomiting, abdominal cramps and watery diarrhoea. In the majority it is an unpleasant short-lived illness, the worst being over within 48 hours. In the very young and the elderly this can be a severe illness mainly due to the occurrence of dehydration.

On occasion the organism can display invasiveness, entering the bloodstream causing a severe febrile prostrating illness, often characterized by bacteraemic shock and renal failure.

Complications

In the invasive bacteraemic illness there is widespread dissemination of the organism and this can result in the occurrence of pneumonia, meningitis and osteitis.

Diagnosis

This is confirmed by the isolation of the organism from the faeces and, in the severe cases, from blood culture. Very occasionally some of the offending foodstuff may be available for culture. Phage typing can sometimes demonstrate the common source of a widespread outbreak.

Treatment

Most cases respond well to rest in bed for 48 hours, attention being paid to restoring fluid loss. Where vomiting is troublesome, cyclizine 1 ml intramuscularly is often effective, and two tablets of diphenoxylate hydrochloride 2·5 mg plus atropine sulph. 0·025 mg six-hourly is useful in controlling the diarrhoea.

In the ordinary 'non-invasive' case antibiotics should not be used. This policy helps prevent the development of transferred or multiple resistance in the Enterobacteriaceae.

Where there is severe dehydration, intravenous therapy with 5 per cent glucose in normal saline, or Hartmann's solution should be instituted as soon as possible. In the older age group dehydration can quite quickly become irreversible and therefore the situation should be regarded as a 'medical emergency'.

Where there is evidence of invasiveness or bacteraemia antibiotic therapy should be commenced. Chloramphenicol is the drug of choice, the adult dose being 500 mg six-hourly, and in cases of such severity it is added to the intravenous fluids.

Following recovery from the acute illness, many patients continue to excrete the Salmonella organisms in the stools for 3 to 6 months. Although the organisms may be sensitive *in vitro*, antibiotics seldom shorten the period of excretion.

Staphylococcal food-poisoning

In contradistinction to the Salmonella variety of food-poisoning, that due to Staphylococcus is an intoxication not an infection.

When foodstuffs, usually confectionery, cooked meats and dairy products, are contaminated with certain strains of *Staphylococcus aureus* potent enterotoxins are formed on incubation. The ingestion of this material is followed by the abrupt and often violent onset of prostration, abdominal pain, nausea, vomiting and in some cases diarrhoea. The patient may present in a severely shocked condition with subnormal temperature and may be mistaken for an acute abdominal emergency. The interval between eating the contaminated food and the onset of symptoms is short, usually in the order of one to five hours. When an outbreak occurs in an institution, a restaurant or a family this short incubation period is almost diagnostic. Although the illness is often severe, its duration is short—usually less than 24 hours—and fatalities are rare.

Since the condition is due to toxins, antibiotics are unnecessary, and treatment is directed towards maintaining hydration and electrolyte balance. The laboratory diagnosis depends on the isolation of *Staphylococcus aureus* from samples of the food consumed, vomitus and faeces. In an outbreak, careful enquiries from the victims, and those not affected, will indicate the most likely items on the menu to be incriminated. As the common source of infection is usually a food-handler, these persons should be examined and swabs taken from hands, nose and any purulent lesions. After comparison of the phage types of all staphylococci obtained, the causative strain, the item of food contaminated and the food-handler responsible can be determined.

Education of food-handlers is essential in the prevention of this disease. Persons with skin sepsis (especially infected wounds of the hand) or purulent nasal discharges should either be excluded from the kitchen or should be supplied with rubber gloves, face masks, etc. Equally important is the refrigeration of foodstuffs after preparation if immediate consumption is not intended.

Clostridial *(C. welchii)* food-poisoning

In many respects this disease is similar to staphylococcal food-poisoning. Although type A strains of *Clostridium welchii* of the heat-resistant variety are usually incriminated, it is now clear that heat-sensitive strains can also cause the disease.

The usual food source of the organism is cooked meat, especially stews, mince pies and beef gravies that have been contaminated with soil or faecal material. After incubation at kitchen temperature multiplication of the organism takes place.

The disease is usually mild, of less than one day's duration. The clinical features are similar to those of staphylococcal food-poisoning. However, in the majority of cases they tend to be milder, vomiting is absent and diarrhoea almost constantly present. The incubation period is longer, usually 10 to 12 hours after ingestion of the contaminated food. This longer incubation period and the lack of vomiting are helpful in differentiating this form of food-poisoning from the staphylococcal variety. The diagnosis may be confirmed by the examination of the offending foodstuffs and the faeces of the clinical cases for type A strains of *C. welchii*. This involves semiquantitative bacteriological techniques under anaerobic conditions.

Treatment is directed to the maintenance of fluid and electrolyte balance. The majority of patients recover spontaneously without medical treatment.

This is a preventable disease. As the usual cause is faecal contamination of cooked meats, the importance of hand-washing after defaecation should be emphasized to food-handlers. The source may in some cases be due to faecal contamination of fresh meat in the slaughterhouse. The adequate cooking of large cuts of meat and prompt refrigeration of fresh- and cooked-meat products would prevent most outbreaks of this not uncommon disease.

Botulism

This extremely rare form of bacterial intoxication is usually associated with the ingestion of inadequately processed cans or jars of fruit, vegetables or fish. The organism which produces the toxin is *Clostridium botulinum*, or *C. parabotulinum*. Usually about two-thirds of those affected die in three to seven days after the onset of symptoms. The toxin affects the central nervous system, giving rise to symmetrical cranial nerve paralysis. Specific treatment is available in the form of intravenous and intramuscular botulism antitoxin. Diagnosis is usually confirmed by the demonstration of the toxin in blood and the suspected foods. Attempts to isolate the organism from faeces and suspected food should also be made.

VIRAL AGENTS IN INTESTINAL DISEASE

The role played by viruses in intestinal disease is as yet unclear. Enterovirus infection can on occasion upset gastrointestinal function, although this appears to be rare when one considers the prevalence of these viruses, especially amongst children. Echo 18 infection associated with diarrhoea has occurred in outbreaks. Adenoviral infection, although commonly causing respiratory infection, may also be accompanied by a mild diarrhoeal illness. Outbreaks of this variety have in particular been due to adenovirus 15.

Both enteroviral and adenoviral infections cause mesenteric adenitis of varying degree. The enlarged lymph glands can predispose to intussusception.

DISEASES ASSOCIATED WITH ALTERATION IN INTESTINAL FLORA

As has already been discussed the small bowel is relatively free from bacteria and colonization of its contents will occur only if there is a breakdown in the defence mechanisms listed below:

> Maintenance of an adequate flow rate
> Gastric acid production
> Bile production
> Antibody excretion (doubtful).

The most important factor in preventing the accumulation of a resident flora is undoubtedly the maintenance of an adequate flow-rate through the small intestine. Thus colonization of the lumen is rarely a primary phenomenon, and is usually associated with some abnormality giving rise to a diminution in flow rate. These abnormalities may be localized, as in jejunal diverticula, blind loops, enterocolic fistulae, and proximal to obstructive lesions, or generalized, as in intestinal ileus or after gastric surgery. Gastric operations are the commonest predisposing causes of colonization of the small intestine in modern clinical practice.

The colonization of the small intestine that develops is not random. With a mild degree of stasis one finds an increase in the numbers of organisms normally found in that site, e.g. yeasts and aerobic lactobacilli, and in addition other organisms usually associated with the upper respiratory tract, e.g. neisseriae, diphtheroids, staphylococci, and haemophilus species. However, when marked stasis is present the flora comes to resemble that of the colon, with coliforms and anaerobic species such as clostridia, veillonellas, bacteroides and anaerobic lactobacilli. It is usually in association with a 'colonic' type of colonization that clinical disease becomes evident. This may vary from mild diarrhoea to a varying degree of malabsorption. In severe cases the malabsorption may be of such a degree that the patient develops severe malnutrition.

Treatment should be directed wherever possible to alleviating the primary cause of stasis. Where this is impractical, long-term antibiotic therapy with appropriate antibiotics may be undertaken.

DISEASE ASSOCIATED WITH SUPPRESSION OF INTESTINAL FLORA

Although the maintenance of a normal intestinal flora does not appear to be essential for health its suppression by broad-spectrum antibiotics may lead to an overgrowth by organisms which are resistant to antibiotics. *Staphylococcus aureus* can give rise to a severe, sometimes fatal, 'cholera-like' illness. To a lesser extent similar syndromes have been reported with *Pseudomonas aerugenosa* and *Candida albicans*. The occurrence of these diseases is fortunately rare, but when they occur in premature infant and neonatal units they may constitute a major problem.

Two other diarrhoeal illnesses have been ascribed to suppression of the normal flora, namely 'antibiotic diarrhoea', and 'traveller's diarrhoea'; neither has readily yielded to investigation. In the former, some cases are undoubtedly due to sensitivity of the patient to the antibiotic, and the disorder completely resolves when the antibiotic is stopped. In others the diarrhoea may persist for several weeks without any known cause. Evidence is now available to suggest that 'traveller's diarrhoea' may be due to the acquisition of *Escherichia coli* which are not normally considered pathogenic in individuals normally resident in the area visited. When a visitor acquires this organism a mild diarrhoeal illness follows, the organism often suppressing his own *E. coli* strains. As in gastroenteritis of infancy, the mechanism is probably the production of enterotoxin by the 'foreign' strain.

THE PRINCIPLES OF MICROBIOLOGICAL DIAGNOSES OF INTESTINAL INFECTION

The specimens examined by the laboratory in a case of suspected intestinal infection will vary depending on the clinical picture presented by the patient. Faecal specimens should be submitted from all patients presenting with diarrhoea. Blood cultures should be examined in all febrile cases. If there is evidence of associated malabsorption, jejunal aspirates may also be submitted.

In the laboratory, specimens are examined macroscopically, as the character of the stool may give a clue as to the pathogen which may be present. Blood and mucus are often present in Shigella and amoebic infections, 'rice-water' stools are characteristic of staphylococcal enterocolitis, and pale bulky stools may suggest the possibility of a malabsorption syndrome.

Microscopic examination of bowel contents is performed to determine the presence of protozoan parasites, pus cells and red blood cells. The presence of large numbers of Gram-positive cocci may suggest a staphylococcal gastroenteritis. Fluorescent antibody techniques are sometimes employed, using antibody conjugated to fluorescent dyes, specific to the common intestinal pathogens.

Specimens are inoculated into selective and standard media, and after a suitable incubation period colonies with characteristics resembling known pathogens are tested for biochemical activities. Where applicable these are screened for agglutinability with specific antisera.

Blood cultures are of prime importance especially during the first two weeks of an illness resembling enteric fever. In many of these cases stool culture may be negative during this period.

Infections limited to the intestinal lumen do not produce a readily demonstrable humoral immunological response. In the enteric fever group (*Salmonella typhi, S. paratyphi* and occasionally other salmonellae) the organism crosses the bowel barrier giving rise to an immunological response. Antibodies are formed to somatic components (O antigens), flagellar components (H antigens) and capsular components (Vi antigens) when these are present. These antibodies have the ability to agglutinate suitably prepared suspensions of salmonellae containing known antigenic groups. This is the basis of the Widal reaction. The patient's serum is normally tested against *Salmonella typhi, S. paratyphi* (A, B and C) O and H antigens, a non-specific Salmonella H antigen and where applicable Vi antigen of *Salmonella typhi*.

The presence of high antibody titres (1:80 or greater levels) to O and H antigens is indicative of active infection. High H antigens alone usually indicate TAB vaccination or past infection. Titres against the

Vi antigen are indicative of carriage of *Salmonella typhi*. Although high titres are significant, the finding of a rising titre is of greater diagnostic importance.

Although the Widal reaction is at present the only serological test employed routinely in laboratory investigation of intestinal infection, the complement fixation test for *Entamoeba histolytica* can be useful in difficult cases of amoebic disease. It is usually only in cases where spread outside the intestine has occurred, e.g. liver abscess, that significant titres are found. This test is only carried out in certain selected reference laboratories.

9. Crohn's Disease

T. J. Thomson and Stuart Young

In 1932, Crohn, Ginzberg and Oppenheimer described an apparently new clinical entity involving the terminal ileum which they called 'regional ileitis'. This was not the earliest report of the condition. Reports go back to Morgagni in 1769, and Dalziel reported a series of cases of 'chronic interstitial enteritis' from Glasgow in 1913. Other nomenclature, including regional enteritis, right sided colitis, segmental colitis and granulomatous colitis has only led to confusion, and it is recommended that for the sake of simplicity, the term Crohn's disease be used.

Crohn's disease can involve any section of the gastro-intestinal tract, but the lesions occur most commonly in the ileum or colon, alone or in combination. The incidence is low (1·5—2/100,000 per annum). The aetiology is unknown. It is possible that the aetiological factors are multiple, and include environmental, genetic and immunological factors. This disease may present initially at any age but in the small bowel the incidence is highest during the second and third decades, and where the large bowel alone is involved, after middle age. In small bowel disease there is no significant difference in the sex incidence but where the large bowel alone is involved there is a preponderance of females.

Clinical presentation

The essential lesions in Crohn's disease are discrete areas of inflamed, thickened bowel, adjacent lymphadenopathy, and narrowing of the lumen, often associated with adhesions and fistulae. The course of the disease is usually subacute or chronic, with relapses and remissions. The condition of 'acute ileitis', discussed on page 172, runs a self-limiting course. Crohn's disease of the ileum in its early subacute form may simulate this condition.

The commonest presenting symptom of Crohn's disease of the bowel is abdominal colic; it is almost invariably present when the disease involves the terminal ileum and/or the proximal colon. Diarrhoea is also common during the course of the disease, and blood may be seen in the faeces. When the lesion begins in the distal colon, rectal bleeding, often associated with diarrhoea, is an early complaint. General malaise, lethargy, anorexia and loss of weight are usually present in the established case. With the development of stenosis, vomiting and the other signs of intestinal obstruction may appear.

Diagnosis

The history of intermittent abdominal pain, diarrhoea, with possibly rectal bleeding, in a young adult, accompanied by loss of well-being, should suggest a diagnosis of Crohn's disease.

Physical examination reveals that many patients have evidence of recent weight loss, appear ill and are pyrexial. Commonly there is anaemia and elevation of the E.S.R. Finger clubbing is often present. Certain systemic manifestations such as uveitis, erythema nodosum and arthritis may occasionally be seen. On abdominal examination there is often tenderness over the affected segment of bowel, which may feel thickened, and on occasions a firm mass may be palpated in, for example, the right iliac fossa in ileal disease.

The presence of an external abdominal fistula or of chronic perianal ulceration are further signs of diagnostic value. When the large bowel is involved, ulceration or infection around the anus is encountered in a large percentage of cases, and may even precede the onset of intestinal symptoms. The most common lesion is an anal fissure which characteristically has thickened undermined edges and is shallower and broader than a simple anal fissure; it may extend both outwards and upwards in the anal canal, and such lesions may be multiple. In these cases pain is not usually severe, in contrast to simple fissure. Other lesions in this region occurring in Crohn's disease include perianal or ischiorectal abscesses, which may give rise to chronic fistulae.

Rectal examination and sigmoidoscopy should be done in every patient when a diagnosis of Crohn's disease is suspected. The rectum is involved in only about 50 per cent of patients with colonic disease, in contrast to patients with ulcerative colitis, 95 per cent of whom have rectal involvement (p. 208). When the rectum is involved, the wall may feel nodular and firm, or the examining finger may be impeded by a stricture.

The characteristic sigmoidoscopic appearance of Crohn's disease is due to areas of oedematous mucosa being raised up by inflammation in the submucosa, each small area being delineated by linear ulcers extending into the gut wall. This produces a 'cobblestone appearance'. The walls eventually may become rigid and indistensible. Changes, however, are often patchy, with intervening areas of apparent normality, in contradistinction to ulcerative colitis where the inflammatory appearances are confluent. Biopsy should always be taken and may give the characteristic histological picture of Crohn's disease (p. 203).

Radiology. Should the clinical picture suggest that there is disease involving the terminal ileum, barium enema examination should be performed. In addition to observation of the large bowel, the radiologist will pay attention to the position, shape and distensibility of the caecum. If barium passes back into the terminal ileum particular attention will be paid to the mucosal pattern for evidence of ulceration or fissuring, and to the size of the lumen. The classical 'string' sign (Fig. 9.1) may be demonstrated in the terminal ileum on this examination. It is routine practice also to perform a barium meal and follow-through examination, as this may show lesions at a higher level in the gastro-intestinal tract. Several discrete areas of disease may be identified—the so-called 'skip' lesions of Crohn's disease.

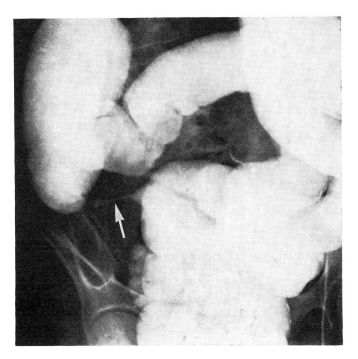

Fig. 9.1 The classical 'string' sign in Crohn's disease of the terminal ileum.

Colonic disease may be identified by barium enema. Mucosal involvement may be recognised by a shaggy irregular outline to the bowel; fissuring by spikes radiating from the lumen. Internal fistulae may also be seen, but they are often difficult to demonstrate.

Biopsy of diseased tissue is all-important in confirming a diagnosis of Crohn's disease. The tissue may be taken from a perianal lesion, from rectum or colon on sigmoidoscopy, or from bowel or affected lymph node at operation.

The most reliable diagnostic finding is the presence of a sarcoid reaction. In this there are focal aggregates of epithelioid cells with giant cells of the Langhans peripheral type, and a poorly demarcated outer zone of lymphocytes. Central caseation does not occur in Crohn's disease. Examination of surgical specimens will reveal such granulomas in about 60 per cent of patients. For the rest, diagnosis must depend on appreciation of a combination of histological features—transmural inflammation, focal aggregates of lymphocytes and fissuring ulceration passing from the mucosa into or even beyond the bowel wall. Such fissures are not, however, a specific feature of Crohn's disease, as a similar appearance can be seen in very acute ulcerative colitis and in malignant lymphoma of the gut.

Differential diagnosis and special investigations. Special investigations are not usually required in order to confirm the diagnosis of Crohn's disease in a typical case where an appropriate history is obtained and the clinical examination, X-ray findings and histology are all consistent with this diagnosis. In cases where doubt exists, further tests are necessary. Tuberculosis of the ileo-caecal region, rectum or perineum may require exclusion. The Mantoux test has been found to be negative in about 70 per cent of patients with Crohn's disease, and a negative test virtually rules out a diagnosis of chronic tuberculosis. X-ray of the lungs may demonstrate active pulmonary tuberculosis; caseation in follicles seen on histology would exclude Crohn's disease; final proof of a tuberculous aetiology might be obtained by culture of tissue material or by guinea-pig inoculation.

Sarcoidosis may cause confusion on histological examination of biopsy material and also by the fact that the Mantoux reaction is negative in 60 to 70 per cent of cases. However, Crohn's disease is not associated with the other manifestations of sarcoidosis and in the latter, intestinal involvement is extremely rare.

When the presenting symptom is haemorrhagic diarrhoea, the other principal diagnosis to be considered is ulcerative colitis (p. 208). The differentiation may prove difficult. Patients are encountered showing clinical and histological features of both diseases, but in the majority of cases, histological appearances of rectal biopsies and/or the demonstration of 'skip lesions' on barium enema examination will clinch a diagnosis of Crohn's disease.

Diverticular disease (p. 243), carcinoma of the colon (p. 220) and ischaemic colitis have all to be considered in the differential diagnosis of localised Crohn's disease of the large bowel. In all four conditions fresh blood may be passed per rectum and the patients are usually over 50 years of age. The site of involvement, the appearances on colonoscopy, and the detailed X-ray appearances are useful guides in coming to a diagnosis.

Complications

The local complications occur as part of the disease process and include intestinal obstruction at any level, chronic abscess formation outwith the wall of the bowel, free perforation, which is indeed relatively rare, fistulae, which may develop internally between loops of bowel, between intra-abdominal organs or penetrate the skin surface, haemorrhage, and urological complications such as ileo-vesical fistula and obstructive uropathy due to involvement of the ureter in retroperitoneal spread of inflammation. A more general effect leading to progressive deterioration of health may result from malabsorption from the small intestine (p. 82).

Distant complications are usually encountered in the eyes, joints and skin, while changes in the liver and an increased incidence of cholelithiasis have also been reported in patients with Crohn's disease. Carcinoma complicating Crohn's disease, irrespective of the site of the primary lesion, is now well documented. There appears to be some association of carcinoma with long-standing small bowel disease, but the position as regards large bowel disease is less clear.

Treatment

There is no specific treatment for Crohn's disease. Details of management must depend on the level and extent of the gastro-intestinal lesion, the severity of the symptoms and the fitness of the patient.

Patients with moderate or severe symptoms should be treated in bed and given a diet of high calorific value (2,500 to 3,000) and of low residue, the latter in an attempt to reduce the hazard of intestinal obstruction. Where there are already signs of obstruction, intravenous feeding with high calorie nutrient fluid should be given. Any abnormality in levels of serum electrolytes and urea should at the same time be corrected by intravenous infusion. Anaemia, if present, should be treated by oral iron supplements or, if severe, by blood transfusion, as it is desirable to obtain and maintain a haemoglobin level of about 14 g per cent. Should there be evidence of malabsorption of vitamin B_{12} or folic acid, these drugs should be given.

Colicky abdominal pain and diarrhoea can be very distressing to the patient. For treatment of the former, paracetamol should be given in the first instance, but the use of more potent analgesics such as pentazocine 50 mg orally or 30 mg intramuscularly may be required. The diarrhoea may be relieved by codeine phosphate in an oral dose of 15 to 30 mg thrice daily. Adreno-cortical steroids are worthy of trial in the treatment of Crohn's disease. During severe attacks, some patients respond dramatically to oral prednisolone in a dose of 40–60 mg daily in divided doses. As soon as a satisfactory response has been achieved dosage should be reduced to 5 to 10 mg per day and, where possible, finally withdrawn. Topical application by means of retention enemata as in ulcerative colitis (p. 215) will frequently bring about temporary improvement in active disease of the distal colon. Sulphasalazine (p. 215) is widely used for maintenance therapy although there is uncertainty about its mode of action or its value.

Azothiaprine alone or in combination with adrenocortical steroids has recently been employed in the treatment of patients with entero-cutaneous fistulae. Some dramatic successes have been reported, but at present the mode of action of this drug is unknown, and it should only be used with caution when other measures have failed.

Surgical treatment. Since there is a high risk of recurrence after any surgical procedure, there is usually reluctance to advise operation un-less conservative measures fail. One must recognise, however, that the majority of patients will at some time require operative treatment for the complications of the disease. Deterioration of a patient's condition as the result of malabsorption, complete obstruction of the intestine, abdominal abscess or fistula, and frequently occurring bouts of abdominal colic, fever and bowel disturbance will hasten a decision to have recourse to surgery.

At operation the two main alternatives are either to bypass the affected segment of intestine or to resect this along with a margin of apparently healthy intestine proximal and distal to the lesion, restoring continuity by end-to-end anastomosis. The margin of safety is never easy to establish in either case as mucosal and submucosal involvement can be present without visible evidence at serosal level and inadequate clearance may partly account for the frequency of recurrence at the site of anastomosis. There is no doubt that a bypass procedure will offer a period of respite to the patient with complete or subacute obstructive symptoms, and it is just under these conditions with dis-tended loops of adherent bowel that resection can be most hazardous. There is evidence, however, that following adequate resection, the incidence of recurrence of symptoms requiring further surgery is much lower over any given period than after a bypass procedure, although the post-operative mortality is usually slightly higher. The choice of procedure therefore is made in the operating theatre and is based on the extent and complexity of the condition, bearing in mind the patient's clinical condition. It can be particularly difficult in those patients who have extensive involvement in continuity or at intervals along the small bowel. Extensive resection of the small bowel can but add to the degree of alimentary insufficiency which may be already present.

Treatment in the case of large bowel disease is worthy of separate consideration. As mentioned above, cortico-steroids frequently bring about temporary improvement, particularly in acute disease, and can be used topically to given relief of symptoms in ano-rectal disease, but this is often with little objective improvement. Diversion of the faecal stream is not helpful as disease tends to progress in the defunctioned bowel. Limited resection and anastomosis does seem justified by a low recurrence rate. Where involvement is more widespread in the large bowel and the small bowel is unaffected or affected only in its terminal segment, procto-colectomy with ileostomy as in ulcerative colitis may be the treatment of choice, but there is always the danger that Crohn's disease may develop subsequently more proximally in the small bowel. Where involvement of small bowel is more widespread in the presence of large bowel disease, conservative management should be maintained as long as possible.

The decision regarding surgery therefore must be made only after full consideration of all relevant features in the individual patient. In view of the continuing possibility of recurrence at any site in the alimentary tract, the long-term prognosis should always be guarded.

FURTHER READING

Kyle, J. (1972) *Crohn's Disease*. London: Heinemann.

Morson, B. C. (1971) Histopathology of Crohn's disease. *Scandinavian Journal of Gastroenterology*, **6,** 573–575.

Smith, I. S., Young, S., Gillespie, G., O'Connor, J. & Bell, J. R. (1975) Crohn's disease in Clydesdale 1961–70: epidemiological aspects. *Gut*, **16.1.** 62–67.

Young, S., Smith I. S., O'Connor, J., Bell, J. R. & Gillespie, G. (1975) Crohn's disease in Glasgow area 1961–70: surgical management and results. *British Journal of Surgery*, **62,** 528–534.

10. Ulcerative Colitis

T. J. Thomson and Douglas Roy

Ulcerative colitis is a non-specific inflammatory process of unknown aetiology, confined to the large bowel. The rectum is involved in almost all cases and the disease may spread in direct continuity to involve the whole of the colon from anus to ileocaecal valve. In these cases the mucosa of the terminal ileum is also sometimes affected, but this is secondary to the disease in the colon, is known as 'back-wash' ileitis, and always resolves when the colon is removed or the disease becomes quiescent. Crohn's disease (Ch. 9), on the other hand, is commonly a patchy, segmental disease which may affect the small intestine in addition to the colon.

It is convenient to classify the extent of the colitis according to the areas involved, proctitis, (affecting rectum only), left-sided colitis (to the middle of the transverse colon) and extensive colitis (affecting the whole colon).

Pathology

The typical, though not pathognomonic, lesion in ulcerative colitis is the crypt abscess. This consists of a mass of neutrophil polymorphs, lymphocytes and eosinophils packed into the deepest part of the intestinal crypts forming small abscesses (Fig 10.1*a*). These abscesses coalesce, leading to detachment of the overlying epithelium and to the formation of ulcers. In parallel with the destruction of mucosa by this process there is evidence of regeneration of mucosa which may produce heaped up areas of epithelium with the naked-eye appearance of polyps (Fig. 10.1*b*). These are the pseudopolyps so often seen in long standing disease and are not the same as the adenomatous polyps which may be seen in the otherwise normal colon or in familial intestinal polyposis.

The disturbance of the mucosal pattern is associated with an increased liability to the occurrence of carcinoma. The risk is significantly increased in extensive colitis (affecting the whole colon) in relatively young patients in whom the disease has been present for ten years or more. When cancer does occur it is often multicentric and usually very invasive.

The destructive aspect of the disease process may lead to paralysis of the colonic musculature leading to gross distension of the large bowel (toxic megacolon) and to perforation. In the early stages of the disease the colon returns to normal in remission but eventually fibrosis of the colonic wall leads to irreversible changes with loss of normal haustrations and thinning of the mucosa.

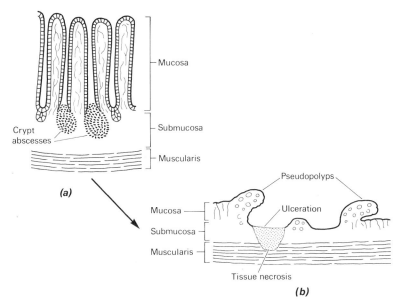

Fig. 10.1 Crypt abscesses (*a*) coalesce, the mucosa is shed leaving ulcers (*b*) which may penetrate the muscularis. At the edges of the ulcers there may be epithelial proliferation leading to the formation of pseudopolyps.

Aetiology

The aetiology of this condition is unknown despite much investigation in recent years. The oldest theory is that it is due to an infection by bacteria or a virus, but no specific one has been incriminated. A few patients have been shown to have an allergy to milk and the disease may remit when milk and its products are excluded from the diet. Allergy to other unknown factors has been suggested but proof of this is lacking. Certain features of autoimmune disease can be demonstrated but these may arise as a result of tissue destruction rather than as a cause of it. Finally, psychological factors certainly play a part in the natural history of the disease in that stress may be followed by exacerbation of the illness in some cases, but there is no proof that they initiate the disease.

Clinical presentation

This varies widely, from slight looseness of the bowel causing little but social inconvenience to the patient, to a fulminating prostrating illness in which the patient is toxic, dehydrated and pyrexial, with watery bloodstained effluent pouring almost continuously from the rectum. In the mild cases the continuing loss of blood may produce anaemia. In the severe case, in addition to the anaemia, there may be serious loss of protein and electrolytes, notably potassium. There may be pain in the hypogastrium or left iliac fossa preceding defaecation, but this is not usually a prominent symptom.

In view of the wide spectrum of symptoms and signs which may make up the clinical picture in this syndrome, it is necessary to attempt to grade the severity of the illness into 'mild', 'moderate' and 'severe' colitis (Table 10.1). This classification allows comparison between different cases by ensuring that observers are using a common terminology.

Table 10.1   Clinical classification of ulcerative colitis

Signs	Severe	Mild
Diarrhoea (motions in 24 h)	Six or more	Four or less
Blood in stools (macroscopic)	Obvious	Small amounts
Temperature (mean)	100°F (37·8°C) or more	Normal
Heart rate (mean)	More than 90/min	Normal
Haemoglobin	75% or less	Mild anaemia
E.S.R. in 1 h	Above 30 mm	Below 30 mm

'Moderate' colitis is the term given when these signs are intermediate between 'severe' and 'mild'. This classification has proved very useful in clinical practice, and it is also a convenient basis on which to outline therapy of a disease in which there is such a wide range of morbidity. The majority of patients suffer from the chronic intermittent form of the disease, with complete freedom from symptoms between attacks; others have chronic continuous symptoms, whereas a few have only one attack with no recurrence. Patients with disease confined to the rectum (proctitis) have a relatively good prognosis.

Diagnosis

How is the diagnosis of ulcerative colitis made? This is essentially a clinical bedside problem. The most important single factor is awareness of the possibility. A history of diarrhoea, perhaps alternating with constipation, but almost invariably with mucus and often with blood in the stools, is alone sufficient to suggest a diagnosis of ulcerative colitis. Many patients are referred to hospitals treating infectious diseases, because the initial attack of colitis has been ascribed by the patient to an item of diet. Culture of the faeces to exclude known pathogenic bacteria is an essential early step in the diagnosis. In the acute case, if the result of one examination is negative, the diagnosis of ulcerative colitis should be considered until this is proved wrong. A search for amoebic dysentery should also be made, even although there is no definite history of direct exposure to this disease. The macroscopic appearance of the faeces is of value, not only as a clinical sign affecting prognosis, but also because it helps to exclude gross steatorrhoea, which occasionally comes into the differential diagnosis. Rectal examination should then be carried out to exclude carcinoma of the rectum and also as a preliminary to the most important single diagnostic investigation in colitis —namely, sigmoidoscopy. As at least 95 per cent of patients with ulcerative colitis have involvement of the rectum, sigmoidoscopy commonly puts the diagnosis beyond doubt. The most reliable index of inflammatory activity is the state of the mucosal blood vessels. A convenient sigmoidoscopic classification based on the vascularity is as follows.

Normal: The individual blood vessels can be seen in the mucosa.

Grade I colitis: There is loss of a discrete vascular pattern and a diffuse blush of the mucosa is seen with, on occasions, petechiae and contact haemorrhage.

Grade II colitis: The mucosa has a dark red colour with haemorrhagic flares rather than petechiae, and the mucosa is usually granular or roughened in appearance.

Grade III colitis: This shows intense congestion of the mucosa with overall 'weeping' of blood; the appearances have been likened to that of an over-ripe strawberry.

A biopsy of the rectum should be taken on the first occasion when a sigmoidoscopy is performed and is of particular value in confirming rectal involvement when the mucosa looks relatively normal. It does not need to be repeated each time a sigmoidoscopy is performed. Certain changes in the cells may indicate increasing instability of the epithelium and predict the onset of malignancy elsewhere in the colon. Detection of these changes demands an experienced pathologist for accurate interpretation.

Barium enema examination is of value in ulcerative colitis, not only in establishing the diagnosis, but also in defining the extent of the disease. This investigation is not without hazard in the acute case, where it may cause exacerbation of the symptoms of the colitis; or where there is marked dilatation and thinning of the bowel wall, infusion of barium could lead to perforation of the bowel. The X-ray appearances are varied, but include spasm or irritability of the colon, loss of haustration and, on occasions, ulceration of mucosa may be seen. In the chronic case the fibrosis which has followed on repeated bouts of inflammation results in shortening and narrowing of the affected area of the colon. Pseudopolyposis representing mucosal islands adjacent to areas of denuded mucosa may be seen. Some of these changes are illustrated in Figure 10.2.

The usual diagnostic criteria are a typical history, absence of known pathogenic organisms, and characteristic changes on sigmoidoscopy.

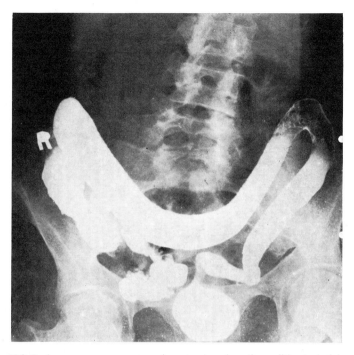

Fig. 10.2 Barium enema appearances in extensive ulcerative colitis: typical loss of haustrations, some shortening of the colon, narrowing in pelvic colon.

The results of these investigations can be available within 24 hours of first seeing the patient. Barium enema can then be carried out in order to demonstrate the extent of the disease. Delay in reaching the correct diagnosis may result in rapid deterioration of the patient's condition, with corresponding worsening of prognosis.

It is useful in day-to-day clinical practice to be able to classify the individual patient in terms of (i) clinical severity, (ii) sigmoidoscopic grading and (iii) extent of disease.

Complications

The complications of ulcerative colitis may be classified as (*a*) local, when these are in or adjacent to the bowel, and (*b*) distant or systemic complications.

The most serious local acute complications are dilatation of the colon, perforation of the colon and massive haemorrhage. Tracking of infection may occur in the paracolic region, giving rise uncommonly to pelvic abscess, fistula-in-ano or rectovaginal fistula. Stricture of the colon, although common in ulcerative colitis, rarely causes obstruction. The latter suggests the development of carcinoma in the diseased bowel. Carcinoma is more common in patients with ulcerative colitis than in the general population. The type of disease which is particularly prone to this complication is extensive colitis involving the whole colon, especially when it begins in childhood; the incidence of carcinoma increases with the duration of the disease.

The systemic complications are diverse and it is difficult to relate some of them causally to the colonic disease. These include pyoderma gangrenosum, conjunctivitis and iritis, arthritis and ankylosing spondylitis, and deep venous thrombosis. Fungal infections of the mouth and perianal region may occur. Disordered hepatic function is common in this disease and established hepatic cirrhosis is an accepted complication. The presence of severe systemic complications may be an indication for surgical treatment of the colitis, even when the colonic symptoms are themselves relatively mild.

Treatment

The treatment of ulcerative colitis can be conveniently considered under the headings of (1) supportive medical measures to combat the effects of the disease, (2) adrenocortical steroids, (3) sulphasalazine and (4) surgical operation.

Supportive measures. Close co-operation and understanding between the patient, physician and surgeon must be both soundly based and effective. It must be remembered that ulcerative colitis is often a chronic condition and always a fickle one. Changes in the course of the disease in the individual patient may occur rapidly, and it must be explained to the patient that early treatment of any relapse is imperative. He should understand in broad terms the possible natural history of the disease. The physician and surgeon should examine the patient together at frequent intervals, and certainly daily during a severe attack. When an indication for surgical treatment arises the implications must be fully explained to the patient.

For all patients being treated in hospital, a daily clinical assessment is essential. A record of bowel movements should be kept, showing the number of motions, the consistency of the faeces, the presence or absence of blood and the time when it was passed. In addition, repeated measurements should be made of haemoglobin and serum electrolyte concentrations. The abdomen should be carefully examined for the presence of abdominal distension, the bowel sounds should be noted and liver dullness should be assessed. Changes in these may occur within a few hours in the severe case, and it is only possible to assess their significance by repeated examination.

The diet should be of high calorific content, up to 3000 calories each day, and this should include 100 to 120 g of protein as there is a loss of protein in the faeces. The food should also be of a low residue type, and this can conveniently be prepared by passing it through a fine-mesh sieve. In view of the difficulty of administering such a diet to patients who may have anorexia, it is sometimes useful to include concentrated protein preparations, such as 'Complan', either with other foods or by the use of a nasogastric tube; the latter may be most conveniently given during the night with the addition of sedation, e.g. 5 mg of nitrazepam. The diet otherwise should be as varied and interesting as possible. Subclinical deficiency of essential vitamins is to be expected, both due to intestinal hurry and to secondary small intestinal malabsorption, which has been shown to be present in some patients suffering from ulcerative colitis. A multivitamin preparation should be given orally or parenterally each day to all patients with moderate or severe grades of the disease. A few patients with ulcerative colitis have been shown to be sensitive to milk and milk products. Withdrawal of these from the diet has been followed on occasions by remission of symptoms of the colitis. It is therefore valuable to assess the effect of withdrawing milk products from the diet in the individual patient. The ultimate test of its significance, however, lies in the deterioration of symptoms on reintroducing milk to the diet.

Dehydration and abnormal levels of serum electrolytes should be corrected by the administration of appropriate fluids orally or intravenously. Particular attention should be paid to the level of serum potassium, as this ion may be lost in large amounts in the faeces. The details of daily requirements of fluids and electrolytes must be dictated by the biochemical results.

Blood transfusion should be given as often as is required to maintain the haemoglobin level between 13 and 14 g per cent. This improves the patient's wellbeing, supplies additional protein and ensures that he is more able to withstand any sudden catastrophe in the illness, e.g. acute haemorrhage or the urgent need for surgical operation. The insidious onset of anaemia is not uncommon in this disease, and repeated estimations of the haemoglobin level should be made.

Many symptomatic remedies have been advocated in the treatment of ulcerative colitis. Although it might seem rational to prescribe antidiarrhoeal agents, these are usually of little value except in the mild case. The diarrhoea is an index of the course of the illness. However, during remission of the disease, when the patient may have a tendency to loose bowel motions, codeine phosphate in a dose of 30 to 60 mg by mouth two or three times daily may give symptomatic relief. Should constipation occur during a remission, a suitable preparation is emulsion of liquid paraffin with magnesium hydroxide in a dose of 4 to 16 ml daily. The prescribing of general sedatives to patients with ulcerative colitis is common practice. This is probably based on the concept that psychological factors are of major consequence in this disorder, but there is, as yet, no acceptable proof that this is the case. Only if the patient is unduly nervous and distressed, or if there is insomnia, should appropriate sedative or hypnotic drugs be prescribed, and then in full therapeutic doses. Antibiotics should not be prescribed routinely in the treatment of ulcerative colitis. It is well known that superficial colonic infection can be lessened by oral administration of streptomycin or tetracycline, but there follows the danger of staphylococcal enteritis or fungal overgrowth. In the event of the development of extracolonic infective complications, the appropriate antibiotic should be given parenterally.

What is the place of psychotherapy in the treatment of colitis? The thesis that psychological disorder can precipitate the onset of colitis remains unproven, but it seems likely that relapses can be precipitated by mental stress. It follows that relief of the latter is an important aspect of the treatment. Formal psychotherapy is rarely indicated, but sympathetic understanding and co-operation between doctor and patient are invaluable.

Adrenocortical steroids. Adrenocortical steroids are of decisive benefit to many patients with ulcerative colitis. Varied routes of administration are used under differing circumstances. Orally, the drug of choice is prednisolone in a dose of 40 to 60 mg per day in divided doses. The parenteral route is employed when nausea and vomiting are troublesome or when it is suspected that absorption from the small intestine is inadequate. Under these circumstances prednisolone 21-phosphate is given intramuscularly or in an intravenous drip infusion, in a dose of 20 mg twice daily. Topical application of adrenocortical steroid to the mucosal surface of the colon can have a beneficial effect. For patients treated in hospital, the dose of hydrocortisone hemisuccinate is 100 mg dissolved in 120 ml of water or saline, which is introduced into the lower bowel slowly over a period of 30 minutes. With the patient lying in the lateral position, the buttocks are elevated on one pillow and a fine plastic catheter is passed high into the rectum. The rate of flow is controlled by a drip infusion set to one drop per second. This slow rate allows the patient to retain the infusion usually without difficulty and the fluid has been shown to exert its effect as high as the middle of the transverse colon; this method of administration is particularly suitable in proctosigmoiditis and left-sided colitis. The solution of hydrocortisone hemisuccinate must be freshly prepared before use. A commercially available solution of 20 mg of prednisolone in a plastic bag carrying a nozzle for insertion into the rectum may be used instead of the drip method. A suppository of prednisolone, containing 5 mg of the active drug, can be used in the treatment of proctitis.

Intramuscular injections of adrenocorticotrophic hormone (ACTH) have been shown to be useful in some cases of relapse when prednisolone therapy has failed; the complications of steroid therapy are, however, more common with ACTH and the incidence of recurrence on withdrawal of the therapy is also higher than in the case of prednisolone.

Sulphasalazine. Another agent of proved therapeutic value in the treatment of ulcerative colitis is sulphasalazine. Chemically it is salicylazosulphapyridine, a substance which has been shown to have a special affinity for elastic and fibrous tissue. It is given orally in the form of tablets containing 0·5 g and is said to be taken up selectively in the submucosa of the colon, where the sulphapyridine is slowly released. A suitable dose is 0·5 to 1·5 g six-hourly. Side-effects from this drug include nausea, vomiting, headache and skin rashes. Heinz-body anaemia may occur, and agranulocytosis has been reported rarely. Suppositories of sulphasalazine, each containing 0·5 g, may be used for the treatment of proctitis.

It can be seen that there is a wide range of treatments in ulcerative colitis, and a guide to suitable regimens in differing circumstances is given in the following paragraphs.

Proctitis or proctosigmoiditis

This can prove a most intractable condition and treatment may last for many months. In addition to the supportive measures described on page 213, prednisolone suppositories of 0·5 g are given twice daily, the duration of treatment depending on the response; this should be assessed at least monthly by sigmoidoscopy. Many patients with this condition require constant psychological support and reassurance that cancer is not present.

Mild and moderate colitis

The mild or moderate type of case where the colitis is more extensive, either left-sided or involving the whole of the colon, requires a different approach. Supportive therapy is given and rectal hydrocortisone hemisuccinate in a dose of 100 mg in 120 ml of saline is given by intrarectal drip twice daily for 7 to 10 days. Sulphasalazine is given orally in addition, in a dose of 6 g per day, while milk and milk products are withdrawn from the diet. Repeated assessment, both of the number and form of the bowel motions, and of sigmoidoscopic appearances, is necessary. This therapy can be continued so long as improvement is taking place. The steroid can then be withdrawn and, if there is no relapse the sulphasalazine dosage can be reduced to 1 g four times a day, which should be continued for at least one year. There is good evidence that long-term treatment with sulphasalazine reduces the relapse rate in ulcerative colitis.

If there is no improvement on the above regime, oral prednisolone, 40 mg daily in divided doses, should be added, and in many instances this is followed by remission of symptoms in 7 to 14 days. In this event, the dose of prednisolone should gradually be reduced and then withdrawn; there is no place for long-term maintenance oral steroid therapy in this disease. Should the condition not improve on these therapies, the whole question of surgical treatment requires to be considered.

Severe colitis

The treatment of the severe case presents an urgent challenge. In the fulminant case with profound toxaemia, watery bloody diarrhoea, severe prostration and dehydration, intensive medical treatment is started forthwith. Anaemia and electrolytic disorders are promptly corrected. Prednisolone in a dose of 60 mg daily is given by intramuscular injection, in addition to rectal hydrocortisone by infusion, provided the patient can retain the fluid. From the outset the physician and surgeon should jointly assess response to treatment at frequent intervals; there is a strong likelihood of these patients requiring operation with a few days. Ideally, the surgical treatment should be postponed until the acute phase of the colitis has passed, but this is not always possible. In the patient whose condition is not truly fulminant and the question of surgical operation is not so urgent, treatment with oral or parenteral prednisolone and rectal hydrocortisone is given, in addition to full supporting therapy. There will almost certainly be symptomatic improvement because of the correction of the anaemia and the protein depletion; also the appetite may be improved because of the steroid therapy. However, it is imperative to have objective evidence before deciding that there is significant improvement in the colitis. Daily clinical assessment and repeated sigmoidoscopic examinations are helpful in this respect. A further guide is given by noting how much supplemental therapy is required in order to maintain the levels of haemoglobin and electrolytes. If there is no improvement on this treatment within two weeks, surgical operation is indicated.

Prior to surgical treatment, the implications of the operation, namely a permanent ileostomy, are explained to the patient. A patient with an ileostomy who is of the same sex and comparable social status should be invited to discuss the matter privately with the patient. In this way, many of the natural fears and anxieties associated with the prospect of an ileostomy can be allayed.

Surgical treatment may be indicated in the following situations.
1. Fulminating disease which fails to respond within a few days to adequate medical treatment. Delay should be avoided as acute dilatation and perforation are liable to occur quite rapidly. Severe haemorrhage may also develop and necessitate emergency colectomy. It is better to anticipate these complications of fulminating disease rather than be forced to deal with them by emergency procedures.
2. Chronic incapacitating disease. To decide on surgery in this group of patients requires careful assessment of the social situation of the patient and of his, or her, ability to cope with an ileostomy. Duration of disease is especially important in relation to the risk of malignant change and decreasing the likelihood of permanent remission.
3. Complications. The complications of fulminating disease have already been mentioned. Many of the chronic complications respond to medical therapy but, when they do not, colectomy may be required irrespective of the severity of the colonic disease.

4. Cancer. If there is a suspicion that malignant change has already occurred then colectomy is, of course, indicated. It has already been pointed out that younger patients with total colitis, moderately severe symptoms of ten years' duration or more, are particularly liable to malignant change. This is, therefore, a factor in deciding to advise colectomy for patients who are already being considered for surgery because of chronic incapacitating disease.

Ileostomy alone is now rarely performed. To cure the disease the colon must be excised. It would be desirable to retain the rectum so that the ileum could be joined to the rectum and ileostomy avoided. Unfortunately, this is only possible in a few cases where the rectal disease is not severe and where there is little destruction of the mucosa and wall of the rectum. In most cases the standard surgical treatment is a one-stage total proctocolectomy with the establishment of a permanent eversion ileostomy in the right iliac fossa.

The form and function of the ileostomy are of great importance. Its success depends on being able to fit a bag over the stoma by means of a flange which adheres to the skin. The ileal output is about 400 g per day, requiring the bag to be emptied two or three times and changed every day or so. There are many excellent appliances on the market and the patient should be encouraged to choose the one that suits best. The ileostomy stoma must be situated so that the bag can be easily attached and concealed by clothing; in particular, it must be clear of

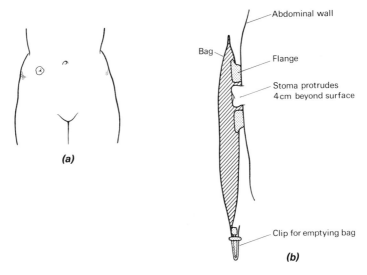

Fig. 10.3 (*a*) Ileostomy in right iliac fossa below belt line. (*b*) Ileostomy flange and bag attached to the abdominal wall with a special adhesive. The bag may be disposable or washable.

the line of the belt of skirt or trousers. It should protrude at least 4 cm from the surface so that the ileal fluid pours easily into the bag and does not macerate the skin round the stoma (Fig. 10.3).

Ileostomies are not without their problems and recently attempts have been made to fashion a reservoir with a mucosal valve from the terminal ileum which lies behind the stoma. This reservoir can be emptied two or three times a day by passing a catheter through the stoma and the wearing of a bag avoided. It is too early yet to assess the success of this procedure but it looks promising.

Ulcerative colitis constitutes a formidable challenge to medical science. The management of this disease will only be satisfactory when diagnosis is made at the earliest possible moment, when there is full co-operation between the patient and the several doctors responsible for his case, and when total proctocolectomy is carried out as a positive decision when indicated, rather than as a last resort after prolonged medical therapy. After total proctocolectomy the patient is free from the risk of recurrent colitis and has a normal life expectancy.

FURTHER READING

British Medical Journal (1974) Continent ileostomies. *British Medical Journal*, iii, 592.
de Dombal, F. T. (1974) Ulcerative colitis, epidemiology and aetiology, course and prognosis. *British Medical Journal*, i, 649.
Goligher, J. C., de Dombal, F. T., Watts, J. McK. & Watkinson, G. (1968) *Ulcerative Colitis*. London: Bailliere, Tindall and Cassell.

11. Tumours of the Intestine

Douglas Roy and F. D. Lee

CARCINOMA

Although carcinoma of the large bowel is one of the most prevalent malignant tumours encountered in this country, carcinoma of the small bowel is rare. In either situation the tumour is an adenocarcinoma of variable differentiation.

Carcinoma of the large bowel is usually a disease of older people. Little is known of its causation, although it is notable that its incidence is greatest in industrialized countries. Known predisposing conditions, such as ulcerative colitis and polyposis coli, may lead to carcinoma in relatively young individuals (i.e. less than 40 years). It is impossible to estimate how often carcinoma may arise in polypoid adenoma (p. 232) or villous papilloma (p. 234), and in most instances a recognizable predisposing cause cannot be detected. There is, however, increasing evidence that the prevalence of carcinoma of colon is related to diet. Where diet is high in protein and refined carbohydrate and low in bulk the prevalence of carcinoma of colon is high. Where the diet is bulky and largely vegetarian (as in most developing countries) the prevalence is very low. In this latter group the transit time of the intestinal contents is short and it may be that this diminishes the effects of carcinogenic substances in the diet or formed in the lumen of the intestine. Organisms of the bacteroides group of anaerobic gram negative bacteria are able to alter bile salts to substances known to be carcinogenic in animals. These organisms are present in greater numbers in the large intestine of people on low residue diets.

The rectum is the site most often involved, especially in men. The sigmoid colon is the next most common site, followed by the caecum and ascending colon; other areas are less commonly affected and the flexures rarely. Tumours complicating ulcerative colitis have a slightly different distribution, with a relatively high incidence in the proximal and transverse colon.

The tumour may present either as a 'ring stricture' or as a fungating mass with central ulceration and raised, rolled margins. Gelatinous 'colloid' variants are occasionally found. The bowel proximal to the tumour may show signs of obstruction, such as dilatation, hypertrophy or pressure (stercoral) ulceration; perforation may result from this. The caecum can accommodate large tumour masses, and growths in this site tend to cause toxic effects and anaemia rather than obstructive features. The tumour may spread (1) by direct infiltration to adjacent structures, such as stomach, bladder or pelvic wall; (2) by lymphatics to the pericolic and mesocolic lymph nodes ('transcoelomic spread' to other sites, such as the ovaries is now thought to be simply another manifestation of lymphatic spread); (3) by the bloodstream, usually to the liver.

Histologically the tumour is usually a moderately well-differentiated mucin-secreting adenocarcinoma; occasionally it is a mucoid carcinoma. In addition to direct involvement of adjacent structures, this tumour tends to spread by lymphatics at an early stage, while blood spread, especially to the liver, is often delayed. In surgical resections the degree of spread determines the prognosis to some extent, and can be assessed by Dukes' classification:

(a) Tumour involves mucosa and submucosa only: good prognosis.
(b) Tumour has completely penetrated muscularis propria: moderate prognosis.
(c) Metastatic tumour in lymph node: poor prognosis.

Obviously the pathologist must examine the tumour carefully and make a diligent search for lymph nodes in the resection. The presence of liver metastases does not necessarily imply a hopeless prognosis, since the metastasis might be solitary and potentially resectable.

Carcinoma of the small bowel possesses much the same morphological and behavioural characteristics as colonic carcinoma. Since the contents of the small bowel are liquid, obstruction has to be virtually complete before it becomes symptomatic. The prognosis is thus less favourable, since the tumour tends to present at a relatively late stage with lymph node metastasis already established.

Clinical features

Carcinoma of the colon is usually ulcerated and therefore bleeds. If the tumour is on the right side of the colon, the haemorrhage will usually only be detected in the stool on testing for occult blood, but the loss of blood may produce an iron deficiency anaemia. If on the left side of the colon or in the rectum anaemia will also occur, but it is more likely that blood will be visible in the stool.

Mucus is produced both from the crater of the ulcer and from the surrounding mucosa. If the tumour is on the left side of the colon or in the rectum excess mucus will be readily seen in the stool. If situated in the right side of colon the mucus may be so mixed with faeces as to pass undetected.

As these tumours encircle the bowel they will produce obstruction. This happens sooner on the left side than on the right side, because the lumen is narrower and the faeces firm. At first, obstruction is partial and intermittent, producing episodes of abdominal colic and constipation alternating with diarrhoea. The patient with rectal carcinoma commonly complains of the sensation of incomplete emptying of the bowel; there may be a serosanguinous discharge from the rectum. Should complete obstruction occur the systemic effects ensue (p. 174), and, if untreated, gangrene and perforation of the obstructed bowel may follow.

Spread occurs by the lymphatics and blood. The liver may become infiltrated and palpable, ascites may occur, but spread beyond the abdominal cavity is uncommon. At first loss of weight is hardly noticeable, and by the time it occurs the tumour has probably spread beyond the bowel wall.

Early clinical signs are few unless the tumour is in the rectum where it can be palpated. Anaemia can be an early sign. In the thin abdomen a tumour in the caecum or transverse colon or sigmoid colon may be felt, but this is not usual at an early stage. With the onset of obstruction, the caecum will become palpably distended. When the colon cannot be cleared of faeces following a bowel lavage, this raises the suspicion of partial obstruction by tumour. Finally the signs of complete obstruction will develop.

Investigations

Tumours between the rectosigmoid junction and the anus should be detected by sigmoidoscopy (Fig. 11.1). Since colonic tumours may be multiple, sigmoidoscopy should be done routinely even when the presence of a lesion in the proximal colon has been confirmed by barium enema.

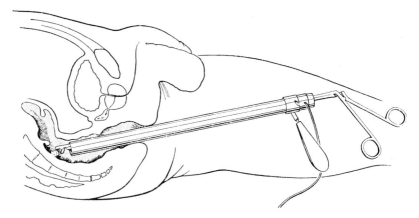

Fig. 11.1 Sigmoidoscope just below the rectosigmoid junction (usually 15 cm from the anal margin). A malignant ulcer is biopsied, and there are polyps higher in the rectum and sigmoid colon.

X-ray examination with the conventional barium enema identifies the presence of the majority of colonic tumours, but greater accuracy in detection is possible by use of 'air contrast' techniques. These involve the introduction of gas in addition to the contrast medium into the bowel.

Occult blood in the stool is an almost constant finding, but testing for this is only of value when the result is positive.

The E.S.R. is of little value as an indication of the presence or absence of a tumour, as a normal reading does not exclude the diagnosis of tumour.

Attempts have been made to identify malignant cells in colonic washings, but results have been disappointing, and the method has no clinical application at present.

An antigenic protein found in the mucosa of foetal colon (carcino-embryonic antigen, CEA) and in the cells of colonic tumours, can be demonstrated in the blood of many patients with colonic carcinoma. Unfortunately it is not specific for colonic tumours and, therefore, is not a diagnostic test of value. However, when a colonic carcinoma is excised the level of CEA in the blood falls and if it rises again this is suggestive evidence of the recurrence of the tumour and the growth of secondaries. It is, therefore, a test of some value in the follow-up of patients after operation.

Examination of the whole colon with a flexible fibre-optic endoscope (colonoscope) has been shown to be practical and to have a high diagnostic accuracy. The instrument can usually be passed as far as the splenic flexure and, often, round to the caecum. Quite small lesions can be detected and biopsied. Occasionally, if colonoscopy is not available, or if it is unsuccessful, the presence of a carcinoma can only be confirmed by laparotomy. This should be advised if clinical suspicion remains after the available diagnostic methods have proved negative.

Treatment

The aims of surgery are:

1. To excise the primary tumour with a sufficient margin above and below to avoid local recurrence.
2. To excise the local tissue into which the tumour might have spread, i.e. ischiorectal fossa or retroperitoneal tissues.
3. To excise as much of the lymphatic drainage of the area as possible in the hope that microscopic secondary deposits in lymphatics and lymph glands are removed.

It is the last of these three aims which dictates the extent of the operation and the amount of bowel which is resected.

Before going on to the details of the definitive procedures, two other aspects of the disease must be considered.

Anaemia. Should severe anaemia be present, e.g. haemoglobin less than 10 g per 100 ml, preoperative blood transfusion is required.

Obstruction. The management of this complication has already been discussed on page 179. Usually it means that the definitive procedure must be delayed and the obstruction relieved by a proximal colostomy, caecostomy or, if the tumour is in the ascending colon, an anastomosis between the ileum and the transverse colon. If the obstruction is partial, colonic washouts should be used to reduce the obstruction.

The definitive procedure

Pre-operative preparation of the bowel should involve (a) mechanical cleansing with purgatives and washouts, (b) fluid diet for three days before operation to reduce faecal bulk and (c) the oral administration of antibacterial drugs. Neomycin has been used for this purpose, but is being superseded by safer drugs such as kanamycin and metronidazole which have a wide activity against both aerobic and anaerobic organisms, and are less liable to promote a staphylococcal enteritis. Mechanical cleansing is the most important of these measures and many surgeons no longer use any oral antibiotic.

There is some evidence that it is possible for malignant cells to become implanted in the line of an anastomosis during operation. As a precaution, it is usual to wash out the lumen of the bowel at operation with 1/500 perchloride of mercury before making an anastomosis.

Tumours in the right colon (Fig 11.2)

These tumours drain into the lymphatics and glands lying along the ileocolic and right colic vessels, therefore these vessels are ligated as far proximally as possible. This inevitably means that the colon from beyond the hepatic flexure to the terminal ileum has been deprived of its blood supply and must be removed. The ileum is then anastomosed to the transverse colon. This is a *right hemicolectomy.*

Tumours of the transverse colon (Fig. 11.3)

These tumours drain into the lymphatics of the middle colic artery which is tied at its origin from the superior mesenteric artery. Therefore the whole of the transverse colon is resected and, after mobilization, the flexures are joined. This is a *transverse colectomy.*

Tumours of the left colon (Fig. 11.4)

Lymphatic drainage is into the lymphatics of the left colic vessels, and they are divided at their origin from the inferior mesenteric artery. The splenic flexure and the descending colon is therefore removed and the transverse colon anastomosed to the pelvic colon. This is a *left hemicolectomy.*

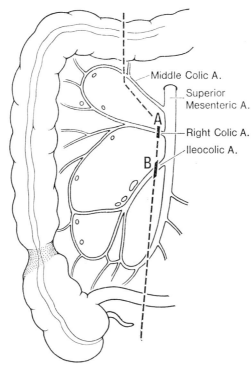

Fig. 11.2 Right hemicolectomy. The right colic and ileocolic arteries are ligated (A and B).

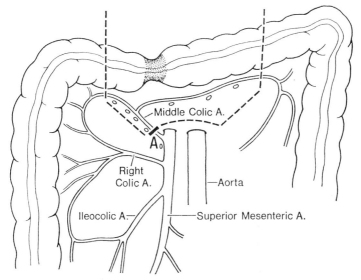

Fig. 11.3 Transverse colectomy. The middle colic artery is ligated (A).

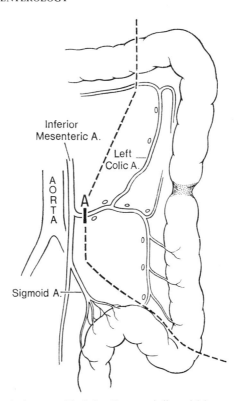

Fig. 11.4 Left hemicolectomy. The left colic artery is ligated (A).

Tumours of the sigmoid (pelvic) colon (Fig. 11.5)

Division of the sigmoid arteries results in the removal of only a limited area of lymphatics, and it is more usual to divide the inferior mesenteric artery just below the left colic vessels. The resection, therefore, extends from the lower descending colon to the upper rectum, the lower rectum being adequately nourished by the inferior and middle rectal vessels. This is a *sigmoid (pelvic) colectomy.*

Tumours of the upper half of the rectum and rectosigmoid junction (Fig. 11.6)

These are tumours lying at least 3 cm above the pelvic peritoneal floor, the lymphatics draining along the inferior mesenteric artery. The inferior mesenteric artery is divided at its origin from the aorta, and the upper line of division of the bowel is in the lower descending colon which is mobilized to be anastomosed to the lower rectum at least 6 cm below the tumour. This is an *anterior resection.*

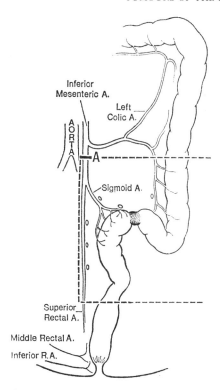

Fig. 11.5 Sigmoid colectomy. The inferior mesenteric artery is ligated (A) just below the left colic artery. The rectum is supplied by middle and inferior rectal arteries.

Tumours of the lower half of the rectum (excluding anal canal) (Fig. 11.7)

As in tumours of the upper rectum the inferior mesenteric artery is divided, but when the tumour is at the peritoneal reflexion or below it, lymphatics drain to the side wall of the pelvis into the internal iliac lymph glands. Therefore, in order to remove the lymph drainage, the lateral ligaments of the rectum, levatores ani muscles and the contents of the ischiorectal fossae must be removed. The lower rectum and anal canal are therefore sacrificed and the patient must have a terminal colostomy of the descending colon in the left iliac fossa. This is an *abdominoperineal excision of the rectum.*

RESECTABILITY AND CURABILITY

If, at operation, there is no obvious sign of spread of the tumour outside the operative field the operation can be regarded as an attempt to cure the patient, although often there is recurrence because microscopic spread has been present. If there are obvious secondary deposits in

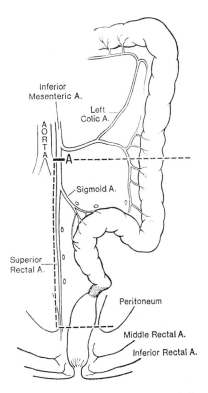

Fig. 11.6 Anterior resection. The inferior mesenteric artery is ligated below (or above) the left colic branch (A). The rectal stump is nourished by the inferior and middle rectal vessels.

lymph glands, on peritoneal surfaces or in the liver the tumour may still be *resectable* and this is worth doing. To remove the tumour is to remove symptoms that may become an increasing cause of suffering, even although the life span of the patient may not be greatly increased. If the tumour is *unresectable* (inoperable) then palliation may be achieved either by *proximal colostomy* or by an anastomosis between the bowel above and below the tumour, for example between the transverse and sigmoid colon in the case of an inoperable carcinoma of splenic flexure.

Colostomy

A colostomy may be performed as a temporary measure to relieve obstruction with a view to later resection of the tumour and closure of the colostomy, or it may be fashioned as a permanent procedure. A permanent colostomy may be required either following resection of the rectum or proximal to an inoperable, obstructing carcinoma.

A colostomy may be in the caecum, transverse or sigmoid colon

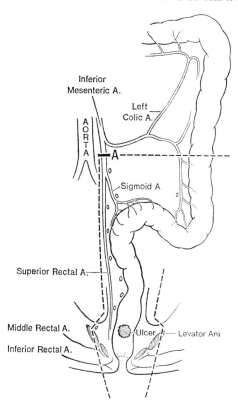

Fig. 11.7 Abdominoperineal excision of the rectum. The inferior mesenteric artery is ligated below (or above) the left colic branch (A). The levators ani muscles, the pelvic fascia covering them and the contents of the ischiorectal fossae are excised with the rectum. An iliac colostomy is required.

(Fig. 11.8) and is usually performed by exteriorizing a loop of colon which may be divided completely so that faeces cannot pass into the distal colon. When the bowel below it has been excised, the divided end is brought out as a direct opening.

If the colostomy is permanent it must be sited carefully so that the patient finds it easy to fit an appliance to it. It should be clear of any bony prominence, such as the anterior superior iliac spine, of the umbilicus and of operation scars. The patient must be reassured, preferably before operation, about his ability to manage the colostomy. The majority of patients can regulate the size and frequency of bowel motions by altering their diet and intake of fluid. Further control can be exercised with methyl cellulose (Celevac), which increases the bulk of the stools, or by codeine phosphate, which slows the passage of the faecal stream. It is desirable that a patient with a colostomy should have

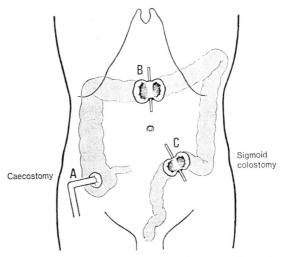

Caecostomy

Sigmoid
colostomy

Fig. 11.8 Caecostomy (A). The bowel is drained with a wide glass tube. Transverse colostomy (B). The bowel is exteriorized over a glass rod. Sigmoid colostomy (C). The bowel is exteriorized in the same way.

well-formed or even constipated stools. Despite all measures, however, some patients have fluid motions, and, if so, the appliance they wear should be adapted to cope with them.

For more detailed advice regarding prevention and management of the various problems associated with a colostomy there are available several excellent booklets, e.g. *The Care of Your Colostomy*, by Goligher and Pollard (published by Baillière, Tindall and Cassell, London).

Prognosis

This depends largely upon the nature of the tumour. The five-year survival rate is probably between 44 and 25 per cent, and the Registrar-General's figures suggest that the lower figure is probably the more accurate if all tumours, treated and untreated, are included. Tumours in the left colon have a better prognosis than those in the right colon, which, in turn, have a better prognosis than those in the rectum. It is possible to predict with some accuracy the prognosis by classifying the cells of the tumour according to Dukes' classification and considering the evidence of spread both to local lymph glands resected with the tumour and through the muscular wall to the serosal surface of the bowel.

Malignant tumours of the anal canal

The important difference from tumours of the lower rectum is that the lymphatic drainage goes to the inguinal lymph nodes as well as to the side walls of the true pelvis and upwards along the inferior mesenteric artery. Therefore, in addition to excision of the tumour, block dissection of inguinal glands on both sides must be carried out. Some surgeons do this only if and when there is evidence of infiltration of these glands, but some prefer to do it in all cases as a prophylactic measure. The evidence either way is, as yet, inconclusive.

Small squamous carcinomas may be locally excised or treated with radiotherapy, but all other malignant tumours should be removed by an abdominoperineal excision.

CONNECTIVE TISSUE TUMOURS

Simple tumours of this type, although seldom symptomatic, are probably much more common than is usually realized. This is especially true of the leiomyoma, but may also apply to other tumours such as the lipoma, the haemangioma and the lymphangioma. Malignant change is unusual, being seen most often in smooth muscle tumours (leiomyosarcoma).

Clinical features

The only clinical importance of these tumours is that they may produce an intussusception, resulting in small bowel obstruction (Fig. 11.9).

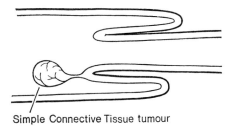

Simple Connective Tissue tumour

Fig. 11.9 A simple connective tissue tumour causing a small bowel intussusception. The tumour is gripped by the bowel wall and is at the apex.

Treatment

If at laparotomy an intussusception of the small bowel is found, other than in the ileocaecal region in children, then it should be assumed that a tumour must be removed to prevent recurrence.

Lymphoma

Although uncommon relative to carcinoma in stomach and colon, lymphoid tumours account for 50 per cent of malignant neoplasms in the small bowel. Most of these tumours are of poorly differentiated types, i.e. reticulosarcoma and lymphosarcoma. These tumours are usually primary in the gut and not as a rule part of a generalized reticulosis. Frequently they are multiple, present by producing small bowel perforation and tend to recur following resection. Initial spread is to the mesenteric lymph nodes. Malabsorption may be a feature, and there is evidence that gluten-sensitive enteropathy predisposes to their development.

The polypoid lymphoid tumours of the rectum (usually found in young adults) are the only benign lesions in this group.

Neoplastic polyps

The term polyp simply means a lesion protruding from an epithelial surface and does not imply any specific pathological process. In the intestine, the most important type is the neoplastic polyp, which is a simple tumour arising from the intestinal mucosa, especially in the large bowel. Histologically these tumours vary in structure, with the adenomatous polyp, consisting exclusively of glandular elements, at one end of a spectrum, and the villous papilloma, composed mainly of papillary fronds arising from the epithelial surface, at the other. Many, however, show a mixed pattern and might exhibit the behavioural characteristics of either of the two main types.

Adenomatous polyps

These tumours might be single or multiple and, although commonly associated with carcinoma, have a more diffuse distribution in the colon than carcinoma, and tend to develop at an earlier age. They are rare in the small bowel. Globular in shape and raised above the mucosa surface upon a stalk, they consist histologically of proliferating glands. Varying degrees of epithelial dedifferentiation especially towards the 'fundus' are typical; this is recognized by nuclear hyperchromatism and loss of cell polarity and may, on some occasions, be so marked as to merit the designation carcinoma *in situ*. Provided, however, that there is no evidence of invasion, most readily seen at the base of the stalk, the prognosis is good. It is thus obvious that excision must include the base of the lesion before such an assessment can be made. The extent to which these tumours become frankly malignant is a disputed matter, but it is unlikely to be greater than 1 per cent.

The controversy about their relationship to carcinoma accounts for the differing attitude of clinicians to them. It is our belief that the risk of carcinomatous change in these polyps has been overestimated in the past. Their prevalence, however, does follow that of carcinoma and they are rare in developing countries where the diet is bulky and carcinoma uncommon.

Clinical features

Commonly these tumours are discovered as a result of investigation for rectal bleeding. Less commonly they may prolapse through the anus or give rise to an intussusception which may be transitory, so that the patient complains of episodes of large bowel colic.

Investigation

If the polyp is in the rectum it can be seen through the sigmoidoscope, biopsied, and, indeed, it may even be removed with a diathermy snare (Fig. 11.10). The introduction of the colonoscope has made it possible to locate and identify adenomatous polyps in any part of the colon. These can then be excised with a diathermy snare both to obtain histological evidence of their nature and also as a form of treatment which avoids the need for laparotomy.

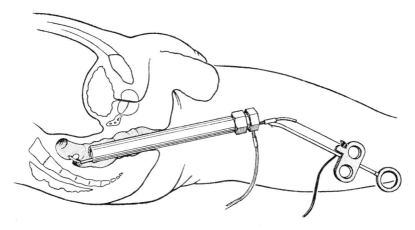

Fig. 11.10 The polyp is viewed through the sigmoidoscope. A snare connected to a diathermy source is tightened round its base to remove it.

However, polyps are often multiple and may be associated with carcinoma elsewhere in the colon. In every case the whole colon must be examined by an air contrast barium enema (Fig. 11.11). It is only after the bowel has been thoroughly emptied by suitable aperients that one can be sure that filling defects are due to polyps and not to faecal masses.

Treatment

This largely depends on the pathologist's report and the clinician's opinion as to the danger of each polyp.

If, regardless of the degree of epithelial dedifferentiation in the polyp, there is no evidence of invasion of the pedicle, then excision of the polyp together with its pedicle and some adjacent mucosa is sufficient. If invasion is, however, present the lesion is regarded as carcinoma and is treated accordingly.

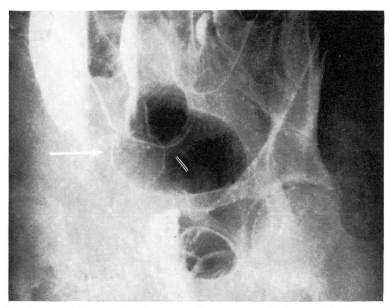

Fig. 11.11(*a*) 'Air contrast' barium enema showing a polyp in the sigmoid colon.

A polyp may be removed by drawing it through the anus if it is low enough, by excision through a sigmoidoscope or colonoscope, or by colotomy following laparotomy.

When the colonic mucosa has produced one or a crop of polyps, it is liable to produce more in the future. These patients should, therefore, be followed up with sigmoidoscopy, colonoscopy and barium examinations for several years, ideally indefinitely.

It is probably true that all polyps under 5 mm in diameter are benign.

Villous papilloma

This tumour is confined to the large bowel, the rectum being most often involved. In contrast to the polypoid adenoma it is a sessile tumour and may arise from an extensive area of mucosa. The surface is distinctly papillary to the naked eye, and histologically the tumour presents a frond-like pattern (Fig. 11.12). The epithelium lining the villous projections often shows extensive mucin secretion, but some degree of dedifferentiation and loss of polarity is usual and malignant transformation is by no mean uncommon. Malignancy is said to be more likely to arise in these tumours than in adenomas, although this might be due to the greater size of villous papillomas at the time of presentation.

Clinical features

The very large mucosal surface of these tumours gives rise to an

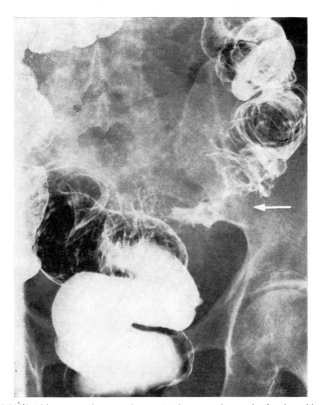

Fig. 11.11(*b*) 'Air contrast' enema demonstrating a carcinoma in the sigmoid colon.

excessive secretion of mucus, water and electrolytes. The patient may suffer from severe watery diarrhoea which contains well-formed faecal masses. If the tumour ulcerates, and this often indicates malignancy, there will also be blood in the stool. The patient may have had diarrhoea for many months before seeking advice because the growth of the tumour is slow.

Some patients can lose so much water and electrolytes that they become dehydrated. Hypokalaemia may develop, producing mental disorder and coma.

Investigation

Eighty per cent of these tumours are within the range of the sigmoidoscope and their characteristic appearance makes diagnosis easy. Biopsies should be taken from several areas of the tumour, but even if they all show a simple pattern some part of the tumour may be malignant. All villous papillomata should be regarded with suspicion. 'Air contrast' barium enema will be required to demonstrate the tumours which lie above the lower sigmoid segment of the colon.

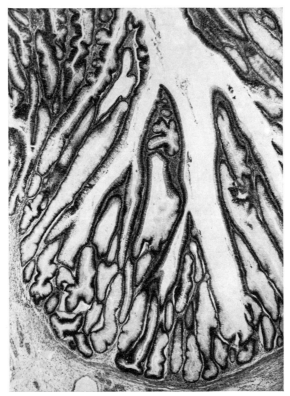

Fig. 11.12 Villous papilloma. This tumour consists of finger-like projections of the lamina propria lined by mucin-secreting epithelium.

Treatment

Any electrolyte disturbance should be corrected and the tumour should be excised completely. If there is no evidence of malignancy on biopsy or at operation the resection of involved bowel can be conservative, but if malignant then the appropriate radical procedure should be performed (p. 226). Occasionally in old people or in the case of small tumours, where adequate biopsies have shown no malignant change, diathermy excision through a sigmoidoscope is justified.

Polyposis coli

This uncommon condition is inherited as a Mendelian dominant of high penetrance—which means that the actual number of observed cases in a family closely approaches the expected number. The entire colon may be involved and enormous numbers of polyps (up to 5000) may be present. Histologically each lesion presents the appearance of a polypoid adenoma (p. 232) with varying degrees of epithelial dedifferentiation. The development of carcinoma is almost invariable and usually takes place 10 to 15 years after the onset of the disease and often before the age of 40 years. Polyposis coli can, however, present for the first time in late adult life.

Clinical features

These polyps do not usually appear until the second decade of life, when the patient will begin to complain of diarrhoea with increasing quantities of mucus. Fresh blood is not usually seen and if present is only in small amounts, unless a carcinoma has developed. If another member of the family is already affected, the significance of the symptoms should be immediately recognized, but they may also occur in cases without a family history, the patient being the first one in the family to be affected by the genetic mutation. The hereditary nature of the disease should be explained to the patient so that other members of the family can be carefully examined at regular intervals.

Treatment

The aim is to prevent the development of carcinoma which is almost certainly going to occur sooner or later. The only way to prevent this with certainty is to excise the colon and rectum leaving the patient with an ileostomy. However, if the rectum does not bear too many polyps it is acceptable to excise the colon and upper one-third of the rectum, anastomosing the ileum to the lower rectum, the rectum having been cleared of its polyps by diathermy. The patient must then be followed up for life so that any further polyps in the remaining rectum can be removed by diathermy through a sigmoidoscope.

Juvenile polyp

This lesion may be quite large and frequently shows surface ulceration. Histologically it consists of dilated cysts lined by flattened or well-differentiated epithelium and embedded in intensely inflamed lamina propria. It is probably hamartomatous in origin and not truly neoplastic.

Clinical features

These benign tumours present in young children by bleeding or prolapse through the anus.

Treatment

Simple excision is all that is required.

Metaplastic polyp

These common lesions, often multiple, appear to the naked-eye as small pale, sessile polyps only a few millimetres in diameter, and are usually found incidentally. Histologically they show a curious 'feathery' alteration in the surface epithelium, and the mucosal crypts are often irregular and hyperchromatic. These polyps do not cause symptoms and have no tendency towards malignant change.

Carcinoid tumour of the intestine (argentaffinoma)

This rare tumour usually arises from the argentaffin cell, which resides in the intestinal epithelium, and indeed in the epithelium of other structures of endodermal origin, e.g. respiratory tract and stomach, and belongs to the APUD (amine precursor uptake and decarboxylation) system of cells, which are thought to be of neural crest origin and to subserve an endocrine function. Carcinoid tumours are usually recognisable to the naked eye by their bright yellow colour.

The appendix and ileum are most often affected. In these sites the tumour has a characteristic histology, the cells usually exhibiting the argentaffin reaction which is probably a reflexion of their capacity to secrete 5-hydroxy-tryptamine (5-HT, serotonin). In stomach and colon the tumours are often atypical histologically. Appendiceal carcinoids are almost always benign despite histological evidence of invasion, hence the term 'carcinoid'. On the other hand ileal carcinoids, which are often multiple, usually behave as malignant tumours, and metastasize to the mesenteric lymph nodes and liver. The malignancy is, however, of a low grade and patients may survive, with metastases, for prolonged periods. These tumours secrete 5-HT, or its percursor 5-hydroxytryptophane, and possibly other substances, such as bradykinin.

Clinical features

Although these interesting tumours secrete 5-HT many of them present with local symptoms and signs before sufficient amounts of this hormone have been secreted to produce systemic manifestations—the carcinoid syndrome.

Local manifestations

About 60 per cent of the tumours occur in the appendix and present the picture of appendicular 'colic' or acute appendicitis, and, if they have not already given rise to secondary deposits, are unlikely to be diagnosed before laparatomy. Of those that occur in the small intestine about half will present with intestinal obstruction. A few occur in the colon and rectum where they are said to be particularly benign; they occur rarely in the stomach, ovary, testis or lung.

Carcinoid syndrome

This requires a sufficient mass of tumour tissue to produce large quantities of 5-HT and therefore the tumour is usually malignant. Since 5-HT is destroyed in the liver (and in the lung) by the enzyme amine oxidase, the carcinoid syndrome is usually associated with massive liver metastases which can secrete directly into the systemic circulation.

(a) *Carcinoid 'flush'*. This is usually regarded as being episodic, but it may be persistent. The face and the upper part of the body are particularly affected. The flush is often 'blotchy' in appearance with areas of cyanosis. It is due to vasodilatation, and is usually made worse by the ingestion of alcohol. As the flush occurs tachycardia develops and the blood pressure, after an initial fall, rises above the preflush level. There is, therefore, an increase in cardiac output.

This flush does not seem to be caused by 5-HT alone, but appears to require the presence of another agent, probably also produced by the tumour, and possibly bradykinin, to produce an alteration in the reactivity of the skin vessels. We do not yet know all the substances with physiological activity which are produced by these tumours.

(b) *Abdominal manifestations*. These are unrelated to obstruction, although obstruction may alter their pattern. Colicky abdominal pain and distension occur, and diarrhoea with watery, unformed motions leads to potassium loss and dehydration. Barium given orally passes rapidly through the small intestine. The accelerated passage of bowel contents leads to malabsorption which can often be demonstrated by the usual tests. The muscle of the bowel wall is hypertrophied, and there is dilatation above the tumour if there is an element of obstruction. These changes seem to be the result of direct stimulation by 5-HT.

Secondary masses in the abdomen may be palpable and deposits in the liver may also be felt. Auscultation over the abdomen confirms the impression of increased bowel activity.

(c) *Cardiac lesions*. Cardiac lesions mainly affecting the right side of the heart tend to occur late in the syndrome. It has been shown that the concentration of 5-HT in the blood falls after passage through the pulmonary bed where it is inactivated by an amine oxidase, so that the left side of the heart is largely protected. The pulmonary and tricuspid valves are distorted and their cusps fuse, resulting in lesions which are usually stenotic, although incompetence of the tricuspid valve may occur. Right ventricular hypertrophy develops.

Once cardiac changes occur they are likely to be progressive and the patient may die of heart failure. An 'injection-type' systolic murmur heard at the left sternal margin is the most common clinical indication of the lesion in the pulmonary valve, and enlargement of the heart may be demonstrated radiologically. Catheterization will show a rise in the right ventricular pressure and low pressure in the pulmonary artery.

(d) *Other features*. Asthmatic attacks may occur and be precipitated by handling the tumour; bronchospasm can occur during operation.

Oedema and oliguria have been reported and some patients may pass urine which becomes burgundy-coloured after standing in the light for a few minutes; this colour is thought to be due to the production of indole during the formation of 5-HT.

It is interesting that 5-HT does not pass the blood-brain barrier, so that these patients do not develop the psychological changes that might have been expected from the known effect of this substance on the cells of the cerebrum.

Diagnosis

While the clinical features and radiological study of small bowel pattern may allow a presumptive diagnosis to be made, estimation of 5-hydroxyindole acetic acid (5-HIAA), a metabolite of 5-HT, in the urine is a reliable index of the presence of tumour tissue. Excretion of 2 to 10 mg of 5-HIAA per 24 hours is regarded as normal. This test may also be used to detect recurrence of the tumour after surgery.

Treatment

(a) *Surgical.* The object is to carry out a wide resection of the tumour and its lymphatic drainage. Sometimes a diagnosis is only made on pathological examination of the excised appendix, and if there is no evidence of tumour tissue near to the line of excision, and likewise no gross evidence of lymph node enlargement in the ileocaecal area, most surgeons would not advise re-exploration of the abdomen. However, where pathological examination revealed tumour near the base of the appendix or there was any uncertainty regarding localized lymph node enlargement, a formal right hemicolectomy would be advised. Even when there are widespread deposits of tumour it is worthwhile removing as much tumour tissue as possible in an attempt to prevent development of the carcinoid syndrome. Patients may live for many years despite secondary deposits, and are most likely to die from the cardiac lesions.

(b) *Medical.* It would be most useful if there were a drug available which would antagonize the actions of 5-HT. Unfortunately, such antagonists have serious physiological and psychic side-effects and some which are active in animals are inactive in man. Phenol acetic acid interferes with the metabolism of 5-HT and has been used with some success. Anticholinergic drugs may reduce the diarrhoea, and chalk and opium may also be helpful. There is, however, at present no drug therapy which satisfactorily controls the systemic effects of 5-HT.

Peutz-Jegher syndrome

This rare condition is inherited as an autosomal dominant with high penetrance. It is mainly characterized by melanosis of the skin and mucous membranes (only the latter persisting into adult life) and the development of polyps, usually in the small bowel, although sometimes in the stomach and colon. The intestinal polyps are, unlike the polypoid adenomata (p. 232), highly differentiated and all the epithelial elements of normal mucosa—absorptive epithelium, goblet cells, argentaffin cells and Paneth cells—are represented in normal proportion. This would suggest that they are hamartomas, i.e. tumour-like malformations, rather than true tumours. The early belief that malignancy is common (due to the fact that some polyps appear to be embedded initially in the intestinal musculature) is almost certainly incorrect. True malignant change (in the small bowel at any rate) is extremely rare.

Clinical features

The numerous polyps in this rare condition affect mainly the jejunum. They may cause no symptoms at all, and then the only clinical feature to be demonstrated is the melanotic pigmentation around the lips and in the mucous membrane of the mouth. If they do cause symptoms these present as episodes of acute or subacute obstruction, or anaemia due to loss of blood from ulceration of the surface of the polyps.

Treatment

If treatment is required because of haemorrhage or recurrent obstruction no attempt is made to resect all the bowel affected by polyp formation. As malignancy is rare an extensive resection is not necessary and might lead to malabsorption. Small segments of bowel may be resected if they are packed with polyps, or an enterotomy can be performed and large polyps excised.

FURTHER READING

Calman, K. C. (1975) Tumour immunology and the gut. *Gut*. **16,** 490–500.
Lancet (1971) Treatment of colo-rectal cancer. *Lancet*. ii, 537.
Lancet (1974) Beware of the ox. *Lancet*. i, 791–792.

12. Diverticular Disease of the Colon

M. Kennedy Browne

Anatomy and physiology

An understanding of the pathogenesis of diverticular disease in the colon requires some basic knowledge about its muscle wall, blood supply and motility patterns. The smooth muscle of the wall of the colon is arranged in two layers, an inner circular and an outer longitudinal. The longitudinal layer is concentrated into three thick bands, the taeniae coli. One, the mesenteric taenia, lies adjacent to the mesentery, while the other two, the antimesenteric taeniae, lie 120° apart (Fig. 12.1). The outer layer is considerably shorter than the inner one so that the circular muscle is plicated in a concertina-like fashion to form a large number of saccules called haustrations. The circular muscle fibres are arranged in the form of a loose meshwork rather than a solid wall.

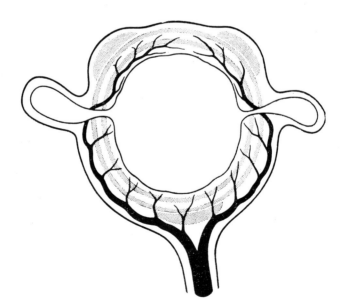

Fig. 12.1 Cross-section of colon showing correlation between position of diverticula and the site for penetration of the arterioles through the muscularis.

The artery to a segment of colon travels through the mesentery until it reaches the junction of mesentery with colon where it divides into two branches. These travel round the segment between the serosa and muscularis to the midpoints between the mesenteric and antimesenteric taeniae, at which point they penetrate the muscularis to enter the submucosa.

Transport of material in the colon is dependent upon the development of rings of contraction between haustrations, followed by contraction of the smooth muscle in such segments. When interhaustral rings contract a segment is isolated from the rest of the alimentary tract so that contraction of the smooth muscle in its wall produces a rise in pressure at this site. If this is followed by relaxation of one of the two rings enclosing a segment, the increased pressure results in propulsion of the colonic contents, as shown in Figure 12.2a.

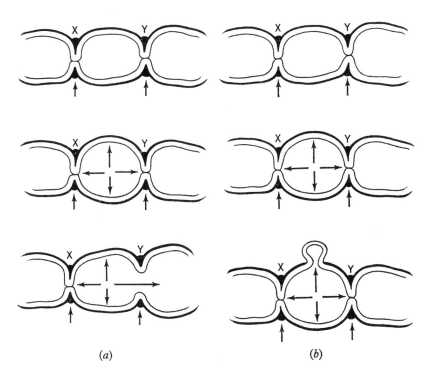

(a)   (b)

Fig. 12.2(a) Normal motility patterns in the colon. Contraction rings are formed at x and y followed by contraction of the muscle in segment xy resulting in an increased intraluminal pressure. Relaxation of segment y results in contents being propelled in that direction. (b) Abnormal motility patterns in the colon. Contraction rings are formed at x and y followed by contraction of the muscle in segment xy. Failure in relaxation of either x or y results in increasing intraluminal pressure leading to herniation of the mucosa through the muscularis.

Pathology and pathogenesis

Diverticular disease of the colon is characterized by the herniation of mucosa through the muscularis to form flask-shaped saccules lying between the mesenteric and antimesenteric taeniae. The saccules are found most often and in greatest numbers around the sigmoid colon but may involve any part of the colon. Extensive diverticular disease of any part of the large bowel without involvement of the sigmoid colon, however, is rare. Infection of diverticula may occur and spread to surrounding tissues.

Surveys have shown that the condition is one of middle or old age. It is rare below the age of 40, but radiological surveys suggest that diverticula exist in approximately 35 per cent of those over 60. There is a slight female preponderance over the age of 60, but there is an equal sex incidence below this age. The disease is much less common in Africans than in European communities. This may be related to the higher roughage of the African diet and not to any genetic predisposition. This is suggested by the fact that in the United States of America the incidence is similar for Caucasians and Negroes.

Examination of sections of colon affected by diverticular disease shows gross thickening and shortening of the taeniae coli resulting in increased folding and congestion of the circular muscle layer; there is also true hypertrophy of circular muscle fibres. Such changes have been found at the earliest stages of diverticular disease, suggesting that increased muscle wall activity could well play a part in the formation of diverticula. It is also noteworthy that saccules occur between the mesenteric and antimesenteric taeniae in close relation to perforation of the muscularis by branches of the mesenteric arteries. This would suggest that herniation occurs through points of greatest weakness. The proximity of the diverticula to large blood vessels would explain the severity of bleeding sometimes encountered in this condition.

Recent studies combining manometry with cineradiography have done much to support the possibility that diverticular disease may be due to a disordered motility pattern in the large bowel (Fig. 12.2b). Under resting conditions the activity in healthy and diverticular colon is almost identical, but in diverticular disease there is an abnormal response to the administration of morphine or prostigmine. Each of these drugs produces marked segmentation of the affected apart of the colon, followed by contraction of smooth muscle and marked increase in intraluminal pressure in the segments. It is tempting to suggest that such stimuli as food, drink or emotion may initiate the same pattern of disordered activity. A similar disturbance of motility has been encountered in the irritable colon syndrome. This is one of the commonest upsets in colonic function and although previously thought to represent the earliest stages of diverticular disease, there is no real evidence to support this. The basic lesion underlying such bowel dysfunction has not yet been adequately explained.

Clinical features

In the past, diverticular disease of the colon has been classified into diverticulosis and diverticulitis. In diverticulosis sacculation of the bowel is uncomplicated, whereas in diverticulitis there is inflammation of the saccules. Recent work has shown that many radiological and pathological features, formerly thought to be pathognomic of diverticulitis, may occur in the earliest stages of uncomplicated diverticular disease, so that the distinction between diverticulosis and diverticulitis is almost impossible. This being so, the two conditions are better grouped under the single heading of diverticular disease.

Diverticular disease is often asymptomatic and will remain unidentified unless a barium enema is performed in the investigation of some unrelated condition. In many patients symptoms are mild and may take the form of flatulence, diarrhoea or constipation, never severe enough to warrant seeking medical advice. Some patients complain of either diarrhoea or constipation as the predominating feature, whereas others may suffer from intermittent bouts of both. Lower abdominal discomfort is a common symptom. This may be continuous or may be related to defaecation or to meals. Such features can be directly related to disordered activity of the sigmoid colon and it is possible that they may precede the development of diverticula in many subjects. Similar symptoms are found in spastic colon. Alternating constipation and diarrhoea are common, as are distension, flatulence and pain. Unlike diverticular disease, however, all investigations will prove to be negative.

The majority of cases of diverticular disease do not proceed beyond this stage, but in about 25 per cent more acute attacks occur which may complicate previous symptoms or appear unheralded. Symptoms in this group include malaise, anorexia, nausea or vomiting, severe lower abdominal pain and marked constipation or profuse watery diarrhoea. There is often pyrexia, with marked guarding and tenderness in the left iliac fossa. Polymorphonuclear leucocytosis and elevation of the E.S.R. are common.

The condition which most commonly gives rise to problems in differential diagnosis is carcinoma of the sigmoid or descending colon. Both conditions can give rise to lower abdominal discomfort, anaemia, diarrhoea or constipation and a palpable abnormal mass in the left iliac fossa. There are, however, several differentiating features. Pyrexia is more commonly associated with diverticular disease than with carcinoma. Anaemia is associated with both diseases, but in carcinoma this is usually related to mild continous blood loss whereas in diverticular disease haemorrhage may be episodic and profuse. It should be recognized that both diseases occur in the same age group so that a dual pathology may be encountered. The frequency with which asymptomatic diverticular disease occurs in elderly patients should also put the clinician on his guard against too readily accepting the demonstration of a few diverticula in the sigmoid colon as an explanation for all of a patient's alimentary symptoms. He should also appreciate that carcinoma may develop after the onset of diverticular disease, so that with each exacerbation a fresh assessment and investigation of the diagnosis must be made.

Radiology

Radiological investigation is essential for the accurate diagnosis of diverticular disease. In the more acute stages this may not be possible and several weeks may elapse before a barium enema can be performed. The barium enema shows several characteristic features:

1. A short segment of colon, usually sigmoid colon, may be narrowed and show hypersegmentation due to spasticity of the bowel wall.
2. Diverticula may be obvious as barium-filled saccules (Fig. 12.3).
3. The involved segment may show a 'saw-toothed' effect (Fig. 12.3).

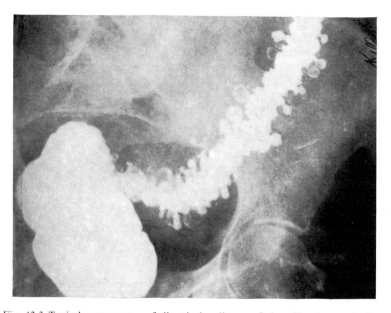

Fig. 12.3 Typical appearances of diverticular disease of sigmoid colon on barium enema examination: non-inflamed diverticula filled with barium; 'saw-tooth' appearance of inflamed or spastic segment.

Current manometric and cineradiographic evidence suggests that the 'saw-toothing' represents a prediverticular stage in which mucosa has only partially penetrated the lattice-work of circular smooth muscle.

A distinction must be made between narrowing of a segment due to spasticity and that due to stenosis. This may sometimes be difficult during the course of a normal barium enema, and in this situation the parenteral administration of an anticholinergic agent can be of value. Such a manoeuvre products relaxation of a spastic segment of bowel, but has no effect upon a stenotic area.

Sigmoidoscopy is part of the routine investigation of patients with diverticular disease. The mouths of diverticula are rarely seen, but the presence of increased sacculation and spasticity may provide indirect evidence of their presence. The main value of sigmoidoscopy lies in the exclusion of other lesions such as carcinoma or ulcerative colitis, which may co-exist with diverticular disease.

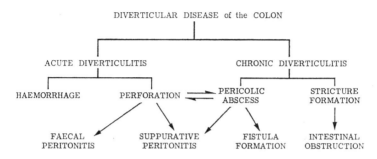

Fig. 12.4

Complications

The complications of diverticular disease of the colon are all inflammatory and are summarized in Figure 12.4. In an acute attack of inflammation there is an exacerbation of the signs and symptoms. The patient has an increase of pain in the left iliac fossa accompanied by diarrhoea, pyrexia, a rise in the leucocyte count and in the E.S.R. Examination reveals a tender, palpable sigmoid colon. In favourable circumstances, or with prompt medical treatment, these symptoms will subside leaving the original complaints as before; in some cases each attack leaves increasingly thickened colon with worsening symptoms and steady progression towards stricture formation. As has been pointed out, the diverticula occur in the bowel at the point of entry of the blood vessels, which therefore lie in intimate relation to them. During a bout of acute inflammation there may be erosion of a blood vessel at its point of entry into the bowel, resulting in a sudden severe haemorrhage. This complication tends to occur more often in older patients and it may occasionally be the presenting symptom. There is profuse rectal bleeding of red blood with associated shock and collapse. The haemorrhage usually stops as suddenly as it starts and rarely requires surgical intervention, but blood transfusion may be required. Apart from these dramatic episodes of bleeding there is often a slow continuous loss of blood, rendering patients anaemic.

During acute inflammation a diverticulum may rupture, resulting in generalized peritonitis. This may be suppurative and present as a pelvic peritonitis of unknown origin, or the prodromal symptoms of pain in the left iliac fossa may indicate the source. The peritonitis differs in no way from that due to any other infective process, e.g. acute appendicitis, and carries a similar mortality. If, however, faecal material escapes into the peritoneum a most severe form of peritonitis develops, accompanied by profound shock and cardiovascular collapse, which closely resembles the effect of the release of endotoxin into the circulation. The mortality of this condition has not improved markedly with modern resuscitative techniques and antibiotics, and remains at over 50 per cent.

Chronic diverticulitis applies to a bowel which has been subject to repeated bouts of inflammation, with resultant fibrosis and adhesion to surrounding structures. This in itself may cause signs of subacute obstruction or merely an increase in the symptoms found in uncomplicated diverticular disease. The final obstructive picture may be precipitated by a superimposed acute attack which leads to a pericolic abscess occluding the already narrowed lumen. When the colon has been the site of repeated attacks of inflammation, adhesions have usually developed and rupture of a diverticulum leads to the formation of a localized abscess. The patient exhibits the signs of suppuration with a high swinging fever, tachycardia, leucocytosis and raised E.S.R. He complains of pain in the left iliac fossa, with vomiting and perhaps diarrhoea or constipation, and examination reveals the presence of a tender mass in the left iliac fossa. This inflammatory mass may resolve and the underlying lesion can be resected several weeks later. On the other hand, the abscess may rupture, leading to suppurative peritonitis. More commonly, however, the abscess ruptures into a viscus which has become adherent to it, resulting in fistula formation, e.g. to the ileum, transverse colon or bladder. Rarely, either spontaneously or following on surgical drainage, the abscess may open on to the skin surface to form an external faecal fistula. As is to be expected from anatomical considerations, a vesicocolic fistula is one of the commonest varieties and it is most dramatic in its presentation. The flow is always from colon to bladder and the complaint is of pneumaturia, or the passage of faecal material in the urine. The history is diagnostic and further investigations rarely add any new information. A severe cystitis is present but cystoscopy rarely demonstrates the fistula and barium enema is likewise unhelpful. Nevertheless, these investigations should be carried out to exclude carcinoma as the causative factor. Fistulous connexions to other parts of the bowel result in a short circuit. This may cause malabsorption, weight loss, diarrhoea, and general debility.

Other complications are those general upsets associated with any infective lesion of the large bowel, pruritus ani, anaemia and general debility, but cutaneous eruptions do not occur with diverticulitis.

In the more rarely encountered right-sided diverticulitis or solitary diverticulum of the caecum, the inflammation produces changes indistinguishable from appendicitis and its complications, and many of the so-called 'caecal ulcers' may be inflamed diverticula.

Treatment

A clearer understanding of the aetiology in diverticular disease has led to the development of a more rational scheme of therapy. Treatment varies with the severity of the condition.

When symptoms are chronic and mild, particular attention should be given to altering the motility pattern of the large bowel. This may be achieved to some extent by the administration of anticholinergic agents. Propantheline hydrobromide is the most widely used in diverticular disease. It has both an anticholinergic and a ganglion-blocking action. The normal oral dosage is 15 mg three times daily, but when this is not effective it may be increased to 30 mg three times daily. With the larger dose, side-effects related to the drug's anticholinergic activity are encountered fairly often. These include dryness of the mouth, blurring of vision, and difficulty with micturition. Some authorities recommend a small regular dose of Senokot instead of antispasmodics.

The development of high pressures within segments of bowel is dependent upon the complete closure of interhaustral rings, and measures designed to interfere with such closure may prevent the generation of high pressure. This may be achieved by distending the lumen of the colon by hydrophylic bulk-forming substances such as methylcellulose granules, Normacol or Fybogel, or by the administration of unprocessed bran. The impalatable nature of these materials may be disguised to some extent by mixing it with food eaten at each of the three main meals. Faecal bulk may also be increased by the introduction of a high roughage diet. This management of diverticular disease is completely different from the older, less satisfactory, regimen which employed liquid paraffin and a low roughage diet in the hope that these would reduce colonic irritation. This therapy still has a limited application when the disease has produced marked inflammation and stenosis.

A similar regime of increasing the bulk of the colonic contents is of value in the treatment of the irritable bowel syndrome. Dicyclomine HCl and phenobarbitone may be used for the pain so common in this condition, but antispasmodics are often disappointing and better results may be achieved with diazepam or tricyclic antidepressants. Associated diarrhoea is best treated with codeine phosphate and constipation with a mild laxative.

In the acute episode of diverticular disease the main objectives of therapy are relief of pain, reduction of colonic spasm, and the control of infection. Though a potent analgesic may be necessary, morphine should be avoided since this has been shown to induce and potentiate the hypersegmentation and increased colonic pressure encountered in diverticular disease. Pethidine is a useful alternative analgesic. Anticholinergic drugs are also of value in this situation. When there are signs indicating the presence of infection, a suitable antibiotic should be given. Either ampicillin or tetracycline, given in a dose of 500 mg four times daily, is usually effective. When the illness is associated with vomiting these drugs may have to be given parenterally; gastric suction and the intravenous administration of fluid and electrolytes may be necessary. When the disease is limited to the sigmoid colon and when symptoms are sufficiently troublesome, surgical treatment is indicated. The standard operation is excision of the affected segment with end-to-end anastomosis of the remaining bowel. Recently it has been suggested that reduction of the pressure in the diseased segment may arrest progress of the disease. To achieve this reduction in pressure the operation of sigmoid myotomy has been introduced; this is analogous to cardiomyotomy in achalasia of the cardia.

The complications of diverticulitis require surgical treatment. Perforation and peritonitis demand immediate exploration and, indeed, a specific diagnosis often cannot be made until the laparotomy. In the presence of faecal peritonitis the peritoneal cavity is irrigated with saline containing antibacterial agents, e.g. kanamycin or noxytiolin. Often it is impossible to close the perforation, but, if possible, it is over-sewn and covered with omentum, the abdomen is drained and the prudent surgeon adds a proximal transverse colostomy to divert the faecal stream.

The high mortality associated with this condition is related to bacteroides infection and release of endotoxin. The antibiotic treatment of choice is therefore a combination of lincomycin and gentamicin given intravenously. Hydrocortisone should be given in large doses, of for example 4 g in the first 12 hours followed by 2 to 4 g daily until the temperature has settled and the cardiovascular status is satisfactory.

After a suitable period, e.g. six weeks, the abdomen is reopened and an elective procedure is performed, following which the colostomy can be closed. Re-operation should not be unduly postponed as the distal defunctioned bowel tends to narrow and this makes subsequent anastomosis difficult and fistula formation more likely.

When the patient presents with a pericolic abscess and signs of intestinal obstruction, the diagnosis may lie between carcinoma and diverticulitis; at laparotomy, it is often difficult to differentiate between the two conditions. While some surgeons advise immediate resection for carcinoma, this may be difficult in the presence of obstruction and foolhardy in the presence of infection and frank pus. The method which is safe and has stood the test of time is to create a proximal defunctioning colostomy. This allows the patient to recover while further investigations can be done to establish the diagnosis. Bowel continuity can be restored subsequently at formal resection of the segment while, in the 'bad risk' case, the simple colostomy can be left permanently.

In the case of vesicocolic fistula the infection of the urinary tract may be controlled by antibiotics, while the bowel is 'sterilized' with antibacterial agents. A laparotomy can then be performed in the hope of closing the fistula in one stage. The fistula is often very small, so that simple closure of the bladder wall after mobilization of the colon, with perhaps an omental patch, may be adequate, and the diverticular disease can be dealt with by resection or myotomy. The more conservative approach is to initiate treatment by a proximal defunctioning colostomy, allow six weeks for the inflammatory changes to subside, then resect the affected bowel and close the fistula. The colostomy is then closed at a third stage. The 'safe' approach entails a lengthy period of treatment in hospital and three separate operations, each carrying a risk. The risk of ascending pyelonephritis, which influenced treatment so much in the past, is by no means always a reality and is now controllable by antibiotic therapy.

If a faecal fistula develops following drainage of an abscess or after anastomosis, then it is unlikely to close spontaneously and is likely to recur even after closure of a defunctioning colostomy. The axiom that a fistula will always close if there is no distal obstruction, should dictate the immediate treatment of such fistulae for a limited period, and if resolution is not occuring, then excision of the fistula with the associated bowel is indicated and a new anastomosis is made, using healthy bowel. If the fistula involves another loop of bowel, resection of the involved portion of bowel is the treatment of choice.

Summary

Diverticular disease of the colon is now visualized as a neuromuscular disorder of the bowel, resulting in thickening of the muscular layers and disordered segmentation. This results in protrusion of mucosa through the weak points in the bowel wall at the entry point of the blood vessels. Inflammation follows with aggravation of the symptomatology and the development of more or less serious complications. The management in the majority of uncomplicated cases is medical. Elective operations are being advised more frequently than in the past for those whose symptoms fail to respond to conservative measures.

FURTHER READING

Cummings, J. H. (1973) Dietary fibre, progress report. *Gut*, **14**, 69–81.
Misiewicz, J. J. (1974) Muscular disorders of the colon. *Hospital Medicine*, **11**, 91–202.
Painter, N. S. & Burkitt, D. P. (1971) Diverticular disease of the colon: a deficiency disease of western civilisation. *British Medical Journal*, ii, 450–454.

13. The Anal Canal and Anus

Shedden Alexander

ANATOMY

The anal canal is the terminal portion of the bowel; the anus is the opening to the exterior (Fig. 13.1). The canal runs from the anorectal junction to the anal verge, and measures $1\frac{1}{2}$ inches (3·5 cm) in length. At its upper end it commences where the balloon-like ampulla of the rectum narrows; this coincides with the angle formed by the rectum and the anal canal, and with the level of the muscular diaphragm of the pelvic floor, the levator ani muscle. Posteriorly lies the coccyx with some fatty, fibrous and muscular tissue intervening. Laterally on each side is the ischiorectal space, a fat-filled area lying between the anal canal and the side wall of the true pelvis. The ischiorectal space is bounded inferiorly by skin and superiorly by the levator ani. Running medially across the space from the lateral walls are the pudendal vessels and nerves. Anteriorly lies the perineal body, with the bulbous urethra and posterior border of the urogenital diaphragm in the male, and the lower vagina in the female.

ANAL CANAL MUCOSA

The principal features of the internal aspect of the anal canal, from above downwards, are: the columns of Morgagni, the anal valves, the pecten, the intermuscular groove, and the anal verge itself. The columns of Morgagni, eight to twelve in number, are longitudinal folds of mucosa. The anal valves are transverse folds of mucosa which unite the lower ends of the columns and thereby form crypts, the openings of which face upwards. The resultant ring of mucosa is called the pectinate, or dentate, line. The upper part of the anal canal is lined by cuboidal cells which merge into the simple columnar epithelium of the rectum. The only glands present in the anal canal are the small straight anal glands, which open into the anal crypts. Just below the pectinate line is found the transition from columnar to squamous epithelium. The epithelium of the lower anal canal differs from true skin, in that it is moist and hairless, but it merges gradually into the true perianal skin at the anal verge.

The different character of the mucosa of the anal canal above and below the mucocutaneous junction has important clinical implications; malignant lesions of the upper and canal are nearly always adeno-carcinomas, while in the lower anal canal squamous carcinomas are found; the mucosa above the junction is insensitive to pain in contrast to that below it; the lymphatic drainage above the junction is to the lymphatics within the pelvis, while the lymphatic drainage below the junction is towards the inguinal nodes.

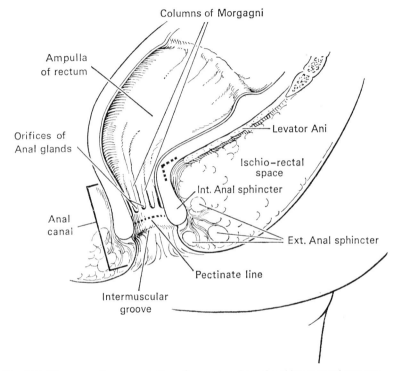

Fig. 13.1 Diagrammatic representation of normal anal canal and lower rectal structure.

ANAL CANAL MUSCULATURE

The internal sphincter encircles the upper part of the anal canal. It consists of smooth muscle and represents the thickened continuation of the circular muscle coat of the rectum. Its upper border coincides with the anorectal junction, and at the lower border there is a circumferential intermuscular groove. This is an important surgical landmark in the operation of haemorrhoidectomy.

External to the internal sphincter is the fibromuscular termination of the longitudinal muscle of the bowel. This fibromuscular sheet blends with fibres of levator ani muscle, and gains attachment to the anal verge and perianal skin through a series of fan-like condensations radiating from its lower end. These condensations form the anal intermuscular groove which separates the internal from the external sphincter. The external anal sphincter consists of bundles of voluntary muscle fibres disposed circumferentially around the anus. The fibromuscular termination of the longitudinal muscle which is attached to the perianal skin is known as the corrugator cutis ani, and is responsible for the radial folds of skin around the anus.

The levator ani is a voluntary muscle sheet which arises from the wall of the pelvis, and is attached to the outer smooth muscle of the anal canal. Its most medial fibres are responsible for the angulation which is found at the anorectal junction. During defaecation the levator ani relaxes, the anorectal ring disappears, and the angle between rectum and anus is reduced.

BLOOD VESSELS

The blood supply to the anal canal is via the superior, middle and inferior rectal vessels. The superior rectal vessels are derived from the inferior mesenteric, the middle rectal from the internal iliac, and the inferior rectal from the pudendal vessels. A free anastomosis between these arteries takes place in the submucous plexus.

On the venous side there is also a submucous plexus, from which the principal drainage is upwards through the superior rectal veins. As these veins are in the left lateral, right anterolateral and right posterolateral positions, haemorrhoids usually occur at these three sites. The internal haemorrhoidal plexus is an important watershed between portal circulation (superior rectal veins) and systemic venous circulation (middle and inferior rectal veins).

LYMPHATICS

Lymphatics from the upper part of the anal canal run into iliac nodes in the pelvic walls and mesenteric nodes in the root of the pelvic mesocolon, and thence to the para-aortic nodes. Lymphatic drainage from the lower anal canal is first to the inguinal nodes.

NERVES

The mucosa above the mucocutaneous junction is innervated by the autonomic system, through the pelvic parasympathetic outflow. This zone is thus insensitive to pain and temperature. Below the mucocutaneous junction the epithelium receives a somatic innervation, which is derived from the pudendal nerves and, like true skin, is sensitive to pain and temperature.

PHYSIOLOGY

CONTINENCE

Smooth muscle tonus in the internal anal sphincter is chiefly responsible for normal continence. This is an intrinsic property, and persists when all connection with the central nervous system is severed. The levator ani muscle and the external anal sphincter are of secondary importance in maintaining continence, but when they become flaccid, as a result of old age, multiple childbirth, or other trauma, there is a tendency for the rectum to prolapse through the anus.

EVACUATION

The act of defaecation is a reflex involving voluntary and involuntary muscles of the anal canal and the terminal bowel. The stimulus for defaecation is either distension of the rectum or peristaltic activity in the upper intestine. The principal reflex centre is in the sacral part of the spinal cord. As the balloon-shaped rectum contracts, the levator ani relaxes, thus causing the anorectal ring and angle to disappear. The internal anal sphincter is 'taken up', similar to the cervix uteri during parturition, and the external anal spincter relaxes. Voluntary inhibition of defaecation can be effected by contraction of the levator ani muscles.

Congenital anomalies of the anal canal

Embryology

The definitive anal canal is formed during the third month of intra-uterine life from the lower end of the hindgut, and the primitive cloaca. The urorectal septum grows down towards the cloacal membrane separating the primitive cloaca into a posterior rectum and an anterior bladder. Failure of this part of development results in vesicorectal and rectovaginal fistulae. About the same time the cloacal membrane disappears, but when this disappearance of the posterior part is incomplete a persistent anal membrane and imperforate anus result. Atresia of the primitive rectum may leave a considerable gap between the definitive rectum and the exterior. The lower end of the anal canal is completed by the anal tubercles, maldevelopment of which results in congenital anal fistulae into the perineum, scrotum or vestibule. Total absence of these tubercles results in failure of development of the anus, with no muscular tissue and no external evidence of an anus.

Congenital malformation of the anal canal occurs in about 1 in 5000 births, and almost all are types of imperforate anus. In the commonest type the blind lower end of the rectum is separated by some distance from the anal membrane, but all degrees of severity between this and partial stenosis of the canal may be found. The majority of the more severe grades of imperforate anus are associated with rectal fistulae.

Additional congenital abnormalities are found in about a quarter of all cases, e.g. cardiac defects, absence of oesophagus or small intestine, or hare-lip and cleft palate.

Clinical management

In the clinical management of imperforate anus it is important to know whether an anal sphincter is present or not. If there is even the slightest evidence of a dimple at the site where the anus should be it can be presumed that an anal spincter exists. Radiological examination with the child inverted reveals the distance between the gas-filled rectum and the perineal skin. In the more severe abnormalities the presence of *Bacillus proteus* or *B. pyocyaneus* in the urine usually indicates the presence of a fistula.

When a fistula is excluded, and an anal dimple is present, conservative surgery is indicated, and incision of the membrane, with regular bouginage for several months, is usually sufficient. When fistulae are present, a diversionary colostomy is performed as a preliminary to reconstruction. Total absence of the anus requires specialized plastic reconstruction.

Haemorrhoids

True internal haemorrhoids result from congestion of the internal haemorrhoidal venous plexus in the anal submucosa (Fig. 13.2). Several aetiological factors have been implicated, e.g. heredity, constipation, straining at stool, chronic diarrhoea, pelvic congestion associated with pregnancy, enlargement of the prostate, retroversion of the uterus and uterine fibroids, tumour of the rectum and portal hypertension.

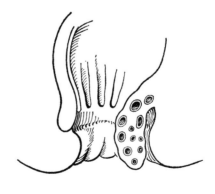

Haemorrhoid

Fig. 13.2 Haemorrhoid is a prolapse of mucosa of the anal canal, with distended veins within the prolapsing area.

Pathology

The haemorrhoidal veins distend and become varicose, losing their elasticity and bulging into the lumen of the anal canal. The venous plexus lies just above the pectinate line, where the mucosa is normally slack and offers little resistance. Because of the disposition of the superior rectal vein into one left lateral and two right lateral tributaries, the anal varicosities form in three corresponding positions (p. 254). Not infrequently there are small secondary haemorrhoids. In advanced cases the haemorrhoids merge one with another, to result in a circumferential bulging of the anal mucosa, amounting to partial prolapse. Redundant skin tags tend to form at the anal verge in positions corresponding with the haemorrhoids.

Haemorrhoids are liable to bleeding during defaecation as a result of minor trauma to their thin walls. They are also liable to prolapse.

When viewed through a proctoscope a haemorrhoid appears as a bright red or purple swelling covered by mucosa.

Mucus is secreted by the engorged mucous membrane, and may cause irritation of the perianal skin, leading to pruritus ani. With the passage of time a pedicle forms, allowing the haemorrhoid to prolapse through the anus. Spontaneous reduction usually occurs at the end of defaecation, but when the pedicle is long, manual reduction by the patient may be necessary. Constriction of the pedicle by spasm of the external anal sphincter may occur after defaecation. Occlusion of the blood supply in this way gives rise to strangulation of the haemorrhoid.

Clinical features

Bleeding during defaecation is the commonest and usually the earliest symptom. The history often goes back for years, and haemorrhoids are one of the commonest causes of anaemia. Haemorrhoids are common in adults of both sexes, and rare in children. When bleeding is the only manifestation, haemorrhoids are referred to as 'first degree'.

Prolapse during defaecation occurs later in most cases, but may be the only symptom, occurring without bleeding. At first the haemorrhoid reduces spontaneously at the end of defaecation, and this occurrence is referred to as 'second degree'. If manual reduction is required it is called 'third degree'. Permanently prolapsed haemorrhoids are referred to as 'fourth degree'. Haemorrhoids may undergo gradual spontaneous resolution after an interval, as a result of fibrosis.

Pruritus ani due to the accompanying mucous discharge is a common feature of haemorrhoids. Pain does not occur unless a haemorrhoid thromboses or becomes strangulated, or is accompanied by a painful lesion such as an anal fissure.

The diagnosis is made by inspection and proctoscopy. In the absence of prolapse, inspection may initially reveal no abnormality, but the haemorrhoid may come into view when the patient is asked to strain. The diagnosis of 'first degree' haemorrhoids in most cases can only be made by proctoscopy. The instrument is introduced to its full extent, the obturator removed, and, as the proctoscope is withdrawn, the bright red or purple haemorrhoid comes into view.

In middle-aged and elderly patients the association between haemorrhoids and a tumour of the lower bowel should be kept in mind, and sigmoidoscopy should always be performed.

Complications

Severe haemorrhage may occur following defaecation. Anaemia is common.

Strangulation of the prolapsed haemorrhoid may occur as a result of spasm of the external sphincter. This is accompanied by considerable pain. Unless reduced within a few hours, either by gravity or by manual reduction, thrombosis often follows.

Rarely thrombosis may occur in a 'first degree' haemorrhoid, but it is commoner in prolapsed haemorrhoids. There is usually a considerable degree of oedema, and a thrombosed haemorrhoid is extremely painful and tender. In the absence of strangulation most thrombosed haemorrhoids undergo spontaneous resolution, but occasionally ulceration or sloughing may occur.

An acute condition which in many ways resembles the thrombosis of internal haemorrhoids, and which can cause diagnostic confusion, is that referred to as either 'thrombosed external haemorrhoids' or 'perianal haematoma'. In this condition there is the sudden appearance of a spherical, tense, tender deep-blue collection of thrombosed blood in the subcutaneous tissue close to the anal verge. This probably results from minor damage to small blood vessels at this site below the pectinate line, and separate from the internal haemorrhoidal plexus.

Suppuration is a relatively rare complication of haemorrhoids, and it is usually confined to thrombosed haemorrhoids, or follows injection treatment or surgical operation. A local abscess may result, but the much more dangerous condition of ascending infection of the portal vein, known as portal pylephlebitis, may occur, accompanied by fever, rigors, acute malaise and jaundice.

Treatment

When the haemorrhoids are small and do not prolapse, bleeding may be prevented simply by avoiding constipation. In all other cases treatment is by injection or surgical excision.

Injection treatment. Probably more than half of the patients with haemorrhoids seen in a surgical clinic are suitable for injection treatment. Haemorrhoids which bleed, but do not prolapse, are ideal, but many which do prolapse are also worth a trial with injection, provided that the mucosa over the pedicle is not unduly redundant. The objective is to induce fibrosis of the submucous areolar tissue by the injection of a sclerosant; the vessels are obliterated and the haemorrhoid shrinks.

Through a proctoscope the sclerosant is injected by a special syringe and guarded needle, into the upper part of the pedicle. One to 5 ml of a 5 per cent solution of carbolic acid in almond oil is usually employed. The injection is painless since it is made above the mucocutaneous line, and there is no special after-treatment. The patient is seen two weeks later, and the haemorrhoids re-injected as necessary; two or three repeat sessions may even be required.

Two recently introduced alternative simple ways of treating haemorrhoids are (1) the application of tight rubber bands around the pedicles, using a special applicator through a proctoscope as an outpatient procedure, and (2) forcible anal dilatation under general anaesthesia.

Operation. The objective is to excise the haemorrhoid with any associated skin tags, with transfixation ligation of the pedicle. After operation there may be a delay of several days before the bowels move, and some assistance by olive oil enema or mild laxative may be required. Haemorrhage may occur in the early postoperative period. This may respond to the local application of gauze soaked in 1 in 1000 solution of adrenaline hydrochloride; re-exploration may be required to control more severe bleeding. Stenosis of the anal canal due to fibrosis is rare, but can be prevented by prophylactic dilation. Haemorrhoidectomy wounds are better left open to granulate.

Treatment of strangulated haemorrhoids. When seen within a short time of onset of the strangulation it may be possible to reduce the prolapsed haemorrhoid by manual pressure, with or without a general anaesthetic.

In most cases thrombosis and swelling make reduction impossible and attempts to do so only aggravate the condition. Two courses are then open: (1) to perform an immediate haemorrhoidectomy or (2) to treat conservatively with bed rest and the local application of cold compresses. As a routine the latter is probably safer, but if it seems possible to perform a haemorrhoidectomy without obliterating entirely the mucocutaneous ring, this procedure has the advantage of rapid cure of the condition, and prevention of the risks of local gangrene and slough formation.

Anal fissure

An anal fissure is a superficial linear ulcer at the anal verge, lying radially to the anus and usually in the midline posteriorly (Fig. 13.3). It occurs in adults and affects the sexes equally.

Aetiology

The usual location, in the midline posteriorly and less commonly in the midline anteriorly, is attributed to the fact that the external anal sphincter leaves the anus less well-supported at these two points.

The precipitating cause of an anal fissure is trauma by the passage of a hard faecal mass. Frequently there is a history of constipation. The acute fissure may heal, but many recur and become chronic because of spasm of the underlying internal sphincter which prevents free lymphatic and venous drainage.

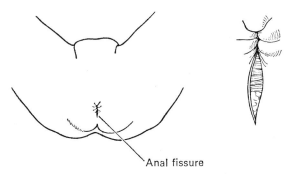

Anal fissure

Fig. 13.3 Diagram of typical posterior anal fissure. Circular muscle fibres of the lower end of the internal anal sphincter visible in enlarged view on the right.

Pathology

An early fissure is a vertical tear on the squamous epithelium of the pecten and anal verge, with usually a small 'sentinel' skin tag at its lower end. Later the internal sphincter is exposed in the base of the fissure and sphincter spasm is more marked. In long-standing cases the muscle fibres of the sphincter are replaced by fibrous tissue with stenosis, induration and oedema of the anus. Perianal infection and fistula-in-ano may occur at any stage.

Clinical features

The characteristic symptom is pain during or after defaecation. Anticipation of pain leads to excessive anal sphincter spasm, which in turn exacerbates the condition. A serous discharge and pruritus ani may be present. The stools may be streaked with blood and haemorrhoids may also be present. Digital examination of the anus and proctoscopy without anaesthesia are not advised because of pain.

Differential diagnosis

Perianal haematoma, prolapsed thrombosed haemorrhoid and perianal abscess are easily distinguished by their appearances. Idiopathic pruritus ani with secondary cracks of the anal skin is distinguished by the lack of anal spasm or tenderness. Septic complications of ulcerative colitis and Crohn's disease give rise to broad, often multiple anal fissures and inflammation of the surrounding skin. Carcinoma of the anus gives a history not unlike that of anal fissure and may look like a chronic anal fissure, but induration is more notable and extends more into the anal canal. A syphilitic fissure may closely resemble an anal fissure;

dark-ground microscopy of exudate or diagnostic serological tests for syphilis will usually separate the two conditions. Other rare conditions which may cause diagnostic difficulty include tuberculous fissure, and idiopathic stenosis of the sphincter.

Treatment

In the early case, in which induration is not prominent, the objective of treatment is the avoidance of constipation, and the reduction of anal spasm and pain by the application of a simple anaesthetic ointment, e.g. 1 to 2 per cent lignocaine.

If the fissure recurs or is associated with much anal spasm, dilatation of the anal sphincter under general anaesthesia is the treatment of choice.

A chronic fissure with much induration, or one which has not responded to one dilatation of the anus, requires operative division of the internal sphincter. An incision is made through the base of the fissure to include the circumferential muscle of the lower part of the internal sphincter. The 'sentinel' skin tag is excised at the same time, and if the simple nature of the fissure is in any doubt or if the muscle is entirely replaced by fibrous tissue in the fissure base a triangular excision of the fissure is performed. The resultant wound usually takes four to seven weeks to heal, during which period daily baths should be taken.

Perianal suppuration

Two forms of suppuration are commonly encountered in the vicinity of the anus: perianal abscess and ischiorectal abscess (Fig. 13.4). Both forms are commoner in women than in men. If inadequately treated, perianal suppuration may lead to a fistula-in-ano.

Aetiology

In the absence of a predisposing lesion in the anal canal, the focus of infection in most cases of perianal suppuration is the anal crypts which lie deep to the anal valves at the lower end of the columns of Morgagni. The anal glands open into these crypts and obstruction of, or trauma to, their ducts gives rise to stasis and predisposes to infection. Minute mucosal tears from hard faeces also play a part. The commonest infecting organism is *Escherichia coli*.

In a small percentage of cases a predisposing local lesion of the anal canal is present, such as an anal fissure or ulcerated haemorrhoids; in others Crohn's disease or ulcerative colitis may predispose to the suppuration.

Classification

The usual classification is into perianal, submucous, ischiorectal and pelvirectal abscess (Fig. 13.4).

Perianal abscess lies within the external anal sphincter, and lateral spread into the ischiorectal fossa is limited by the corrugator cutis ani. A submucous abscess is confined within the wall of the anal canal. Ischiorectal abscess is situated in the ischiorectal fossa. Pelvirectal abscess is an ischiorectal abscess which has penetrated the levator ani and come to lie in relationship to the peritoneal floor of the pelvis.

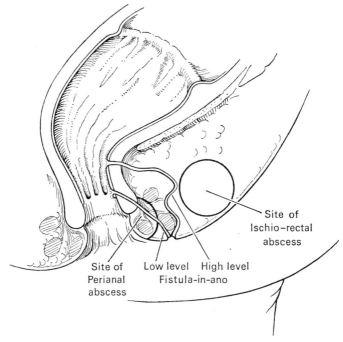

Fig. 13.4 Diagram to show the various locations of perianal abscesses and fistulae.

Symptoms

The patient complains of throbbing pain around the anus, aggravated by coughing, sitting and defaecation. With a large ischiorectal abscess there may be accompanying pyrexia and general loss of well being. The diagnosis may be obvious on inspection. Where there is doubt, the presence of an abscess may be confirmed by gentle digital examination. Testing for fluctuation and proctoscopy usually require general anaesthesia. Occasionally it may be difficult to demonstrate fluctuation in indurated ischiorectal or pelvirectal abscesses.

Treatment

The objective in all cases of perianal suppuration is to evacuate the pus and secure adequate drainage; general anaesthesia is required. The abscess is incised over the area where it 'points', whether it be the skin of the buttock or the anal canal mucosa, pus evacuated, and any loculi broken down with the finger. In perianal and ischiorectal abscesses some deroofing of the abscess is performed to ensure adequate drainage. The depths of the wound are gently probed for an internal fistulous opening, and if none is present the wound is allowed to heal by granulation tissue and spontaneous epithelialization. With a large ischiorectal wound this may require a period of up to three weeks in hospital, during which twice daily baths are taken.

Most pelvirectal abscesses are secondary to intra-abdominal suppuration such as appendicitis, diverticulitis or pelvic inflammation, which may require to be dealt with by later operation through the abdomen.

Fistula-in-ano

A fistula-in-ano is a fistulous track communicating between the anorectal canal and perianal skin. There may be several external openings, but usually only one internal opening. The track is lined by granulation tissue and its wall is composed of tough fibrous tissue. Nearly all fistulae are the result of perianal suppuration. The possibility of a fistula being tuberculous should always be kept in mind as also should the possible co-existence of ulcerative colitis, Crohn's disease, carcinoma of rectum or lymphogranuloma.

The fistula is classed as 'high level' if it penetrates the levator ani (Fig. 13.4). Thus an internal opening above the anorectal ring or a deep sinus left by a pelvirectal abscess makes the lesion 'high level'. All other fistulae-in-ano are 'low level'. A fistula-in-ano with the external orifice anterior to the transverse meridian of the anus (with the patient in the lithotomy position) usually has a straight track into the anal canal, while one posterior to the meridian usually has several external openings, the tracks of which are disposed in horseshoe fashion on the inferior aspect of the puborectalis muscle.

Clinical features

The patient gives a history of perianal suppuration and complains of a painless discharge with or without pruritus ani. There may be symptoms to suggest associated intestinal disease.

The external opening or openings may be inconspicuous and only seen after a bead of pus is expressed by palpation, or there may be a little pink or red nodule of granulation tissue covered with thin epithelium, or a small healed scar to mark the site. The indurated track may be palpable either externally or with a finger in the anal canal. The internal opening of a posterior fistula is usually midline. The gentle passage of a probe through the external opening, with a finger in the anal canal to guide its tip, demonstrates the entire fistula. At this stage it will be evident whether the fistula is 'high level' or 'low level'. Proctoscopy may show an internal opening which has not been clearly demonstrated by palpation or the passage of a probe and may help to distinguish between high and low level fistulae.

Treatment

The object of treatment in all fistulae-in-ano is to lay open the track, and curette the granulation tissue. This method ensures that no pockets of infection are left to cause recurrence. A probe is passed along the fistula to emerge at the anus and the intervening tissue is incised down to it. In 'low level' fistula there is no danger of incontinence since the anorectal ring remains intact. If multiple tracks are present each requires to be carefully located and laid open. 'High level' fistulae cannot be completely laid open because of the risk of incontinence after division of the anorectal ring. Instead they are treated by coring out the track from the ischiorectal fossa. A defunctioning colostomy is often necessary if there is a higher internal communication. Healing may be speeded up by split skin graft. Primary closure of fistulae wounds has been employed successfully after antibiotic dusting of the wound.

Pilonidal sinus

A pilonidal sinus refers to any subcutaneous sinus which contains hair. The commonest site is in the midline over the coccyx, but it may occur in other sites such as the webs of the fingers, the sole of the foot, the umbilicus or the axilla.

Aetiology

The condition is encountered most often in young adult men, being four times commoner in men than women. The cardinal feature of a pilonidal sinus is that any hairs found within the sinus are loose. Hair follicles in the wall of the sinus have never been demonstrated. In many cases, notably barbers, these loose hairs do not arise from the patient himself. In other cases, although the pilonidal sinus is commoner in hirsute males and may occur in hair-bearing skin areas, the hairs present have arrived there by curling over and penetrating the skin surface, the pointed end directed towards the blind end of the sinus. The condition may therefore be said to be acquired. A familial tendency can be explained by the inheritance of wiry hair.

Pathology

The principal opening of the common type of pilonidal sinus is in the midline of the natal cleft, and represents the original point of penetration of a hair through skin. The track in relation to this opening is always lined by epithelium for a variable depth. Often there are other skin openings due to the discharge of multiple pockets of suppuration to the surface. These other tracks are lined by a mixture of epithelium and granulation tissue. Loose hairs may be recovered; not infrequently they are embedded in granulation or scar tissue and foreign body giant cells are common. The track ends blindly before reaching the sacrum, and it is not directed towards the anorectal canal. Secondary infection causes formation of the abscesses which may rupture through the original midline track or produce secondary sinuses lateral to the midline.

Clinical features

In uninfected cases the patients complain of an irritating discharge over the coccygeal region; discomfort is aggravated by sitting. There may be a history of abscesses which may have ruptured spontaneously or been incised surgically. If the lesion is infected the patient complains of a painful throbbing sensation at the bottom of the spine.

On examination there is a sinus opening in the natal cleft with or without other midline or secondary lateral openings. An abscess presents as a hot, tender fluctuant swelling, with possibly a purulent discharge from the sinus.

Treatment

When infection is present measures are aimed to control infection before attempting to eradicate the sinus. Hot baths may be sufficient if drainage has already been established, and a systemic antibiotic may abort an early infection. If all hairs and granulation tissue can be removed at this stage some will resolve spontaneously and require no further treatment. A fully developed pilonidal abscess requires surgical incision and drainage. The majority will require definitive treatment after infection has settled.

Surgical excision. Under general anaesthesia, skin and subcutaneous tissue are excised in a vertical ellipse *en bloc* down to sacrum and over the whole area affected by the sinus openings. Recurrence is most usual in the lower part of the wound, and it is necessary in most cases to include skin and subcutaneous tissue as far as the margin of the external anal sphincter. A large wound is unavoidable if recurrence is to be avoided. Provided there are no pockets of infection, and haemostasis has been adequately controlled, the wound may be closed by suture. There is a high percentage of breakdown of this primary closure, and many surgeons prefer to leave the wound open to granulate from its depths and heal with secondary intention.

As an alternative to this operation some surgeons have used the instillation of a sclerosant, such as phenol, into the sinus track under general anaesthesia. Some success has been reported, but the method is still under trial.

Rectal prolapse

Prolapse of the rectum is a circumferential descent of the rectum through the anus (Fig. 13.5). The condition is described as partial or complete, depending on whether mucosa only or the whole rectal wall prolapses.

Rectal prolapse occurs at all ages of adult life and in children. The majority of adults are women, not necessarily women who have borne children. Children are more likely to have a partial prolapse and older patients a complete prolapse.

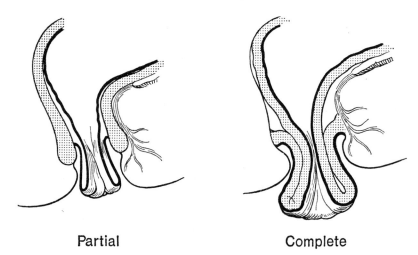

| Partial | Complete |

Fig. 13.5 Rectal prolapse. Partial prolapse involves only the mucosa and submucosa of the anal canal and rectum; in complete prolapse the muscle layers are also involved.

Aetiology

Partial prolapse occurs in children because of their relatively poorly supported anal canal and their irregular bowel habits. Partial prolapse in young and middle-aged adults is often related to haemorrhoids or fistulae repairs, and in women to obstetrical tears. When haemorrhoids are large and so numerous as to encircle the wall of the anal canal a partial prolapse is produced. In older patients partial prolapse is associated with a slack external anal sphincter which is usually idiopathic, but occasionally is secondary to organic disease.

Complete prolapse is produced by incompetence of the sphincters, and is often associated with an unusually deep rectovesical or rectovaginal pouch of peritoneum.

Clinical features

In children the prolapse occurs during defaecation and may reduce spontaneously or require manual reduction. The child is usually well and is continent.

In adults the prolapse may occur with coughing and exertion as well as with defaecation, and there is often some disturbance of normal continence which occurs at other times as well as when the prolapse is down. The patient may complain of a discharge of mucus and blood.

If the prolapse is not obvious at the time of examination the diagnosis can be made by asking the patient to strain to bring down the prolapse.

PARTIAL PROLAPSE

A partial prolapse consists of a ring of mucosa projecting beyond the anus, by about 3·5 to 5 cm. A prolapse projecting more than 5 cm is almost certainly a complete prolapse. The fact that a partial prolapse consists of only two layers of mucosa is confirmed by palpation. The examining finger cannot pass between the prolapse and the wall of the anal canal at any point, which finding differentiates the condition from a prolapsed rectal polyp or the apex of an intussusception. In children the anal sphincter is normal, but in adults there is considerable slackness of the anal sphincter and the anus is often patulous.

COMPLETE PROLAPSE

A complete prolapse forms a large red swelling at the anus. The mucosa covering the swelling appears thickened and is usually thrown into circular folds. The greater thickness of a complete prolapse is obvious on palpation. The total length of the prolapse is seldom greater than 12 cm from the anal verge. The external anal sphincter and levator ani muscle are grossly deficient in contractile power, and three or even four fingers can be inserted into the anal canal without encountering resistance or causing the patient discomfort. The rectovesical or rectovaginal pouch of peritoneum may descend in the anterior wall of a large complete prolapse, in which case loops of small intestine may be contained within the wall of the prolapsed bowel.

Complications are not common as most patients learn the habit of reducing their prolapse manually. An irreducible prolapse may become gangrenous. Minor ulceration of the tip of a prolapse is not uncommon and may cause some bleeding.

Treatment

PARTIAL PROLAPSE

Partial prolapse in children usually disappears as the child grows older. Treatment is directed to correction of irregular habits of defaecation and this is best done under medical supervision in hospital. Submucous injection of phenol under general anaesthetic, similar to the procedure described for haemorrhoids, fixes a very redundant mucosa in these cases of partial prolapse which do not respond to simple measures.

The treatment of partial prolapse in adults is dependent on the state of the anal sphincter. If the anal sphincter is taut and nearly normal the mucosa prolapse is excised in the manner of a haemorrhoidectomy, taking care to leave at least one mucocutaneous bridge of tissue between each wound. If the anal sphincter is slack this procedure is valueless because the patient's main complaint is of incontinence, and treatment is directed to tighten the sphincter. Continuous electrical stimulation by an electronic implant, the electrodes of which are placed in the external sphincter or alongside the pudendal nerves, should in theory achieve this, but practical experience of this is as yet very limited.

Complete prolapse is usually associated with some degree of incontinence due to impaired sphincter action, and the results of surgery are not entirely satisfactory.

One method of treatment is the insertion of a metallic suture subcutaneously around the anus. This, the Thiersch operation, has been used for over 70 years, but suffers from the disadvantage that the wire fractures or ulcerates through skin and may, if too tight, cause faecal impaction. Rectosigmoidectomy, or amputation of the prolapse, is another old procedure which has stood the test of time, but is also not entirely satisfactory because it does not deal with the abnormally deep pelvic pouch of peritoneum in these cases or the disordered sphincter mechanism, and the recurrence rate is high. An abdominal operation in which the pelvic floor is reconstituted to obliterate the deep pelvic pouch, and the rectum fixed (by polyvinyl alcohol sponge packing), is the operation most commonly practised today—the Roscoe Graham operation or one of its modifications. Abdominal resection of redundant lower bowel with end-to-end anastomosis is the fourth type of surgical procedure which has a place in the treatment of complete rectal prolapse; complete excision of the rectum with a terminal iliac colostomy is rarely required for gross recurrent prolapse.

Tumours of the anal canal

HYPERTROPHIED ANAL PAPILLA

The commonest so-called tumour of the anal canal is the hypertrophied anal papilla. This is usually found at the pectinate line, and may represent the primitive ectodermal membrane separating hindgut from proctodaeum. It is so common as to be considered a normal finding, and is only excised if it causes bleeding or a tendency to prolapse through the anus.

MALIGNANT TUMOURS OF THE ANUS

The commonest malignant tumour involving the anal canal is an adenocarcinoma, and even if the tumour projects through the anus it still has a 50 per cent chance of being an adenocarcinoma. It is always an extension of a low rectal carcinoma and is treated as such, by abdominoperineal resection of the rectum and terminal colostomy.

SQUAMOUS CELL CARCINOMA

This tumour arises in the modified skin lining the lower part of the anal canal and in the perianal skin (p. 252). Growths within the anal canal are more common in women, and those in the skin at the anal verge more common in men. Compared to rectal carcinoma, squamous cell carcinoma of the anal canal is relatively rare. The tumour may arise in a chronic fissure or as a result of previous irradiation.

Squamous carcinoma may take the form of an ulcer with typically rolled edges, or of an irregular warty mass, usually on the anterior aspect of the anus. Spread occurs both intra-abdominally via inferior mesenteric and internal iliac lymphatics, and superficially to the inguinal glands. Patients complain of 'haemorrhoids', pain during defaecation or a discharge from the anus. On examination the typical ulcerating growth confirms the diagnosis, but earlier lesions may be confused with fissure, prolapsed haemorrhoids or anal ulceration due to Crohn's disease. The diagnosis should always be confirmed by biopsy.

MALIGNANT MELANOMA

Malignant melanoma of the anal canal is rare. It presents as a bluish-black soft mass which is liable to be confused with a thrombosed haemorrhoid.

Treatment

Treatment of anal tumours may be by irradiation or surgery, and consultation between radiotherapist and surgeon should always take place. Basal cell carcinoma of the anal verge is effectively treated by irradiation. Surgical cure of other types is by an abdominoperineal excision with a generous resection of perianal skin. The inguinal glands are usually left, unless clinically involved or shown on biopsy to be histologically involved, when bilateral groin dissection is performed at a second operation.

Apart from these organic diseases, a complaint of discomfort or pain in the anal region may be made when the appearance of the anus is normal. In such circumstances the diagnosis may be of proctalgia fugax, coccydynia or psychoneurosis.

Disorders of the perianal skin

Before considering diseases of the perianal skin it is pertinent to consider the climate in which it normally lives. Being situated in a deep cleft with opposed sides, it forms a natural harbour for retaining sweat, mucous discharge and excreta. The temperature of the perineum is higher than the general body surface, this being accentuated by the fact that it is generally clothed. It is abundantly supplied by both eccrine and apocrine sweat glands which give the area a high humidity. Its pH tends to be higher (6·84) than that of the general body surface (5·86 to 6·10). This combination of a closed, hot, humid area, with a tendency to alkalinity, provides ideal conditions for the growth of micro-organisms, both saprophytic and pathogenic. These factors are also responsible for the way in which simple infections in this area (e.g. virus warts) often produce exuberant vegetative lesions which may be extremely resistant to therapy.

INFECTIONS

(a) *Pyogenic.* The perineum is a common carrier site for pathogenic staphylococci, but these organisms rarely cause local disease unless a portal of entry is available through trauma or pre-existing disease. Furuncles and carbuncles may arise by organisms obtaining access to a pilosebaceous follicle. Should pyogenic organisms gain access to the apocrine glands, deep-seated inflammatory nodules develop around the anus, eventually discharging pus and leaving extensive scarring and often persistent sinus formation. This disorder, hidradenitis suppura-tiva, is extremely resistant to therapy and in the fully established case may require wide surgical excision followed by plastic repair. When the body defences are impaired, such as during immunosuppressive therapy, extensive ulceration of the perianal skin caused by organisms not normally pathogenic may be seen. Secondary bacterial infection of the perianal ulcerated lesions associated with Crohn's disease and ulcerative colitis may occur.

(b) *Virus infections.* Such infections are not common in this region although in rare instances the perianal skin may be involved by herpes zoster or herpes simplex. Viral warts or condylomata acuminata are the most frequently encountered virus infection. They are often asso-ciated with similar lesions on the penis or vulva. In some instances they may spread into the anal canal, giving rise to recurrence after the skin lesions have been adequately treated. Clinically they are rec-ognized by their superficial nature, multiplicity, rapidity of growth and lack of induration. They must be distinguished from the broader, flatter, moist condylomata lata of secondary syphilis. If the lesions are not too numerous, painting each with podophyllin resin, 20 per cent in liquid paraffin, may be effective. The intervening skin is protected by Vaseline. The podophyllin is washed off after one to two hours. A brisk inflammatory reaction results, usually followed by disappearance of the lesions. It may, however, be necessary to repeat the treatment if any lesions persist. In extensive cases destruction by diathermy or electro-cautery under general anaesthesia is necessary.

(c) *Mycotic infections.* Fungal infections are common in this area, either due to infection by one of the species of epidermophytes spread-ing from the groin or to invasion of the skin by the yeast Candida.

Invasion of the perianal skin by dermatophytes is usually secondary to tinea cruris, caused either by *Trichophyton rubrum* or *Epidermophyton floccosum*. It is much commoner in males. The lesions are well-demarcated, circinate in outline, scaly and continuous, with similar lesions in the groins and inner aspects of the thighs. The diagnosis is confirmed by finding mycelia and spores in the scales. Local therapy consists of applying magenta paint (B.P.) twice daily. The administration of griseofulvin 1 g daily in divided dosage, for four to six weeks, is advised.

Candida albicans is a normal saprophyte found in the gastrointestinal tract and vagina, but not usually on the skin. The precise mechanisms which result in its becoming a pathogen are not as yet understood. Certain general disorders, obesity, diabetes mellitus and blood dyscrasias such as the leukaemias predispose to its development. Alterations in the normal gastrointestinal flora induced by the administration of antibiotics and the topical applications of corticosteroid preparations are among the commonest precipitating factors.

The conditions of warmth, moisture and friction in the perianal region, groins, axillae, umbilicus and inframammary regions appear ideal for its proliferation and explain its localization to these areas.

Clinically it presents as a moist, glazed, red area, with scalloped edges and with characteristic small crusted or eroded satellite lesions. Itch may be severe. The diagnosis is confirmed by the isolation of Candida from the lesions. This should always be done before therapy is commenced.

The older forms of therapy, such as magenta paint (B.P.), crystal violet or brilliant green, $\frac{1}{2}$ per cent of each in aqueous solution applied twice daily, give excellent results. Newer and more cosmetically acceptable remedies include nystatin ointment or paint (100,000 units per g) either alone or combined with amphotericin B. Treatment for two to four weeks is usually necessary. Underlying disorders such as diabetes and obesity must of course be treated.

NON-INFECTIVE INFLAMMATORY DISORDERS

Contact dermatitis of the perineum may be caused by a variety of agents, the commonest of which are topically applied medicaments. Those most frequently incriminated are antipruritic ointments or creams, antihistamine ointments and creams, and antibiotics. More rarely toilet preparations, cosmetics and contraceptives are the cause. Clinically it presents as an itchy, ill-defined area of dermatitis, exudative in the acute stages, thickened and perhaps fissured in the chronic phase. When due to a medicament a simultaneous contact dermatitis of the fingers used to apply it is often seen. Treatment consists of removing the causative agent once this has been identified. The use of potent topical corticosteroid preparations such as fluocinolone acetonide and beta-methasone valerate has revolutionized the treatment of dermatitis. These preparations are used combined with a hydroxyquinolone to minimize the risk of secondary infections. Lotions are preferable to ointments or creams in this region. Applied two or three times daily they will successfully clear up contact dermatitis within a few days, provided the contactant is removed.

Psoriasis frequently affects the perineum and natal cleft as a dull, somewhat glazed erythema. Examination of the patient will usually reveal typical patches of psoriasis on the other sites of election—elbows, knees, scalp and fingernails. Local treatment is as for psoriasis elsewhere, although the concentration of active ingredients should be reduced.

Seborrhoeic dermatitis in this region may mimic psoriasis closely. The lesions tend to be brownish-red in colour and to show quite large greasy scales at the margins. Typical greasy seborrhoeic patches are usually present on the chest and upper back.

Lichenification or neurodermatitis is the end result of pruritus ani (*vide infra*).

Pruritus ani. Severe itching of the perianal skin is a distressing condition. While it occurs in both sexes it is commoner in the male. Organic disease of the rectum or anus, such as fissure-in-ano, haemorrhoids or proctitis, may be causative in some cases. In others it may be due to a pre-existing skin disease, such as a contact or seborrhoeic dermatitis or an infection with *Candida albicans.* In well over half the cases no definite cause can be found. In this group complex psychosomatic factors appear to be involved, such as overwork, financial stress and sexual frustration. The main complaint is itch, often cyclical in character, being worse in the evening or at night when the patient's mind is less occupied. In the absence of the diseases noted above the repeated scratching produces thickened, white, often excoriated, areas of skin around the anus. In long-standing cases this extends forward to involve the scrotum. Eventually the scrotal and perianal skin becomes chronically thickened, pigmented and with increased surface markings, a process described as lichenification, or chronic neurodermatitis.

The first step in management is to correct or treat any rectal, anal or local skin disorder, either by surgical means or the appropriate local application. Where no cause can be detected the first priority is to interrupt the scratch cycle. While normal hygiene is encouraged, any tendency to overwashing with either soap and water or antiseptics should be corrected. Tissue paper or cotton wool should be advised in place of toilet paper. Local application of one of the more potent corticosteroid lotions, such as fluocinolone acetonide or betamethasone valerate, three or four times daily, effectively diminishes itch. It is advisable to use these combined with hydroxyquinolone to reduce the risk of superadded Candida infection. Sedation with small doses of phenobarbitone or one of the phenothiazines may be necessary. Time must be spent with these patients to encourage them to discuss their worries and frustrations. Long-term therapy is necessary as a rule, but even then relapses and recurrences are frequent.

FURTHER READING

Barron, J. (1963) Office ligation of internal haemorrhoids. *American Journal of Surgery,* **105,** 563.

Eisenhammer, S. (1953) The internal anal sphincter: its surgical importance. *South African Medical Journal,* **27,** 26.

Goligher, J. C. (1967) *Anus, Rectum and Colon.* London: Bailliere, Tindall and Cassell.

Graham-Stewart, C. W. (1962) Injection treatment of haemorrhoids. *British Medical Journal,* i, 213.

Lord, P. H. (1968) A new regime for haemorrhoids. *Proceedings of the Royal Society of Medicine,* **61,** 935.

Maurice, B. A. & Greenwood, R. K. (1964) A conservative treatment of pilo-nidal sinus. *British Journal of Surgery,* **51,** 510.

Milligan, E. T. C. (1942) The surgical anatomy and disorders of the peri-anal space. *Proceedings of the Royal Society of Medicine,* **36,** 365.

Staff, K. W. (1953) Primary closure in proctology. *Postgraduate Medicine,* **14,** 365.

Wells, C. A. (1962) Polyvinyl alcohol sponge prosthesis for rectal prolapse. *Proceedings of the Royal Society of Medicine,* **55,** 1083.

14. Gastrointestinal Diseases in General Practice

J.H. Barber

INTRODUCTION

Disease of the alimentary system accounts for about 11 per cent of the family doctor's workload, or about 1,200 consultations each year in a practice of 2,500 patients. The diseases seen by the hospital specialist are not always representative of the pattern of illness seen by the general practitioner. Morbidity patterns in the community tend to vary with the age of the patient and presenting symptoms can alter with age both in frequency and in the interpretations put on them by both the patient and the doctor. While the family doctor will see about 200 patients each year suffering from gastroenteritis, he will only have two or three patients in his practice with a carcinoma of any part of the intestinal tract. The frequency with which diseases of the gastrointestinal tract are seen in the community is shown in Table 14.1.

Table 14.1 Frequency of varying diseases of gastrointestinal tract in general practice. 'Average' practice of 2,500 patients

Disease	No. of patients seen per year
Gastroenteritis	195
Acute gastritis	50
Constipation	30
Simple dyspepsia	28
Peptic ulcer syndrome	18
Anal fissure	12
Appendicitis	12
Cholecystitis	5
Hiatal hernia	4
Carcinoma of colon	2
Carcinoma of stomach	2
Acute obstruction	1
Perforated peptic ulcer	1
Carcinoma of rectum	1
Carcinoma of oesophagus	one every five years
Intussusception	one every five years
Congenital pyloric stenosis	one every ten years
Coeliac disease	one every ten years

The symptoms usually associated with disease of the gastrointestinal system—abdominal pain, nausea, vomiting and bowel disturbance—are also seen as the presenting symptoms of diseases of other systems. It is important to remember that these symptoms are words which are in every-day use and the doctor should make sure that he establishes precisely what the patient means by terms such as 'diarrhoea' or 'sickness'. The presentation of one of the recognised symptoms of gastrointestinal disease does not necessarily indicate that the patient is suffering from an illness referable to that system.

INFANTS (FIRST YEAR OF LIFE)

Feeding difficulties

Minor upsets due to poor or inappropriate feeding are common. Difficulties occur most frequently with a first baby and are usually the result of the mother's lack of knowledge about her child's food and fluid needs. In this respect feeding difficulties are most common and troublesome when the mother is in her 'teens and particularly when she lives at a distance from parents and relatives. Maternal anxiety, from any cause, can result in an irritable baby who does not feed properly.

Abnormalities of the type and quantity of food given can present in several ways. 'Under-feeding' presents as a fractious child failing to gain weight, sleeping for short spells and waking crying and hungry. Hard scybalous stools leading to constipation or to anal fissure can result from under-feeding or from the introduction of solid food too early in life. Insufficient fluid intake in hot weather can be accompanied by constipation resulting in episodes of screaming towards the end of the feed when defaecation usually occurs. 'Diarrhoea', in the absence of infection, can result if an excessive amount of sugar is added to the milk feed. It can also be due to a certain type of food—notably orange or fruit juice.

Feeding difficulties can also result from oral thrush caused by *monilia albicans*. The infection usually results from the inadequate sterilisation of feeding bottles and teats before each feed. Two drops of a nystatin mixture run into the mouth before each feed is a rapidly effective treatment, but should be continued for not less than five days to ensure that the infection is eradicated. Naturally, the mother must also be taught the correct way in which to sterilise all feeding utensils.

Almost all feeding difficulties respond to simple explanation and advice which are best given by a health visitor.

Diarrhoea

It is important to remember that when the diet consists of milk, an infant will have a semi-solid yellow stool after each feed: this normal pattern may be described as 'diarrhoea' by an inexperienced mother. Abnormalities of feeding can be responsible for diarrhoea but the cause is usually infective. In infants it is characterised by frequent *liquid* yellow or greenish-yellow stools, often passed explosively and accompanied by audible borborygmi and abdominal pain. The baby responds by pulling the knees up over the abdomen and crying 'painfully'. In the infant, dehydration and electrolyte disturbance can develop rapidly and admission to hospital should be arranged as an emergency if there is evidence of fluid depletion. If the child shows no evidence of dehydration all milk or solids should be stopped for twenty-four hours and frequent small feeds of boiled water should be given. There is usually no need for antibiotic therapy. In most cases the baby will be able to resume diluted small quantity milk feeds after about twenty-four hours, with normal feeding the following day.

Infantile colic

This common disorder is most prevalent at about the age of three months. It is characterised by bouts of screaming with the knees held up over the abdomen. In mild cases, the bouts of colic tend to occur after a single feed, often in the evening, but the child is otherwise well and the condition is self-limiting. More severe cases show prolonged and painful crying after each feed and occasional vomiting with a resultant fretful baby and an anxious and disturbed mother. Infantile colic is caused by the child swallowing excessive quantities of air at each feed, either because the feeding bottle is held in such a way as to allow the teat to contain air as well as milk, or because the teat has a hole which is either too large or too small. The condition responds to advice and reassurance to the mother and the correction of any faulty feeding technique.

Pyloric stenosis

This is a rare condition. It is characterised by bouts of projectile vomiting associated with a palpable and sometimes visible pyloric tumour. The condition is uncommon before ten or fourteen days of life and seldom appears *de novo* later than six weeks. If a diagnosis of congenital pyloric stenosis is considered, the nature of the sickness and the presence of a pyloric tumour should be observed while the child is being fed. Treatment is by Ramstedt's operation in which the thickened pyloric muscle is divided longitudinally.

'Posetting'

This is the vomiting of small quantities of milk at the end of each feed, and is common in infants of between two and four months of age. It is usual to find that the child is being given relatively large quantities of milk—seven or eight fluid ounces at each feed—and the vomiting represents an 'overflow' from an overfull stomach. This diagnosis should also be considered in the older infant who, despite large volume feeds, is not satisfied for longer than 2 or 3 hours. In this situation there is an indication to reduce the quantity of the feed and to increase its food value by giving a cereal before the bottle feed. Once the mother understands the cause of the vomiting and its management it ceases to be a problem.

THE CHILD OF 3 TO 12 YEARS

With the exception of acute appendicitis almost all gastrointestinal illnesses in this age group are relatively simple and self-limiting. Only rarely will more serious 'adult' illnesses such as peptic ulcer, intestinal obstruction, non-alimentary diseases or psychosomatic illness present with symptoms referable to the gastrointestinal tract.

Diarrhoea

The commonest cause in children is Sonne dysentery. This condition is most prevalent where standards of hygiene are low and where food can be contaminated by flies and insects. It is particularly common in warm weather. Over-crowding and inadequate toilet facilities are important contributing factors and once infected, a child can infect others in school; minor epidemics are therefore common.

Sonne dysentery presents more acutely and is a more serious condition in the infant and the younger pre-school child. Abdominal pain and fever is followed by profuse diarrhoea in which mucus and occasionally frank blood is obvious. In the older child, the illness is less severe and this is also true when there have been repeated re-infections. When the infection drags on in a subacute form occasional mild diarrhoea may be the only symptom. The diagnosis is suspected from the clinical features, can be confirmed by stool culture, and treatment is determined by the sensitivity pattern of the organism identified.

The health visitor should visit the home as it is important that the mother understands how the infection is transmitted and the ways in which this can be prevented. If the family lives in condemned property or has inadequate toilet facilities, a move to another home may be the only way to ensure that repeated recurrences of the infection are prevented.

Constipation

In the pre-school years, toilet training and the mother's supervision of her child's bowel habit usually ensure that constipation does not become established. After the age of about four, the child becomes more independent, and the possibility of constipation becomes likely as children frequently ignore the call to stool in favour of more interesting activities. Organic causes such as subacute obstruction or congenital megacolon are excessively rare. When established, constipation may present as vague ill-health, anorexia, fatigue or lack of concentration, and only rarely with a complaint of repeated episodes of abdominal pain. The child is seldom aware that he is constipated—indeed he probably does not know what the term means. The diagnosis is easily established: faecal masses can usually be palpated in the left iliac fossa, and their presence confirmed by rectal examination. The condition is treated simply by the re-introduction of proper bowel training, aided by the addition of fruit or roughage to the diet. Occasionally, a mild laxative is necessary in the first few days of treatment. The habitual or repeated use of laxatives is to be avoided.

Severe and long-standing constipation can present with a 'spurious' diarrhoea, when fluid faeces from the bowel proximal to the impacted faecal mass escape at the anus, soiling the child's clothes. Encopresis (involuntary defaecation) can also be the manifestation of a severe behavioural disorder, or of a malabsorptive syndrome of which coeliac disease is the most common.

Anorexia

Anorexia normally accompanies any co-existing infective illness in children and the return of a normal appetite is a sign of recovery. While relatively common in the adult as a symptom of a psychosomatic disease, anorexia in a child is a symptom of organic disease.

Abdominal pain

Diarrhoea from any cause is usually preceded or accompanied by colicky abdominal pain. Infective hepatitis is characterised by upper abdominal right subcostal pain which is related to the development of hepatomegaly. In young children any infective illness can be accompanied by abdominal pain. Other important conditions in children in which abdominal pain is a feature are appendicitis, diabetes, dyspepsia and the periodic syndrome.

1. *Appendicitis.* This relatively uncommon condition is suspected more often than it is proved, but it is a diagnosis which is frequently feared and suggested by parents.

It is uncommon before the age of four but its prevalence increases thereafter and particularly after ten years of age. In the pre-school and younger child the mode of presentation may be atypical and can be masked by the symptoms of an upper respiratory infection which frequently co-exists. In family practice the patient is usually seen early in the course of the illness and the typical features of the established condition may be absent. There is ordinarily tachycardia and mild pyrexia, but the patient may show little systemic upset: he may not look ill, and this in itself can be misleading. Evidence of guarding or of peritonitis is uncommon in the early stage of the illness; the presence of *persistent* low grade central abdominal pain is the most important feature.

Unless there is clear evidence of toxicity, muscle guarding or signs of localised or generalised peritoneal involvement, the patient can be nursed at home under close supervision for a period of up to 48 hours. In many cases the symptoms and signs will resolve within this time. When the illness runs this kind of course, a diagnosis of mesenteric adenitis may be made, but in many cases no definitive cause can be identified. In those patients eventually referred to hospital with appendicitis, the diagnosis becomes increasingly more probable over the first 24 hours.

Following discharge from hospital after operative treatment, the child should stay off school for about four weeks.

2. *Diabetes.* Diabetes in childhood normally presents as an acute illness characterised by keto-acidosis, in which abdominal pain may be a prominent feature.

3. *Dyspepsia.* 'Dyspeptic' pain may result from gastric irritation due to the type or quantity of food ingested, and is usually associated with nausea and possibly vomiting. The episodic bouts of epigastric pain with nausea and vomiting classically associated with peptic ulceration are uncommon in childhood. Where there is a strong family history of peptic ulcer, this diagnosis should be considered. The decision as to whether formal investigation is indicated must vary with the circumstances. Where the pain may be due to dietary indiscretion or a reaction to stress, it may be unwise to advise X-ray examination by barium meal as the mention of 'possible ulcer' may only increase the anxiety in the child and in the parents. In the management of the child with dyspepsia, the doctor should attempt to identify causes of stress and to reduce their effect by explanation and discussion. More specific therapy includes the correction of any gross abnormalities of the diet and the use of an antacid, such as magnesium trisilicate. There is seldom any need for other drugs. If the symptoms of anxiety are marked a sedative such as nitrazepam in a dose of 2·5 or 5 mg thrice daily may be given for the first week or two of treatment. It is important that such treatment does not continue indefinitely and that the child does not thus grow up with a reliance on drugs as the answer to responsibility or stress.

4. *Periodic syndrome.* The periodic syndrome is a manifestation of reaction to stress. It occurs most frequently in children between the ages of 12 and 16 years, during adolescence, and is more common in girls. Episodic attacks of central abdominal pain occur, associated with headache and nausea or vomiting, and these are relieved after a period of sleep. There is a clear association with excitement or stress, but the diagnosis may not be made until several such episodes have occurred and the pattern of the illness becomes obvious. Explanation and reassurance are in themselves therapeutic and there is

seldom any need for more specific sedative therapy. As in other anxiety states in children, care should be taken not to allow the child to develop a reliance on sedative drugs.

THE YOUNG ADULT

Diarrhoea

In the adult patient diarrhoea is usually infective (p. 185) in origin, and food poisoning of one kind or another is the commonest cause. Occasionally, hyperthyroidism may present with a complaint of diarrhoea. The symptom may also result from the abuse of laxative drugs in an obsessional and disturbed patient, and diarrhoea may be the presenting symptom of an anxiety state. Ulcerative colitis (p. 208), Crohn's disease (p. 201) and a malabsorptive syndrome (p. 76) are the other potentially serious diseases.

Dyspepsia

Three broad categories of dyspeptic patient can be identified: those with non-periodic dyspepsia, those with 'ulcer-type' dyspepsia and those with gall-bladder dyspepsia.

Almost all adults will from time to time suffer from dyspepsia resulting from over-indulgence in food or drink or from ingestion of irritants such as alcohol or drugs (p. 67).

The second group of patients is characterised by episodes of dyspepsia in which nausea or vomiting, heartburn and epigastric pain last for periods of one to three weeks. In some patients, anxiety or stress seems to be an aetiological factor. The patient may be able to identify some item of food or drink which seems to provoke symptoms and those with recurrent dyspepsia soon recognise and avoid foods which upset them.

The treatment of the acute attack involves dietary advice and drugs, and time off work is usually necessary (p. 43). It is important to confirm that the patient fully understands the management of the illness and is adhering to the instructions given. In both the acute attack and the subsequent long-term management of the patient, the persistence of symptoms may mean that the patient is unwilling to eat a restricted diet, to avoid alcohol or to reduce his cigarette smoking, preparing to put up with some discomfort rather than to alter his way of life. The indications for admission to hospital are varied, but will include such situations as his being unable to look after himself adequately or when his symptoms persist despite adequate medical therapy. The move to hospital is likely to be followed by recovery if some factor in the home environment, such as stress, has been a causative factor. The patient may be able to limit further episodes of dyspepsia if he can recognise and come to terms with stress.

In general practice there may be disadvantages in seeking X-ray confirmation of an ulcer in all patients. As with the younger child, the diagnosis of an ulcer may be accompanied by an 'invalid' reaction and a barium meal examination or endoscopy should be arranged only when there are reasonably strong clinical suspicions of an ulcer.

The third group comprises those patients with cholecystitis (p. 111).

THE MIDDLE YEARS

When gastrointestinal symptoms present for the first time in the 40 to 65 year age group, conditions such as carcinoma of the stomach (p. 69) or large bowel (p. 220) should be suspected.

Anorexia is an important symptom in adult life, and if progressive or present for more than four weeks, may denote serious pathology. It can be a feature of carcinoma of the stomach, but is also a late symptom of advanced carcinomatosis from any site. Anorexia is perhaps most commonly found as a persistent feature of an infective illness, and influenza can be followed by two or three weeks of almost total anorexia. Endogenous depression in middle and late adult life may also present with anorexia.

Morning nausea and anorexia which disappear later in the day may suggest a diagnosis of alcoholic gastritis. Weight loss is not necessarily present: indeed the quantity of alcohol consumed each day can exceed the patient's caloric requirements. Patients will seldom admit immediately to excessive drinking and an accurate history is often only obtained after several consultations when the confidence of the patient has been gained.

THE ELDERLY

Diarrhoea

Infective diarrhoea is less common in the elderly than in childhood or early adult life. A common cause is abuse of laxatives, many elderly patients feeling the need to have regular bowel movements and a daily purge can become a ritual. This can be exaggerated if the patient is prone to constipation through being relatively immobile or bed-bound or if he is taking regular medication with codeine or a codeine-containing analgesic. The 'spurious' diarrhoea associated with faecal impaction is relatively common, and again much more so in the bed- or chair-bound patient. It is seen particularly following a cerebrovascular accident or 'stroke'.

Constipation

Mention has been made of the association between constipation and drugs or immobility. The diet taken by the elderly patient is frequently abnormal, with a preponderance of carbohydrate foods as they are relatively cheap. Constipation may be aggravated, therefore, by insufficient roughage from meat, fruit or vegetables in the diet. Diminished bowel function can also be a symptom of hypothyroidism.

In the elderly male constipation may first present as retention of urine.

Elderly patients seldom complain of diarrhoea or constipation. Obviously any specific cause should be identified and treated; 'treatment', however, will often consist simply of advice about laxatives or diet. Faecal impaction may require a manual removal or treatment with an enema.

Dyspepsia

The disorders of early adult life can obviously continue into old age and mention has been made of the significance of dyspepsia first appearing in later adult life. The clinical picture of sliding hiatal hernia is given on page 21, but there are some important aspects of this condition when it occurs in the elderly. The symptoms can be exacerbated by a poor or inadequate diet, and by drugs such as aspirin, phenylbutazone or indomethacin taken for arthritis. Enquiry should be made about possible self-medication with drugs. The patient with a hiatal hernia may gradually alter the diet in an attempt to obtain relief of symptoms. By the time medical help is sought, the diet may consist mainly of milk, porridge or soft cereals, and a degree of malnutrition can be present. The oesophagitis may cause bleeding and this together with a diet low in iron content may result in a hypochromic anaemia.

The routine management of patients with reflux oesophagitis is given on page 21. The patient's concurrent drug therapy should be reviewed and all potentially irritant preparations should be withdrawn or replaced. It is sometimes possible, as with indomethacin, to give the drug by rectal suppository if it cannot be tolerated by the oral route. Operative treatment should be considered if medical management fails to control the symptoms adequately.

SOME PROBLEMS OF GASTROINTESTINAL DISEASE IN GENERAL PRACTICE

Most of the illnesses of the gastrointestinal tract that are seen in general practice are self-limiting and relatively trivial in terms of mortality and morbidity. Despite this, the continuing nature of medicine in the community and the way in which illnesses are presented at an early stage, and in an undifferentiated form pose certain problems that are peculiar to general practice.

The management of a long-term illness such as dyspepsia requires two differing forms of approach: the intensive treatment of the acute exacerbation, and the preventive, educative and more comprehensive approach necessary for the long term management of the patient. The first is relatively easy; a patient will readily follow the doctor's instructions during a period when he is in pain or when he is ill, but may be much less inclined to conform in the intervals between such attacks. This becomes more marked when the 'treatment' moves from a regime of specific diet and drugs to the need for a continuing alteration in the patient's eating and drinking habits, where home life and employment may have to become involved, and where the whole life-style of the patient may have to change. This difficulty should be recognised and if such changes are thought necessary the reasons for them should be clearly explained to the patient so that his co-operation and his willingness to follow instructions are based on his understanding of their need. The doctor should appreciate that his advice may be difficult for the patient to follow and he should, therefore, be prepared to accept a compromise rather than to always insist on what he considers to be the optimum management of the patient.

Chronic disease is seldom static, but tends to run a slowly progressive course. The treatments that are necessary at an earlier stage in the illness may not be appropriate some years later and the clinical picture can become more confused by the slow emergence of complications. One of the objectives of the long term management should, therefore, be to identify such complications at the earliest possible stage so that some different treatment, medical or surgical, can be planned rather than be precipitated by a crisis at a time when the outcome is adversely affected. This approach to chronic illness is dependent on the doctor's ability to see such ill-health as a continuing and changing disability rather than as a series of isolated crises.

The way that a patient tells of his symptoms is influenced by many factors, by his knowledge of the disease, by information gleaned· from books or magazines, or by his experience of doctors and the way in which they take a medical history. Unless the patient and the doctor both interpret a symptom in the same way, the information gained from the history can be misleading or inaccurate with the possibility that mistakes even of diagnosis or treatment may occur. The patient can interpret the question 'Do you ever feel sick?' as 'Do you ever vomit?', or 'Do you ever feel unwell?' or 'Do you ever feel angry or disgusted about anything?'. Similarly the question 'Are your bowels regular?' will only produce a meaningful answer if both the patient and the doctor have precisely the same frequency and character of bowel habit! This difficulty over the interpretation of symptoms is not peculiar to gastrointestinal disease, but may be more important when symptoms can have different meanings and implications at different ages. Many of the symptoms of such serious diseases as alimentary cancer are common to diseases of other systems and to much commoner and less potentially important conditions. The identification of gastric or colonic cancer is therefore dependent on the doctor continuing to have an index of suspicion which does not become blunted by the rarity of these conditions in relation to the total amount of alimentary illness that he sees. It is equally important that the doctor does not over-investigate his patient, causing anxiety to both the patient and his relatives, and unnecessary additional work to the laboratories and to his hospital colleagues. How to tread the path between these two extremes is only one of the difficulties associated with the practice of medicine in the community.

Index

Achalasia of the cardia, 25
Acute abdomen, 167–183
Acute intestinal obstruction, 173–181
Adenomatous polyps of colon, 232–234
Adrenocortical steroids in ulcerative colitis, 215
Alcoholic liver disease, 145
Amoebic dysentery, 187–188
    treatment, 188
Amylase, levels in acute pancreatitis, 122
Anal canal and anus, 252–273
Anal canal, congenital anomalies, 255–256
    malignant tumours, 230
    mucosa, 252
    musculature, 253
    physiology, 255
    tumours of, 268–269
Anal fissure, 259–261
Antrectomy, 48
Appendicitis, 170–172, 278
Argentaffinoma, 238
Ascaris lumbricoides, 94
Ascites, 151–152

Bacillary dysentery, 185–187
Bacillus fusiformis, 3
Bile, constituents of, 107
Bile pigment, metabolism, 133
Biliary system, 107–117
Biopsy, peroral, of small intestine, 88–90
Borrelia vincenti, 3
Botulism, 197
Bromsulphthalein retention test, 144
Brown-Kelly-Paterson syndrome, 27
Budd-Chiari syndrome, 158

Cancer of stomach, 69–74
Candida albicans, 7
Carbenoxolone sodium, 46
Carcinoembryonic antigen, 223
Carcinoid syndrome, 238–240
    treatment, 240
Carcinoid tumour of the intestine, 238
Carcinoma of colon, 220–231
    carcino-embryonic antigen, 223
    clinical features, 221

investigations, 222
    treatment, 223–230
Carcinoma of gallbladder, 117
Carcinoma of pancreas, 128–130
Cardia, competence of, 15
Charcoal column haemoperfusion, 155
14C-Glycocholic acid breath test, 86
Charcot's triad, 114
Cheilitis, 5, 8
Cholecystitis, acute, 111
    chronic, 112
Cimetidine, 45
Cirrhosis, classification, 142
    macronodular, 145
Clostridial food-poisoning, 196
Clostridium botulinum, 197
Clostridium welchii, 196
Coeliac disease, 91–93
Colon, carcinoma of, 220–231
Colonization of small intestine, 197–198
Colostomy, 228–230
Congenital biliary atresia, 162
Congenital cystic fibrosis of pancreas, 100
Congenital pyloric stenosis, 276
Crohn's disease, 201–207
    biopsy, 203
    complications, 204
    diagnosis, 202
    radiology, 202
    sigmoidoscopy, 202
    treatment, 205–207
Crohn's disease, malabsorption in, 95

Deglycyrrhizinated liquorice, 46
Dental caries, 1
Dental diseases, 1–4
Diphyllobothrium latum, 94
Disaccharide absorption test, 84
Disaccharide intolerance, 96–97
Diseases affecting salivary glands, 11–13
Diverticular disease of colon, 242–251
    anatomy and physiology, 242
    clinical features, 245
    complications, 247–249
    pathology and pathogenesis, 244
    radiology, 246

Diverticular disease of colon (cont'd)
    treatment, 249–251
Diverticula pharyngo-oesophageal, 28–30
'Dumping' syndrome, 59
Duodenal stenosis, 53
Dysphagia, 16
    sideropaenic, 27

Echinococcus granulosus, 156
Encopresis, 278
Endoscopic retrograde choledocho-pan-
        creatography (E.R.C.P.), 115
Entamoeba histolytica, 157
    in amoebic dysentery, 188
Enteric fever, 191
Exchange blood transfusion, 155

Faecal fat excretion, test, 83
Feeding difficulties, 275
Fistula-in-ano, 263
Flora of alimentary tract, 184
Fluoride, 2
Food-poisoning, clostridial, 196
    staphylococcal, 195

Gallstone ileus, 115
Gallstones, aetiology, 108–109
    clinical presentation of, 111
    radiological diagnosis of, 113
    silent, 111
    types of, 109
Gastrectomy partial,
    Billroth I, 49
    Polya, 49
Gastric secretion, inhibitors of, 45
Gastritis, 67–69
    acute, 67
    chronic, 67
General practice, gastrointestinal diseases
        in, 274–284
Giardia intestinalis, 89
Giardiasis, 189
Gingivitis, 2, 5
Globus hystericus, 19
Glossitis, 5
Glucose absorption test, 80
Gluten, 91–92, 104
Glycogen storage diseases, 165–166

Haematemesis and melaena, 54–59
Haemochromatosis, 159–161
Haemorrhoids, 256–259
    complications, 258
    treatment, 258
Hartmann's solution, 190
Heartburn, 16

Hepatic amoebiasis, 157
Hepatic arteriography, 162
Hepatic cirrhosis, 140–144
    clinical features, 144
Hepatic coma, 153–155
Hepatic scintiscanning, 162
Hepatic vein occlusion, 158
Hepatitis, chronic, 147
    viral, 136–140
Hepatolenticular degeneration, 161
Hiatal hernia, para-oesophageal, 24
    sliding, 21
Homologous serum jaundice, 137
Hookworm infestation, 95
Hydatid disease, 156–157
5-Hydroxytryptamine, 238
Hyperbilirubinaemias, 164

Ileitis, acute, 172
Ileostomy in ulcerative colitis, 218
Infantile colic, 276
Infantile gastroenteritis, 189–191
Infectious hepatitis, 136
Insulinoma of pancreas, 130–132
Intestinal infections, 184–200
Intestinal ischaemia, 97–98
Intestinal obstruction, acute, 173–181
    electrolyte changes, 176–179
    management, 179
Intussusception, 180

Jaundice, 109–111, 134–136
    haemolytic, 134
    hepatocellular, 135
    obstructive, 113–115, 135

Kayser-Fleischer rings, 161

Lactobacillus acidophilus, 154
Leptospirosis, 155–156
Leukoplakia, 8, 6
Liver abscess, pyogenic, 156
Liver biopsy, 142
Liver, tumours of, 161–162
Lundh test, 127
Lymphoma of small intestine, 231

Malabsorption, causes of, 80–81
    clinical presentation, 81–83
    functional anatomy of intestinal mu-
        cosa, 78–80
    radiology, 88
    special investigations, 88
    syndrome, 76–106
    treatment of, 101–106
Malocclusion of teeth, 4

Meckel's diverticulum, 173
Melaena, 54–59
Mesenteric adenitis, 173
Metiamide, 45
Mumps, 11

Neoplasia, oral mucosa, 9

Oesophagitis, reflux, 20
Oesophagoscopy, 17, 18
Oesophagus, Barrett's, 14, 25
  diffuse spasm, 26
  disorders of, 20–36
  foreign bodies in, 35
  functional disorders of, 25–27
  perforation of, 36
  rupture of, 36
  simple strictures, 34
  tertiary contractions, 26
  tumours of, 30–34
Oral mucosa and tongue, 5–10
Osteomalacia, 63
Osteoporosis, 63

Pancreas, 117–132
  anatomy, 117
  carcinoma of, 128–130
  insulinoma of, 130–132
  physiology, 117
  scan, 127
Pancreatic disease, malabsorption in, 94–96
Pancreatitis, acute, 118–125
  aetiology, 119–121
  chronic
    diagnosis, 125
  clinical features, 121–122
  diagnostic aids, 122–123
  pathology, 113
  treatment of, 123–125
Paratyphoid fever, 191
Parotitis, epidemic, 11
Peptic ulcer, 37–65
  clinical presentation, 38–40
  complications, 53–59
  diagnosis, 40
  gastric acid secretion, 41
  medical treatment, 42–46
  perforation of, 53
  recurrent, 52
  surgical treatment, 46–53
Perianal skin, disorders of, 269–273
Perianal suppuration, 261–263
Periodic syndrome, 279
Periodontal disease, 3
Peritonitis, 170

Peutz-Jegher syndrome, 240
Pharyngitis, acute, 17
  chronic, 19
Pharynx and oesophagus, 14–36
Pharynx, diseases of, 17–20
Pig liver perfusion, 155
Pilonidal sinus, 264–265
Pinocytosis, 79
Plummer-Vinson syndrome, 27
Polycystic disease of liver, 164
Polyposis coli, 236
Polyps of intestine, 232–234
Portal hypertension, 147–151
  treatment of, 148–151
Portal vein block, 151
Portal venography, 148
Portasystemic encephalopathy, 153–155
Posetting, 276
Postgastrectomy syndromes, 59–65
Primary biliary cirrhosis, 145–147
Proctalgia fugax, 269
Prostaglandins, 45
Pruritus ani, 272
Pyogenic liver abscess, 156

Ranula, 11
Rectal prolapse, 265–268
Reflux oesophagitis, 20
Regurgitation, oesophageal, 16
Retropharyngeal abscess, 20
Rupture of spleen, 181
Ruptured aneurysm of abdominal aorta, 182

Salivary glands, 11–13
  calculi, 11
  infections, 11–12
  mucocele, 11
  post-irradiation damage, 13
  tumours, 13
Salmonella paratyphi, 194
Salmonella typhimurium, 191–194
Salmonellosis, 194
Salpingitis, acute, 172
Secretin test, 126
Secretin—pancreozymin test, 126
Sengstaken tube, 148
Serotonin, 238
Serum hepatitis, 137
Shigella organisms, 185
Sialoadenitis, acute, 12
Sialoadenitis, chronic, 12
Sjögren's syndrome, 12
Sprue, 93–94
Staphylococcal food-poisoning, 195
Stomach, 37–75

Stomatitis, 5, 7–8
  acute specific fevers, 7
  Candida infections, 7
  drugs, 8
  herpes simplex, 7
  herpes zoster, 7
Sulphasalazine in ulcerative colitis, 215
Swallowing, physiology of, 14

Teeth, developmental abnormalities, 4
Tongue, recurrent aphthae, 5
  geographic, 6
  'leukoplakia', 6
  syphilitic lesions, 6
  trauma, 5
  tuberculous ulceration, 6
Tuberculosis, ileocaecal, 95
Tumours, of the anal canal, 268–269
  of the intestine, 220–241
  of the liver, 161–162
  pharyngeal, 19
Typhoid fever, 191

Ulcerative colitis, 208–219
  cancer in, 212
  clinical classification, 210
  clinical presentation, 209
  complications, 212
  diagnosis, 210

  pathology, 208
  sigmoidoscopy, 211
  surgical treatment, 217
  treatment, 213–219
Urinary calculus, 181

Vagotomy, selective, 48
  truncal, 48
Villous papilloma of colon, 234
Vincent's infection, 3
Viral hepatitis, 136–140
Viruses in intestinal disease, 197
Volvulus, 180
Vomiting, 15, 168
  bilious, 61
  faeculent, 168
  projectile, 168

Waterbrash, 16
Weil's disease, 155
Whipple's disease, 95
Widal reaction, 193
Wilson's disease, 161

Xerostomia, 5
Xylose absorption test, 84

Zollinger-Ellison syndrome, 65–67

NOTES

NOTES

NOTES

NOTES

NOTES

NOTES

Printed in Hong Kong
by Sheck Wah Tong Printing Press